ACTA NEUROCHIRURGICA
SUPPLEMENTUM 30

Advances in Stereotactic and Functional Neurosurgery 4

Proceedings of the 4th Meeting of the European Society for Stereotactic and Functional Neurosurgery, Paris 1979

Edited by
F. J. Gillingham, J. Gybels, E. R. Hitchcock
G. F. Rossi, G. Szikla

SPRINGER-VERLAG
WIEN NEW YORK

F. John Gillingham
Professor of Neurosurgery, University of Edinburgh
Western General Hospital and Royal Infirmary, Edinburgh

Jan Gybels
Professor of Neurosurgery, Academisch Ziekenhuis, Leuven

Edward Hitchcock
Professor of Neurosurgery, University of Birmingham
Midland Centre for Neurosurgery and Neurology
and Queen Elizabeth Hospital, Birmingham

Gian Franco Rossi
Professor of Neurosurgery, Università Cattolica del Sacro Cuore,
Istituto di Neurochirurgia, Roma

Gábor Szikla
Maître de Recherche C.N.R.S., Neurosurgeon, Service de
Neurochirurgie Fonctionnelle, Centre Hospitalier Sainte Anne, Paris

With 159 Figures

ISSN 0065-1419
ISBN-13:978-3-211-81591-5 e-ISBN-13:978-3-7091-8592-6
DOI: 10.1007/978-3-7091-8592-6

Contents

Introduction

Section I. Surgery of Epilepsy

A. Introduction

B. Reports

C. Communications

D. Closure

Section II. Stereotactic Cerebral Irradiation

Section III. Neurostimulation for Pain and Spasticity

A. Pain

B. Spasticity

Section IV. Advances and New Techniques

Acta Neurochirurgica, Suppl. 30, 1—3 (1980)

Introduction

Target Point, Target Volume, "Whole Brain" Stereotaxis: Remarks on Some Present Trends of Evolution in Stereotactic Neurosurgery

Some years ago when the L-Dopa dramatically reduced the number of operations for Parkinsons' disease, Nicholas Zervas wrote in a letter "stereotaxis is at a dead end in this country" (the U.S.). At that time, many colleagues all over the world not only shared this pessimistic evaluation but were inclined to think that the era of stereotactic surgery as such was over, and that societies for stereotactic and functional neurosurgery continued to exist essentially because of intellectual inertia.

During the following years, however, this pessimism gave way to a renewed interest in stereotaxis. It became evident that only a limited concept and practice of this surgery was at a dead end—not stereotaxis itself. The vitality and the attractive power of newer developments in this field are, besides others, shown by the example of our present European meeting with more than 200 participants coming from 23 countries all over the world. However, stereotaxis is taken today in a much wider sense, with a different philosophy. It might be useful to emphasize the main conceptual changes which seem to play a role in this evolution.

1. The target *point* became enlarged and transformed into the target *volume:* such is the case for epileptogenic cortical areas and even more for brain tumors.

2. The field of application of stereotactic methods was progressively extended from some centrally located deep structures to the *entire brain* including the cortex.

3. Multi-probe methods became available, allowing for safe *simultaneous exploration of several brain structures.*

4. *The availability of the CT scan* together with the introduction of computer techniques in the stereotactic procedures increased enormously both our surgical capabilities and the number of patients who might benefit from the precision of stereotactic methods.

0065-1490/80/Suppl. 30/0001/$ 01.00

Thus instead of being synonymous with specific procedures performed at the level of the basal ganglia, *stereotaxis is in fact a general diagnostic and therapeutic concept*, which has as its aim the precise three-dimensional representation of the patient's brain in its entirety. This three-dimensional representation is based on anatomical, neuroradiological and other localizing information, the spatial integration

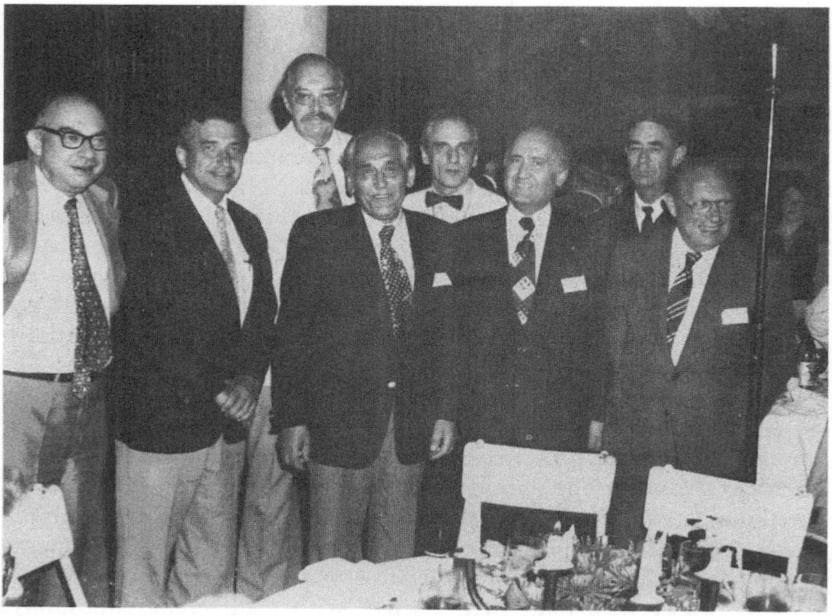

Prof. Jean Talairach with friends and coworkers at the congress dinner in the Royaumont Abbey near Paris. (From left to right: Drs. J. Bancaud, N. T. Zervas, B. Nashold, J. Talairach, G. Szikla, F. Mundinger, P. Tournoux, J. Pecker)

of which allows a more precise "anatomical" approach to the human brain and to the surgical management of localized pathologic processes. Literally, stereotaxis means "orientation in space". Taken in this general sense, all surgical procedures obviously should be stereotactic, at least in their principle!

Two of the main themes of our meeting, namely the topic of the first day, "Surgery of Epilepsy" and that of the second "Stereotactic Cerebral Irradiation" of small brain tumours correspond to this evolution toward a global "whole brain" concept of stereotaxis. The same philosophy inspired the scientific efforts of the stereotactic group of the Sainte Anne Hospital, under the leadership of its promoter, Professor Jean Talairach. This is the reason why the present Meeting is dedicated in honor of his scientific work.

Gábor Szikla
President of the IVth Meeting of the
European Society for Stereotactic and
Functional Neurosurgery

Section I

Surgery of Epilepsy

Acta Neurochirurgica, Suppl. 30, 7—11 (1980)

A. Introduction

Why, When, and How Surgery of Epilepsy?

G. F. Rossi*

With 1 Figure

In the official Congress of the European Society for Stereotactic and Functional Neurosurgery it seems mandatory that at least one whole day be devoted to surgery of epilepsy.

This is probably the oldest field of functional neurosurgery. It was conceived in antiquity, at least three thousand years ago. It entered in the modern surgical era about forty years ago. Progress has been, indeed, remarkable. It has been permitted by the steady advancement of our knowledge of the pathophysiological mechanisms of epilepsy and by the progressive improvement of our diagnostic and surgical techniques. However, we are still faced with a number of problems. The main task of this review will be that of underlining both the advances so far achieved and the problems still to be solved. The outstanding experience of the invited speakers certainly makes possible the fulfilment of this task.

Before starting our reunion I think it would be helpful to give some introduction to the detailed reports which will follow so that we can define some preliminary aspects of the subject under discussion. It appears to me that the best way to do that is that of briefly considering and commenting on the answers which might be given to the following three questions: "why," "when" and "how" in the surgery of epilepsy?

Why Surgery of Epilepsy?

The answer to this first question does not appear difficult. Surgical treatment is considered when the epileptic syndrome is dis-

* Institute of Neurosurgery, Catholic University, Rome, Italy.

0065-1490/80/Suppl. 30/0007/$ 01.00

abling and resistant to pharmacological treatment and because we have to-day sufficient data to prove its therapeutic value. Such an answer is based on the assumptions that when we speak of surgery of epilepsy: 1. we mean surgical treatment of patients in whom the epileptic seizure is the only or the main manifestation of a brain disease; 2. the nature of the brain disease does not require, per se, surgical treatment. Can the answer I have given to this first question be regarded as generally acceptable? Personally, I think it can. However, certain arguments appear to contradict such an opinion.

Let us briefly take into consideration some quantitative data. How many patients might be regarded as possible candidates for surgical treatment? It is difficult to give precise figures. However, an approximate estimation can be considered [1]. Firstly, the prevalence of epilepsy is of the order of 5 per 1,000 persons. Secondly, about 20% of the epileptics are not controlled by medical therapy, in spite of the improvement of pharmacological treatment permitted by the evaluation of drug blood levels. Thirdly, of this 20% of epileptic patients a percentage ranging from 25 to 50% might probably benefit from surgical treatment. This is, indeed, a large number of patients. Thus, such an estimation indicates that in France or in Italy or in Great Britain there are from 13,000 to 26,000 epileptic patients who might be considered for surgical treatment. There is no doubt that they are many more than those which are actually referred to the neurosurgeon.

There are many possible ways to explain this discrepancy between the above theorical estimation and the actual surgical work for epilepsy. Indeed, the first might be that the answer I have given to the question "why surgery for epilepsy" is not shared by many of those involved in the care of the epileptic patient, particularly the neurologists. Does that mean that the answer I have given to the first of my three questions is wrong? Or is it wrong the quantitative estimation of the possible candidates for surgical treatment? Or are there alternative explanations? I hope that these points might be considered by the following speakers and in the discussion.

I suggest that a possible explanation might be found in certain difficulties in answering to the second of the three questions mentioned above, namely "when surgery of epilepsy".

When Surgery of Epilepsy?

One might answer as follows: Firstly, when the length of time necessary for convincing evidence that pharmacological treatment is not sufficient has elapsed. Secondly, when reliable information on the anatomo-functional organization of the epileptogenic process has been obtained. Thirdly, when one has reached the knowledge that the spatial location of the epileptogenic process is such as to allow safe surgical manipulation.

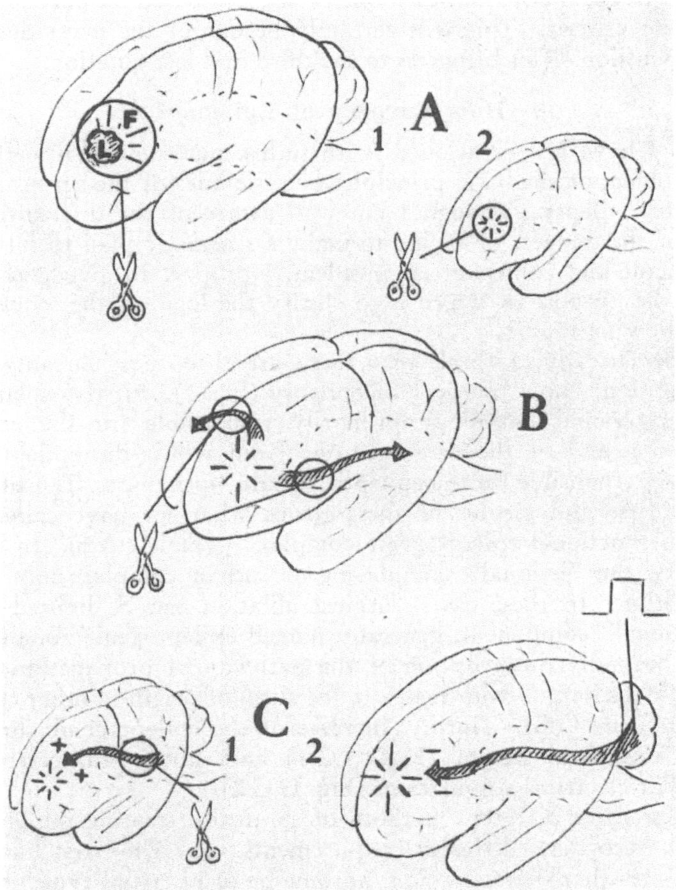

Fig. 1. Schematic illustration of surgical approaches to the treatment of epilepsy. (See text for explanations)

I think that everybody agrees on the first point, though one might discuss how much time is necessary to prove that pharmacological treatment is insufficient. On the other hand, there might be disagreement on the other two points. In fact, the need to undergo the long and often painstaking work necessary to ascertain the answers to the second and third points, as well as the means used for this purpose are dependent on the rationale of the surgical treatment. As will be seen from the reports which will follow, such a rationale is not standardized. The methods used to treat the epileptic patients surgically are many, and each one of them is based on particular and different criteria. This will certainly be one of the main themes of our discussion. This brings us to the third and last question.

How Surgery of Epilepsy?

As I have just mentioned, with such a question we directly face the problem of the basic principles or rationales of the surgical treatment of epilepsy. Though I am well aware of the difficulties and even of the dangers of trying to make a schematic plan to solve such a difficult and controversial problem, I propose to give you a synthesis the purpose of which is to clarify the logic of the sequence of the following reports.

Schematically, I think that there are three possible answers to the question: "how" surgery of epilepsy (Fig. 1). Firstly, ablation of the intracranial pathology primarily responsible for the epileptic syndrome, and of the cerebral zone from which the epileptic discharge—responsible for the epileptic seizure—originates. The ensemble of the first and second of these forms what we have called "the lesional-functional epileptogenic complex" [2] (Fig. 1, A 1). In certain patients, the "lesional" component of such a complex may escape recognition. In these cases, surgical ablation can be limited to the "functional" component, generally named epileptogenic zone (Fig. 1, A 2). Secondly, interruption of the pathway of propagation of the epileptic discharges from their site (or sites) of origin to other cerebral districts (Fig. 1, B). Thirdly, increase of the epileptogenic threshold through cerebral lesions (Fig. 1, C 1) and, above all, cerebral or cerebellar electrical stimulations (Fig. 1, C 2).

These three different methods of surgically treating the epileptic patient recognize different requirements. 1. The first modality necessitates that the epileptic syndrome be of a partial type; that the lesional-functional epileptogenic complex responsible for it be unique; that its spatial location be precisely known, and that it be such as to allow surgical ablation without morbidity. 2. As for the second modality, whether the epileptic syndrome has to be of partial type or not can be an interesting matter of discussion. In the case of partial epilepsy, not only unifocal but also multifocal syndromes can be considered. At any rate, in my view, it is necessary that the main pathways of propagation of the epileptic discharge should be known and that they can be interrupted without morbidity. 3. The third surgical approach seems, so far at least, independent on the characteristics of the epileptic syndrome. However, it requires proof of the existence of structures which have a facilitating or, viceversa, a restraining influence on epileptogenicity, and the evidence that these structures can be safely ablated or, on the other hand, electrically stimulated.

Finally, the therapeutic goals of these three different modalities of surgical treatment of epilepsy are to a certain extent different. Obviously, all of them aim at improving the epileptic syndrome. However, it is the first one which provides the greatest opportunities to completely cure the patient, *i.e.*, to definitively suppress seizures. The other two approaches can rarely reach that goal; their main, or most likely, purpose is that of reducing, not suppressing, seizures.

Of these three surgical approaches to epilepsy only the first two have been employed for a time sufficiently long to permit a critical evaluation of the results. The third approach, and particularly that based on cerebellar electrical stimulation, the last of the surgical means of treating epilepsy, has to be regarded as still in an experimental phase. For this reason, our discussion to-day will consider mainly the first two approaches.

References

1. Robb, P., Focal epilepsy: the problem, prevalence, and contributing factors. In: Advances in Neurology, Vol. 8, pp. 11—22 (Purpura, D., Penry, J. K., Walter, R. D., eds.); Neurosurgical Management of the Epilepsies, pp. 356. New York: Raven Press, 1975.
2. Rossi, G. F., Gentilomo, A., Colicchio, G., Le problème de la recherche de la topographie d'origine de l'épilepsie. Arch. Suis. Neurol. Neurochir. Psychiat. *115* (1974), 229—250.

Acta Neurochirurgica, Suppl. 30, 13—24 (1980)

B. Reports

Surgical Aspects of Temporal Lobe Epilepsy

Results and Problems

Th. Rasmussen*

With 6 Figures

Summary

The Montreal Neuroligcal Institute's experience with cortical resection for medically refractory temporal lobe epilepsy had grown to 1,102 patients as of the end of 1978, 932 in the non-tumoral category and 170 patients with tumors, including a few major vascular malformations. Follow-up data, (complete to date or to the patients' death in over 80% of the patients) shows that 70% of those with 2 or more years of adequate follow-up data (median period 11 years) have experienced a complete or nearly complete reduction of the seizure tendency.

Since the attack pattern frequently does not give evidence as to the lateralization of the epileptogenic area, special EEG techniques are often required to select those patients apt to benefit from temporal lobectomy. Sphenoidal recordings with chronically implanted fine wire electrodes have been particularly useful. Telemetry has enhanced the capability of recording a large number of epileptic spikes during sleep and various daytime activities and of recording spontaneous attacks. An automatic spike detection gadget gives promise of major help in analyzing these lengthy records. The addition of a video tape system, correlated with the EEG telemetry system, aids in determining the side of origin of the seizures. A small number of patients in whom this could not be determined with these various EEG techniques, were studied with stereotactically implanted chronic depth electrodes employing a modification of the Talairach-Bancaud technique. Over ¾ of these patients were shown to have the onset of their seizures to be sufficiently well laterized to warrant temporal lobectomy.

Keywords: Epilepsy; temporal; EEG; telemetry.

Dr. Penfield's first operation on the temporal lobe for focal epilepsy was carried out in 1928, just over 50 years ago [11], but it only

* Montreal Neurological Institute, 3801 University Street, Montreal, Quebec, Canada H3A 2B4.

0065-1419/80/Suppl. 30/0013/$ 02.40

gradually became apparent that epileptogenic lesions involving primarily the temporal lobe represented the most common type of focal epilepsy. Operations on the temporal lobe for focal epilepsy increased steadily in number over the years both at the MNI [1, 12, 16] and in many other neurosurgical centers around the world [14]. During the past 2 decades, operations for temporal lobe epilepsy have consistently accounted for about two thirds of all cortical resections carried out for focal epilepsy by the neurosurgical staff of the MNI.

Although the details of the surgical approach, and management of medically refractory temporal lobe epilepsy at the MNI, along with the results of temporal lobectomy, were reported most recently in some detail in 1975 [14], it seems appropriate on this occasion to summarize briefly the results obtained in reducing the seizure tendency in this series of patients with medically refractory temporal lobe epilepsy. Secondly, data will be presented emphasizing the astonishing variety of brain lesions that can produce seizures of temporal lobe origin. Thirdly, I will comment on the recurring diagnostic problems encountered in studying patients as possible candidates for temporal lobectomy and outline some of the various tactics we have employed in this assessment.

Results of Cortical Resection

1. Total Temporal Lobe Series

A total of 722 patients had been operated upon for temporal lobe epilepsy at the Montreal Neurological Institute by the end of 1972 (Fig. 1). There were 3 postoperative deaths (1938, 1950, 1950), 13 patients died of a variety of causes during the first 2 postoperative years and in 53 patients there was less than 2 years of follow-up data available. There remain, therefore, a total of 653 patients with satisfactory follow-up data of more than 2 years duration in whom the effectiveness of the surgical procedure in reducing the seizure tendency can be evaluated. The follow-up data are complete to date or to the patients' death in over 80% of these 653 patients.

For the purposes of our continuing follow-up analyses and studies through the years, persisting clinical epileptiform episodes are classified on a roughly quantitative basis as auras, minor attacks or major attacks. An episode is classified as an aura if it consists *only* of a sensory phenomenon *without* motor manifestation and *without* interrupting the patient's mental activity or contact with the environment and if the episode cannot be detected by an observer. A patient who has only auras, as just defined, is considered to be *clinically* seizure free in the follow-up analyses, since the social impact of these brief sensory episodes, which rarely last more than a few seconds, is not significantly greater than the presence of persistent spiking in the EEG which sometimes persists as the only remnant of the original seizure tendency. On the other hand, if there is any disturbance of contact with the environment, no matter how brief, or if the episode can be detected by an observer, even though it consists only in a brief twitch of the face or thumb, it is classified as a minor attack.

Seizure free since discharge	158 pts. (24%)	257 pts. (39%)	466 pts. (71%)	653 pts. with follow-up data of 2-38 yrs. median 11 yrs.
Became seizure free after some early attacks	99 pts. (15%)			
Free 3 or more years then rare or occasional attacks	69 pts. (11%)	209 pts. (32%)		
Marked reduction of seizure tendency	140 pts. (21%)			
Moderate or less reduction of seizure tendency	187 pts. (29%)			
Inadequate data	53 pts.			
Deaths in first 2 years	13 pts.			
Postoperative deaths	3 pts.			
Total	**722 pts.**			

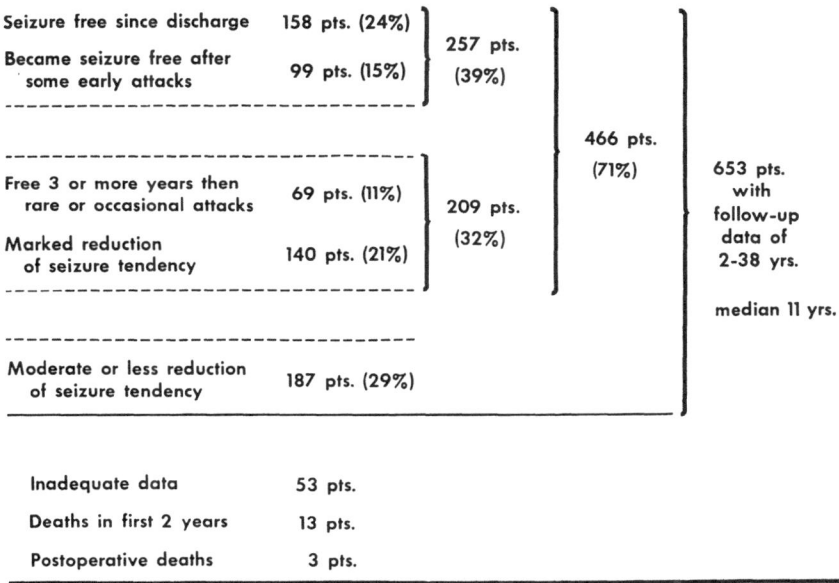

Fig. 1. Temporal lobe epilepsy—results of cortical excision. Patients with non-tumoural lesions operated upon from 1928 through 1972. (From Rasmussen 1979, ref. 14)

Two hundred fifty seven patients, 39% of the 653 patients followed for 2–38 years (Fig. 1), have become and remained seizure free, as defined above, since discharge from the hospital or after having a few attacks during the early postoperative months or years. 69 patients, 11%, have had isolated or occasional attacks after being seizure free for periods ranging from 3 to 25 years. 140 patients, 21%, have had only up to 1–2% as many attacks as compared to the preoperative rate, and not more than 1, 2, or 3 attacks per year. Thus 209 patients, 32%, have had a marked but not quite complete reduction of seizure tendency. Added to the seizure free group, this totals 466 patients, 71%, who have had a complete or nearly complete reduction of seizure tendency following temporal lobectomy [14].

The remaining 187 patients, 29%, have had a lesser reduction of seizure tendency. Some have had only 5–10% as many attacks compared to the preoperative rate, many have had a 40–50 or 60% reduction in number of seizures and a few, little or no reduction.

2. *Etiological Subgroups*

When these same patients are classified into etiological subgroups the results are essentially unchanged [14]. Thus 77% of the 202 patients in the birth trauma group with adequate follow-up data exhibited a complete or nearly complete reduction of seizure tendency. In the postnatal trauma group, 66% of the 103 patients with adequate follow-up data experienced a comparable result, as did 70% of the 104 follow-up patients of the group with postinflammatory brain injury. A similar reduction of seizure tendency was achieved in 61% of the 207 patients in the group with unknown etiology. The results were similar in the small group of patients with various miscellaneous lesions, 71% with complete or nearly complete reduction of the seizure tendency.

When the patients with temporal lobe seizures due to tumours were categorized up to the time of clinical recurrence of the tumour, if that had occurred, the results were again similar, 74% had experienced a complete or nearly complete reduction of the seizure tendency following removal of the tumour, and temporal lobectomy carried out with the special surgical seizure techniques [13].

Our data thus indicate that the effectiveness of cortical resection in reducing the seizure tendency in temporal lobe epilepsy is correlated with the completeness of the removal of the epileptogenic brain tissue rather than with the nature of the lesion or injury responsible for the original brain damage and development of an epileptogenic lesion. Thus we have endeavored through the years to identify and map out the epileptogenic area of the brain as accurately as possible through increasingly lengthy and sophisticated preoperative EEG studies and by cortical electrographic studies at time of operation.

Although half of our cortical resections for focal epilepsy associated with large, multilobe destructive or gliotic lesions of the brain have been carried out in children 15 years of age or younger, only 10% of our temporal lobe operations have been carried out in this age group. When we analyzed the results of these operations, nearly all done under general anaesthesia, we were pleasantly surprised to find that the success rate was essentially the same as that of the total temporal lobe series, 73% with a complete or nearly complete reduction of the seizure tendency [15]. The obvious benefits from the standpoint of the child's psychosocial development of reducing the handicap of recurring seizures as early as possible has become increasingly apparent as we have seen patients for periodic follow-up in whom the operation had been postponed for one reason or another from middle childhood to the early adult years. In recent years, therefore, we have recommended early temporal lobectomy in children when, repeated observations have demonstrated the seizure pattern to be stable, second, when the EEG abnormality is also stable and well lateralized, and third, when maximum tolerable doses of appropriate

Birth trauma, compression or anoxia	260 patients (24%)
Postnatal brain trauma	131 patients (12%)
Postinflammatory brain scarring	161 patients (15%)
Multiple potential etiological factors	80 patients (7%)
Miscellaneous lesions	60 patients (5%)
Unknown etiology	240 patients (22%)
Tumours	162 patients (15%)
Major vascular malformations	8 patients (1%)

Fig. 2. Temporal lobe epilepsy—etiology. 1,102 patients operated upon 1928 through 1978

anti-epileptic medications have failed to keep the clinical seizures under sufficient control to permit the child to take full advantage of the school and social programs available to his peers. Thus a somewhat larger percentage of our temporal lobectomies are now carried out in the 10–15 year age group than has been the case in years past.

Etiology

By the end of 1978 the MNI temporal lobe surgical seizure series had grown to 1,102 patients (Fig. 2). The standard causes of brain scarring or gliosis that becomes epileptogenic, namely birth trauma or anoxia, postnatal brain trauma and postinflammatory brain scarring, together accounted for just over 50% of the series. In 80 patients, 7%, there was more than one significant etiological factor. In most instances these consisted of significant birth trauma followed by a later head injury, or severe febrile convulsion or some inflammatory intracranial episode. Sixty patients, 5%, exhibited a variety of interesting miscellaneous lesions. These will be referred to again below. The etiology was listed as unknown in 240 patients, 22%. It is probable, however, that in many of these the etiology is actually subclinical birth trauma or anoxia. The basis for this belief is threefold: 1. the gross pathological changes encountered during the temporal lobectomy are usually similar to those seen in patients with a definite history of birth trauma or anoxia; 2. the age of onset of the seizures is usually about the same as in these with definite birth trauma, namely early or middle childhood and 3. the skull X-rays of many of this group have shown the typical relative smallness of the involved middle fossa or hemicranium that denotes brain injury sustained at birth or in early infancy. Nevertheless, since these patients did not have definite clinical evidence of having sustained brain injury in the perinatal period, the etiology has been classified as unknown.

There is a small group, 8 patients, with major vascular malformation.

In 162 patients, 15%, the temporal lobe epilepsy was due to a tumour. These patients did *not* have evidence of increased intracranial pressure or advancing neurological deficits. The seizures were the only symptom and these patients thus masqueraded as ordinary seizure problems and were treated as such, sometimes for years. Astrocytomas or other indolent gliomas constituted the majority, 83%. The remainder consisted of a variety of major nodular lesions, cholesteatoma, meningioma, haemangioma, large hamartoma, etc.

The age of onset of seizures in the tumour group was quite variable, ranging from 2 years of age to 60 years of age. It should be noted and emphasized that in 47 patients, 29%, the seizures began before age 16 years. Thus the onset of seizures in childhood does not enable one to rule out the possibility that an indolent glioma might be responsible for the patient's seizure tendency. Both the PEG and angiograms were negative in over 1/4 of these patients. The CT scan is helpful, but may also be normal, particularly in indolent gliomas involving the inferior aspect of the temporal lobe.

The miscellaneous group consisted of a variety of interesting lesions, both congenital and acquired (Fig. 3). The congenital lesions include pial angiomatosis of the Sturge Weber type, both full and forme fruste cases, small hamartomas or angioma calcificans, arachnoid or intracerebral cysts, small vascular malformations, tuberous sclerosis, both full and forme fruste cases, neurocutaneous melanosis and agenesis of the corpus callosum. The acquired lesions are equally varied, immunization complications, anoxic episodes due to a variety of causes, complications of nephritis, diabetes or eclampsia, small vessel disease of the brain, radiation gliosis, parasitic cyst, postpartum or septic emboli, etc.

This list of etiological factors emphasizes the importance of remembering that the so-called classifications of the epilepsies are actually only classifications of the primary *symptom* of the epilepsy. A *diagnosis* is made only when the etiology and the anatomical location of the epileptogenic lesion or area is determined as definitely as possible. The elegance of the term "complex partial seizures" almost inevitably seduces one into believing that this represents a diagnosis rather than merely the description of the patient's symptom. A diagnosis requires the addition to the term, "complex partial seizures", a statement as to the etiology; complex partial seizures due to probable birth injury, due to brain tumour, due to cause unknown, etc., and an indication of the anatomical location of the lesion; right temporal, bitemporal, left fronto-temporal, unlocalized, etc.

Pial angiomatosis (Sturge-Weber, full and forme fruste cases)	11 patients
Small hamartomas, angioma calcifications	11 patients
Arachnoid or intracerebral cysts	6 patients
Immunization complications	7 patients
Anoxic episodes (anaesthesia, toxic fumes, etc.)	4 patients
Complications of nephritis, diabetes or eclampsia	4 patients
Small vascular malformations	3 patients
Small vessel disease of the brain (arteriosclerosis, etc.)	3 patients
Various acquired brain lesions (radiation gliosis, parasitic cyst, post partum or septic emboli to the brain, etc.)	7 patients
Various congenital brain lesions (tuberous sclerosis, neurocutaneous melanosis, agenesis of corpus callosum)	4 patients

Fig. 3. Temporal lobe epilepsy—etiology. Miscellaneous non-tumoural lesions. 60 patients operated upon 1928 through 1978

Diagnostic Problems

The clinical attack pattern of seizures arising in the temporal lobe, as is well known, frequently does not give any evidence as to whether the attacks arise in the right temporal lobe, the left, or in both. Therefore it is necessary as a rule to rely heavily on the EEG to answer this question, and thus provide a basis for recommendation for or against a surgical approach when the patients' seizures cannot be adequately controlled medically. At the MNI we have relied primarily on the repeated recording and localizational analysis of the interictal epileptiform spiking in the EEG as the patient's antiepileptic medication is progressively withdrawn. In recent years the use of chronically implanted flexible fine wire sphenoidal electrodes has been particularly useful, since this permits repeated examinations including sphenoidal recordings to be made without additional discomfort to the patient [6].

The use of telemetry in recent years has greatly increased the capability of recording large numbers of interictal spikes over long periods of time and during various types of daily activity and during various phases of sleep without adding an undue burden and cost to the EEG laboratory[7].

The system set up by Mr. John Ives, our neuroelectronic engineer, and his team, permits the sampling of 16 EEG channels for flexible

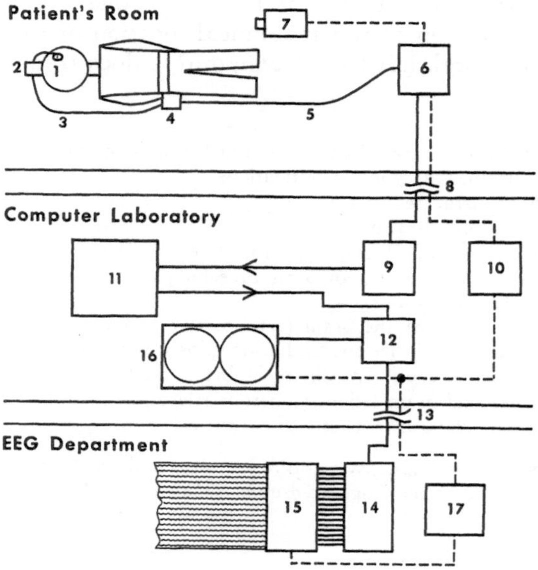

Fig. 4. Block diagram of seizure monitoring system. (From Ives, Thompson, and Gloor 1976, ref. 9)

segments of time and at a variety of preselected intervals. An automatic spike detection gadget developed by Dr. Jean Gottman permits a quantitative analysis of spike localization and lateralization to a degree not possible to date by the traditional eyeball analysis [2, 3]. The usefullness and accuracy of this technique in selecting patients for temporal lobectomy is being studied in detail at present.

Spontaneous attacks have occasionally been recorded since the earliest days of the EEG era at the MNI, and sometimes have provided good localizational and lateralizing information. It is only since the introduction of telemetry however that this has become a *major* aspect of the study of patients with complicated seizure problems. When the recording of attacks is the main aim of the telemetric session [9], the EEG is continually recorded on tape and then erased after 2 minutes have gone by (Fig. 4). If the patient has an aura, or an attack is seen by a nurse or visitor, a button on the bed-side rail is pushed, causing the previous 2 minutes of EEG to be written out, along with the ensuing 3–5 minutes. This system has enabled us to record one or more spontaneous attacks in the great majority of patients in whom this was considered necessary. To date

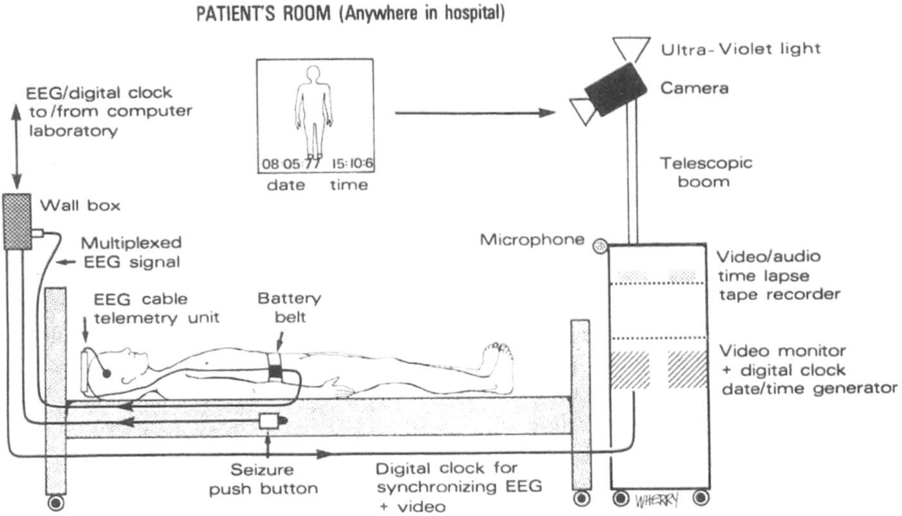

Fig. 5. Mobile video unit, its placement with respect to the patient and its interconnections with existing EEG cable-telemetry system. (From Ives and Gloor 1978, ref. 8)

about half of the recorded attacks have provided clear cut localizing or lateralizing information. In about a quarter of the recorded attacks the onset consists of a bilaterally symmetrical suppression of activity and the recording of the attack does not help in determining the lateralization of the patient's seizure problem. In the remaining quarter of the recorded attacks the brain waves are obscured by muscle artifact and the lateralization of the attack cannot be determined despite replaying the tape using various filters.

Telemetry on an ambulatory or out-patient basis, using a small cassette to record 4 EEG channels is also under investigation. This is employed in patients whose attacks are clinically clearly temporal in origin but the conventional EEG investigation has failed to identify the lateralization of the epileptogenic temporal cortex, and recording of spontaneous attacks is needed [10].

A recent addition to the telemetry system is video monitoring when visualization of the attack and correlation with the EEG record is desired [8]. This system provides for continuous video taping at 3 frames per second, permitting 18 hours of taping before the tape cassette needs to be replaced (Fig. 5). A time marker on the video tape is correlated with a similar time marker on the EEG record so that accurate correlations between the two can be made.

In about 5% of the patients we study at the MNI with more or less typical temporal lobe epilepsy from the clinical standpoint, even this extensive telemetry EEG program fails to tell us whether the attacks are arising in the right temporal lobe, the left temporal lobe, or independently in both temporal lobes. They then become candidates for our chronic stereotactic depth electrode EEG and stimulation program. This is carried out by Dr. André Olivier, one of the younger members of our senior neurosurgical staff, who is also actively involved in all other aspects of the MNI surgical management of medically refractory focal epilepsy. We are deeply grateful to Drs. Talairach, Bancaud, Szikla and Bonis for the gracious and effective assistance they provided to Dr. Olivier when he sought their help several years ago in the early stages of setting up his program.

In the first 18 of these highly selected bitemporal epileptic patients studied by Dr. Olivier, the depth electrode recordings of spontaneous EEG and clinical attacks in 16 were sufficiently well lateralized to warrant temporal lobectomy, which was carried out in 15. In the remaining, 2 patients attacks were recorded arising from each temporal lobe and operation was considered inadvisable. Thirteen of the 15 operated patients now have at least a 2 year follow-up period and the results to date show that 6 patients (46%) have had a complete or nearly complete remission of the seizure tendency.

Finally, a brief comment on positron emission tomography [4], a rapidly evolving technique of great *potential* value in a variety of neurological conditions, including epilepsy (Fig. 6). Its value as a non-invasive method of analyzing regional blood flow and microcirculation in the brain is already well established [17, 18]. Studies on regional blood flow changes in patients with focal epilepsy [5] encourage further investigation of regional cerebral blood flow studies with this new, non-invasive technique as a potential localizing tool in epilepsy. Of even more potential importance, however, is the possibility of measuring regional activity of various aspects of brain function by tagging metabolically active substances with positron emitting isotopes, and thus permitting the delineation of areas of increased or decreased metabolic activity.

Although much basic developmental work lies ahead, the potential effectiveness of this new technique in both clinical and research in-

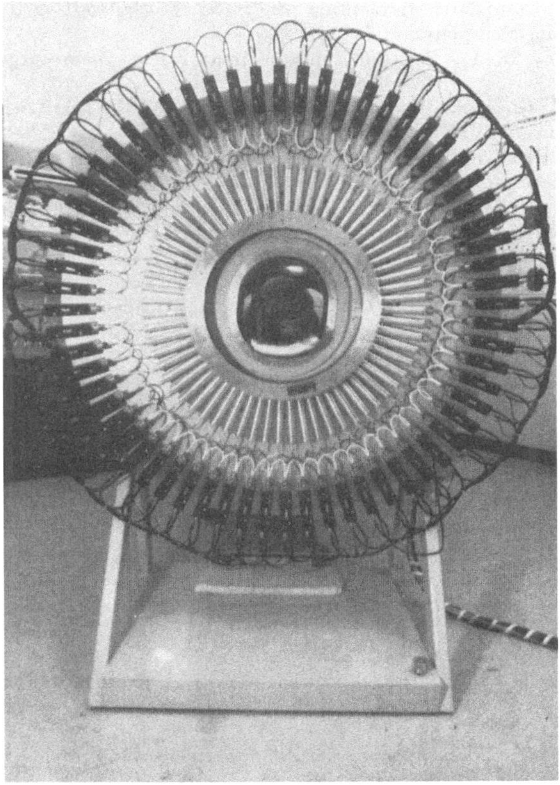

Fig. 6. Positron emission tomography apparatus. (From Yamamoto *et al.*, ref. 18)

vestigations of brain function and dysfunction is exciting to say at the least. Perhaps the EEG, the CT scan and electrical stimulation of the brain, before long, will be joined by another noninvasive clinical and research tool of equal, or even greater importance and clinical usefulness. Positron emission tomography promises to provide further impetus to the tendency for neurosurgery to become progressively more functional in orientation.

References

1. Feindel, W., Penfield, W., Localization of discharge in temporal lobe automatism. A.M.A. Arch. Neurol. Psychiat. *72* (1954), 605—630.
2. Gotman, J., Gloor, P., Automatic recognition and quantification of interictal epileptic activity in the human scalp EEG. Electroenceph. clin. Neurophysiol. *41* (1976), 513—529.
3. Gotman, J., Gloor, P., Schaul, N., Comparison of traditional reading of the EEG and automatic recognition of interictal epileptic activity. Electroenceph. clin. Neurophysiol. *44* (1978), 48—60.
4. Grubb, Jr., R. L., Positron emission tomography. Neurosurgery *2* (1978), 273—280.
5. Hougaard, K., *et al.*, Regional cerebral blood flow in focal cortical epilepsy. Arch. Neurol. *33* (1976), 527—535.
6. Ives, J. R., Gloor, P., Update: Chronic sphenoidal electrodes. Electroenceph. clin. Neurophysiol. *44* (1978), 789—790.
7. Ives, J. R., Thompson, C. J., Gloor, P., *et al.*, Multichannel telemetrycomputer monitoring of epileptic patients. In: Biotelemetry II, 2nd International Symposium, pp. 216—218. Basel: Karger. 1974.
8. Ives, J. R., Gloor, P., A long time-lapse video system to document the patient's spontaneous clinical seizure synchronized with the EEG. Electroenceph. clin. Neurophysiol. *45* (1978), 412—416.
9. Ives, J. R., Thompson, C. J., Gloor, P., Seizure monitoring: A new tool in electroencephalography. Electroenceph. clin. Neurophysiol. *41* (1976), 422—427.
10. Ives, J. R., Woods, J. F., A study of 100 patients with focal epilepsy using a 4 channel ambulatory cassette recorder. 3rd International Symposium on Ambulatory Monitoring. In press.
11. Penfield, W., Gage, L., Cerebral localization of epileptic manifestations. Arch. Neurol. Psychiat. *30* (1933), 1—19.
12. Penfield, W., Jasper, H., Epilepsy and the functional anatomy of the human, p. 521. Boston: Little, Brown and Co. 1954.
13. Rasmussen, T., Surgery of epilepsy associated with brain tumours. In: Neurosurgical Management of the Epilepsies, pp. 227—239 (Purpura, D. P., *et al.*, ed.). New York: Raven Press. 1974.
14. Rasmussen, T., Surgical treatment of patients with complex partial seizures. In: Complex Partial Seizures and their Treatment, pp. 415—442 (Penry, J. K., Daly, D. D., eds.). New York: Raven Press. 1975.
15. Rasmussen, T., Surgical aspects (of temporal lobe seizures in childhood). In: Topics in Child Neurology, pp. 143—157 (Blaw, M. E., *et al.*, eds.). New York-London: Spectrum Publications. 1977.
16. Rasmussen, T., Cortical resection for medically refractory focal epilepsy: results, lessons and questions. In: Functional Neurosurgery, pp. 253—269 (Rasmussen, T., Marino, R., eds.). New York: Raven Press. 1979.
17. Yamamoto, Y. L., Thompson, C. J., Meyer, E., Robertson, J. S., Feindel, W., Dynamic positron emission tomography for study of cerebral hemodynamics in a cross section of the head using positron-emitting ^{68}Ga-EDTA and ^{77}Kr. J. Computer Assisted Tomography *1* (1977), 43—56.
18. Yamamoto, Y. L., Little, J. R., Meyer, E., Thompson, C., Feindel, W., Topographical regional cerebral blood flow by positron emission tomography with Krypton ^{77} before and after vascular by-pass to the brain. J. Neurosurg. In press.

Acta Neurochirurgica, Suppl. 30, 25—34 (1980)

Surgery of Epilepsy Based on Stereotactic Investigations — the Plan of the SEEG Investigation

J. Bancaud*

With 7 Figures

The main references of this report will be the methodology and the results obtained by the Montreal team who brought up the basic problems of this surgery requiring an actual multidisciplinary collaboration (Talairach *et al.* 1974).

After the Second World War most authors, less strict perhaps but willing to follow the Montreal researchers, had to give up their fruitless endeavours which proved to be quite detrimental, in Europe at least, to that type of surgery (Talairach *et al.* 1974).

In 1957, Talairach and I thought that stereotactic investigation and isotopic destruction of certain deep structures might open new prospects beneficial to patients, but we soon lost our illusions (Talairach *et al.* 1974).

In our opinion the surgery of epilepsy has to rely upon a methodology starting from a thorough electro-clinical study of the particular patient and ending by the removal of the cortical structures basically involved in the seizure: in spite of possible common characteristics partial epileptic seizures are different in each individual case (Figs. 1 and 2).

We therefore emphasize the importance of different interrelated stages in the methodological process.

Above all, we believe that the surgical therapeutic decision must be based on clinical, EEG and neuroradiological investigations.

* Unité de Recherches INSERM (U. 97) sur l'Épilepsie, 2ter, rue d'Alésia, F-75014 Paris, et Service de Neurochirurgie Fonctionnelle de l'Hôpital Sainte-Anne, 1, rue Cabanis, F-75014 Paris, France.

0065-1419/80/Suppl. 30/0025/$ 02.00

I. Investigations Prior to Stereo-EEG Exploration

They are most essential and we can only summarize them in the present report.

1. Clinical Assessment

a) Evolution of the Pathological Process

In our practice, the first step taken up by several clinicians is to trace back the main stages of the pathological process.

1. Occurrence and aetiology of the first seizure taking especially into consideration:

age at onset of seizures,
triggering factors,
neurological, somatic, and psychological background,
seizure pattern—duration—time when seizures occur etc.

2. Anamnestic data on the patient and his family which might influence surgical indications and results.

3. The main problem is to reconstruct as accurately as possible the clinical symptoms of the seizures.

a) Importance of subjective phenomena present at the onset of the seizure.

b) History of seizure patterns, in particular:

monomorphic seizures or discreet modifications of symptoms,
semiologic changes:

disappearance of certain signs,
appearance of new signs,
modifications of the chronological sequence of symptoms.

The aim is to assess whether there is a single type of seizure or different types of seizures which might indicate plurifocal epilepsy, taking into consideration the age (maturation).

This should obviously imply repeated interviews with the patient and with his family.

c) Present seizures.

Seizures have to be observed under different conditions:

before and after a progressive withdrawal of drug treatment,
spontaneous seizures or under hyperpnoea,
standing or lying position of the patient etc.

The basic aim of clinical investigation is to interprete the chronological sequence of ictal signs in terms of an anatomo-functional disorganization.

In other words, this means establishing the hypotheses on the origin and the propagation of ictal discharges in the light of literature data on paroxystic or permanent cortical dysfunction in humans, refering to:

epileptology,

traumatic, vascular, tumoural etc. pathology (neurological deficits),

effects of central electrical stimulation, and

our own experience.

Neurology
EEG
Stereotactic neuroradiology

Fig. 1. Prior to stereo-EEG

Clinical history
Seizures
  Age of onset
  Triggering factors
  Different seizure types?
  Chronology of seizure symptoms
Neurologic examinations (pre-ictal; ictal; post-ictal)
Psychologic examination

Fig. 2. Neurology

b) Pre-, Per-, and Post-Ictal Neurological Investigation

1. Importance of this assessment to evaluate surgical possibilities and consequences.

2. Particular importance of the post-ictal examination: the post-ictal deficit is quite often of very short duration. It expresses either:

the lesion at the origin of the seizures,

a transitional functional exclusion of structures involved in the seizure.

3. Mandatory study of manual prevalence and of speech predominance (Wada's intracarotid amytal test).

c) Paraclinical Examinations

Routine examinations, such as standard radiographs of the skull with at least 3 incidences.

d) Psychiatric and Psychological Assessment

In our opinion, this assessment is a major factor to evaluate the indications of the stereo-EEG exploration, of the surgical decision and it is even bearing upon surgical strategy.

2. EEG Studies

a) Interictal EEG (Fig. 3)

It is imperative to take into account the evolution of EEG patterns over a long period: even over a relatively short period, it is necessary to repeat examinations under different conditions.

The purpose of the examination is double:

To suggest or confirm a possible
single,
multiple,
diffuse.
lesional process.

To evaluate either the presence or the absence of localized or multiple or diffuse spikes.

Interictal EEG even in spite of difficulties in interpretation, is an indispensable tool (Bancaud *et al.* 1973).

b) Ictal EEG

In our opinion, recording of actual seizures is a basic factor to determine the presumed origin of discharges, and an essential point in the discussion of indications of stereo-EEG exploration.

Thus, this determination results from a comparison between the clinical seizure pattern and the expression of discharges on the scalp.

In fact, this is much more a methodological than a purely technical problem: the correlation between different clinical signs constituting the seizure and the chronological expression on the scalp of the discharge of the territory or territories involved, must be established as accurately as possible.

This requires precise observation, description (magnetophone) and reconstruction (magnetoscope) in terms of recorded EEG sequences. EEG records are performed with different techniques (conventional and telemetric) under different conditions (patient awake or asleep, before and during withdrawal of drug treatment etc.).

Spontaneous seizures or seizures induced through hyperpnea or through peripheral stimulations must be recorded. These seizures are, in our opinion, the best criterion for a topographic definition of epileptogenic areas in order to plan a stereo-EEG investigation. However, the patient should be submitted to chemical activators (Megimide or Metrazol), especially whenever these activators are used during the stereo-EEG exploration, which is frequently the case.

The validity of these methods certainly would desserve a wider discussion (Bancaud *et al.* 1973).

Once established, this assessment will lead to make a decision on neuroradiological contrast studies and on its stereotactic modalities.

3. Stereotactic Localization

The three main objectives on this investigation are:

1. to discover and to define as accurately as possible the pathological modifications of cortical and sub-cortical structures possibly involved in the seizures,
2. to allows for the implantation of several intracerebral electrodes with a maximal precision and minimal risks,
3. to facilitate the planning of the surgical act.

Inter-ictal	Multiple several EEG's recorded in various conditions
Ictal	spontaneous seizures hyperpnea peripheric stimulations sleep recording chemical activations

Fig. 3. EEG

Choice of structures to be investigated
Acute or chronic investigation
Techniques
  Electrodes
  Recording
  Stimulation
Successive stages of the investigation

Fig. 4. Stereo-EEG

1. Hypotheses on possible origin and propagation of seizure discharges (anatomo-electro-clinical correlations).
2. Surgical considerations (functional risks etc.).
3. Topography of lesions.

Fig. 5. Choice of the structures to be investigated

II. Stereo-EEG Exploration

Its purpose is to define the epileptogenic area; the neurosurgeon will thus be able to prepare the procedure, taking into consideration relations between the possible lesion and this area, together with the functional data evidenced by the exploration of neighboring brain structures.

This method often explained and described in detail will only be summarized here (Bancaud and Dell 1959, Bancaud 1959, Bancaud *et al.* 1963, Bancaud *et al.* 1965, Bancaud and Talairach 1970, Bancaud *et al.* 1973, Bancaud and Talairach 1974, Talairach and

Bancaud 1966, Talairach *et al.* 1962, Talairach and Bancaud 1973, Talairach and Bancaud 1973, Talairach *et al.* 1974).

1. Strategy of Stereo-EEG Exploration (Figs. 4 and 5)

The choice of structures to be explored through intracerebral electrodes is a decisive factor, inasmuch as the obtained data depend largely on this choice. Thus, and in opposition to classical electrocorticography where the data obtained are limited to the surgical field, our method requires coherent and verifiable hypotheses established prior to the exploration.

These hypotheses are based upon data from previous clinical, EEG and neuroradiological investigations. As the chronological organization of the signs constituting a seizure are most significant to determine the epileptogenic area, electrodes will therefore be implanted according to origin and propagation modalities of ictal discharges.

The great diversity of anatomo-clinical correlations characterizing partial seizures makes it impossible to standardize the implantation of electrodes and to consider identical procedures on patients presenting different types of epilepsy.

As stereo-EEG exploration is obviously aiming towards an efficient excision with minimal functional risks, surgical considerations play a major role in the implantation of electrodes.

Finally, the choice of electrode sites must obviously be decided according to the presence and topography of epileptogenic lesions shown by the previous investigations.

Thus, according to this method, hypotheses underlying the choice of electrode position are major factors in interpreting and validating information supplied by stereo-EEG.

The main significance of stereo-EEG is the possibility to check, to invalidate or to confirm these assumptions and, in the latter case, to plan surgery according to them.

2. Acute and Chronic Stereo-EEG Investigations

We do not think that a discussion on the validity of these techniques is of great interest.

In our experience, the so-called chronic exploration is just a prolonged exploration when the information obtained in the operating theatre are not sufficient to consider a successful procedure (impossibility to record a seizure under satisfactory conditions; occurrence of subintrant seizures; possible need of night sleep studies; seizures occurring with a particular background of triggering factors etc.).

But if a prolongated exploration (for a few days) can prove necessary, we certainly do not think that information recorded during an acute investigation, that is shortly after placement of electrodes, is not useful.

Finally, surgical observations and neuropathological data clearly show that lesions resulting from chronic electrodes even with smaller diameters, are more extended than those left by electrodes implanted for a few hours only.

3. Technique of Exploration

These techniques have been described several times and will only be summarized here (Bancaud *et al.* 1965, 1973).

a) Electrodes

Stainless steel, multilead electrodes (5 to 20 successive plots) with different diameters according to the investigation (600 μ to 2.4 mm); the plots are 2 mm long and separated by a distance of 1.5 mm. Recording and stimulation between two successive plots is always bipolar.

Through the modification of the number and intervals of groups of plots, the electrodes are available in different sizes and adapted to the areas to be explored and to the size of the brain.

Their resistance in saline solution is around 15 or 60 kW for acute and chronic electrodes, respectively.

b) Recording

1. *Recording on paper* (Alvar Electronic and after, Siemens)

These recorders include a certain number of channels allowing for a simultaneous recording of the activities of a great number of plots of deep and surface electrodes (EEG) as well as of electrical data facilitating the interpretation (EMG, ECG etc.).

2. *Cathode oscillograph*

The simultaneous recording of 4 channel signals (Pr. Buser) allows for the study of

potentials evoked through peripheral or central stimulation,
correlations between different paroxystic activities,
normal or pathological connections between different structures.

c) Stimulations

1. *Peripheral stimulation,*
somesthesic,
proprioceptive,
visual,
auditive.

2. *Central stimulation.*

They have two objectives:

To achieve a better definition of the functional role of different structures by the evaluation of the induced functional disturbances (motor, sensory etc.).

To reproduce the seizure and/or the symptom-signal.

4. *Investigation Process*

a) Basic conditions of the investigation

These conditions will vary according to the type of exploration: acute or chronic investigation in the operating theatre or in the laboratory of clinical neurophysiology; during a conventional or telemetric recording; the patient being awake or asleep etc.

However, we wish to emphasize the points we feel to be most important in data gathering:

1. It is always imperative to maintain the patient's clear consciousness during the whole exploration as, in our opinion, his description of seizures and of the effect of stimulation is very important. This means that the anaesthesia required for electrode implantation should be superficial and should not influence the record (curarizing agent; synthetic analgesics).

2. As in previous investigations, stereo-EEG requires the close collaboration of clinicians, neurophysiologists and of neurosurgeons. The recording of seizures being a major criterion in the definition of an epileptogenic area, anatomo-electro-clinical correlations should be as precise as possible; they necessitate the help of

two neurologists dictating on a magnetophone the information inscribed on the record,

two clinical neurophysiologists and an experimental neurophysiologist,

three EEG technicians and one technician to record the whole exploration on a magnetoscope.

3. Naturally, this collaboration is also necessary to evaluate the effects of peripheral or central stimulation as well as the results of various activations.

b) Principal modalities of the investigations, data gathering (Fig. 6)

To obtain the information necessary to define an epileptogenic area and therefore the subsequent surgical procedure (see Fig. 6) the setting up of a program the stages of which varying from one patient to the other, according to seizure occurrences, to stimulation effects etc. is required.

However, we find useful a prolonged recording of interictal

activity involving all the plots of implanted electrodes in order to achieve a precise topography of lesions and of "irritative" areas.

The recording of "infraclinical" paroxysms and of seizures is of special significance therefore, a selection will be made according to different factors (for instance the occurrence of spontaneous fits), activation modalities (hyperpnea, peripheral, and central chemical activations, sleep etc.).

1. Interictal activity
   Background activity; slow waves ...
   Sporadic "spikes"
2. Subclinical paroxysms
3. Ictal activity
   Spontaneous seizures
   Hyperpnae
   Peripheric stimulations
   Central stimulations
   Sleep-recording
   Chemical activations
4. Functional localization

Fig. 6. Information recorded by stereo-EEG

1. Lesional
2. "Irritative"
3. Epileptogenic areas
   Chrono-topographic organization
   of ictal discharges related to clinical symptoms

Fig. 7. Localization of epileptogenic area

The evaluation of various functional localizations is one of the most important features of the investigation (evoked potentials, central stimulations etc.).

Finally, during the exploration, the definition of the epileptogenic area might require the implantation of additional electrodes if the location or the number of the implanted electrodes proves to be insufficient.

5. *Localization of Epileptogenic Areas* (Fig. 7)

This is obviously the major problem and most of the surgical procedure will depend on it. We cannot enter into the details of this complex matter here and will just mention the most important elements.

a) The first aim, through the results of the previous examinations, particularly of the stereotactic neuroradiological studies, is to try to determine the extension and the importance of the epileptogenic lesion.

It should however be recalled that the notion of lesion is quite ambiguous, especially in the field of epilepsy.

A lesion that completely destroys the brain cortex is not epileptogenic in itself.

Most epileptogenic lesions induce anatomical changes without total destruction.

Histological anomalies alone cannot explain the genesis of epilepsy even though they may condition it.

b) The second aim is an evaluation of the topography of the interictal spikes and above all, of their relation to seizure mechanisms. The results of the Montreal school as well as animal experiments have clearly shown that some of these spikes play a part in triggering and maintaining epilepsy while some of them are not strictly related to the origin of seizures.

Up till now and even using computerized processing of data, their differentiation is apparently not easy and rather ambiguous.

c) Therefore our main criterion remains the recording of ictal discharges and their interpretation based on anatomo-clinical criteria.

In short we could say that

the topographic origin of discharges may imply a small territory as well as an extended cortical area,

this origin seems to depend on the relative threshold of the structures involved.

in temporal epilepsy, the Ammon's horn and/or the amygdalian nucleus are very often involved due to their low threshold.

According to our experience, in most cases their destruction alone could not cure the patient.

This is why the origin of a discharge is not a satisfactory criterion to define an epileptogenic area.

The best sign characterizing a seizure seems to be at the very onset of the seizure, the three-dimensional organization of the discharge, including consequently the study of its initial propagation modalities.

If these hypotheses have any significance, they mean that it is presently impossible to define the precise limits of an epileptogenic area, provided they actually exist (dilatation and retraction); the point is to consider the excision of the tissue paying a major role in the onset of the seizure.

This in turn implies that the extent of excision cannot be limited to very small cortical areas except in very few cases.

It is however clear that the value of the definition of an epileptogenic area can only be established through the surgical procedure and its results.

Acta Neurochirurgica, Suppl. 30, 35—54 (1980)

Application of Stereotactic Concepts to the Surgery of Epilepsy

J. Talairach* and **G. Szikla****

With 6 Figures

Summary

For the authors, the essential feature of stereotaxis is the *three-dimensional representation of the entire brain,* including the central gray nuclei as well as the cerebral cortex. Stereotactic neurosurgery, which in this conception might be called "global", associates data from *indirect localization* (basic reference lines, proportional grid) to *direct individual localization* (performed by bidirectional, orthogonal teleradiography, with stereoscopy). The obtained high precision radiographic documents allow to establish the three coordinates (X, Y, Z).

This method, also used in localization of tumours and interstitial irradiation of tumours, led to the definition of a *special methodology* for epilepsy surgery (threefold correlation of the clinical seizure patterns, electrical anomalies and the concerned anatomical structures). The stereotactic implantation of several acute and chronic electrodes (stereo-EEG) gives a *3-dimensional* definition of the epileptogenic area and of its propagation pathways. These data, as well as the individual anatomy of the patient's brain are represented by the neurosurgeon on a surgical diagram. *The transfer of these data to the surgical field* is facilitated by the accuracy of the diagram. A double postoperative control is made (photographs—teleangiography).

The described methodology increases the precision of open surgery. It is also used to localize and to remove "incipient" lesions evidenced by the CT scan (accurate anatomical localization—vascularization). In the opinion of the authors, the use of a *common stereotactic geometry* applied to the collection of paraclinical data will lead in the future to an increased precision of surgery and hence, to a better respect of the brain and of its function.

---

* Prof. J. Talairach, Chef du Service de Neurochirurgie Fonctionnelle du Centre Hospitalier Sainte-Anne, 1, rue Cabanis, F-75674 Paris, Cedex 14, France.

** Dr. G. Szikla, Maître de Recherche au C.N.R.S., Service de Neurochirurgie Fonctionnelle du Centre Hospitalier Sainte-Anne, 1, rue Cabanis, F-75674 Paris, Cedex 14, France.

0065-1419/80/Suppl. 30/0035/$ 04.00

Introduction

For many years[14, 15], we have felt that the use of a "global" stereotactic methodology could contribute to the evolution of "classical" neurosurgery and this concept has been especially applied to the surgery of epilepsy[1]. Epilepsy is the subject of the present report which has already been initiated by J. Bancaud, in the preceeding chapter.

Nevertheless, it seems to us that beyond the surgery of epilepsy, this stereotactic methodology finds an increasing place in the surgery of certain brain tumours because of recent developments in diagnostic methods. Indeed, brain tumour surgery has increasingly to deal with lesions diagnosed by the CT scanner at an early stage when patients present with *seizures* as the first and only symptom. In such cases, the aim of surgery is to remove the lesion and to suppress seizures with an emphasis on minimizing functional loss. In order to reduce morbidity, a high degree of surgical precision is obviously required. This in turn implies the necessity of more complete and more precise *three-dimensional* preoperative data which will help to localize both the lesion and the adjacent brain structures.

This information comes from different sources, for example, the CT and gamma scans, the EEG[2] and neuroradiological, neurophysiological and anatomo-pathological studies. Together these will be particularly useful in planning surgical management but necessitate the collection of all data within the same coordinate system, corresponding precisely to the three dimensions of the brain. In other words, the *stereotactic approach*, used, *e.g.*, to perform an intratumoural interstitial irradiation[3, 9, 19] which will be discussed in an other Symposium, *can also guide open surgical procedures*[3, 20].

This report aims at illustrating the contribution of stereotactic concepts and methods to epilepsy surgery from the technical point of view.

The main problem is to establish, as easily and as accurately as possible, a satisfactory correlation between the pattern of the seizure, abnormal electrical activities, and the location of affected brain structures[1, 19].

This threefold correlation is in our opinion indispensable to the definition of an epileptogenic area in three dimensions and the propagation of the seizure towards other structures, and further to establish an adequate plan of the required neurosurgical procedure. For the localization of the three dimensional focus of the seizure, we use a stereotactic technique which might be called a "global" or "whole brain" stereotaxis allowing also three-dimensional localization

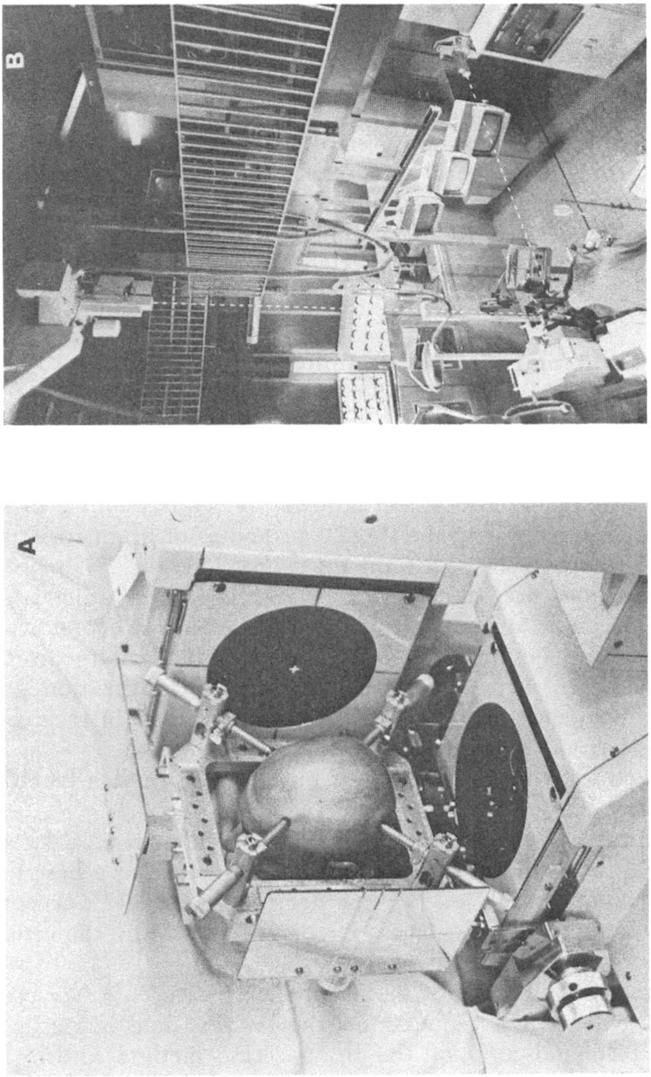

Fig. 1. A. Bidirectional stereotactic angiography: head fixed in the frame equipped with mirrors reflecting laser beam coaxial to X-rays. Film changer. B. Teleradiographic equipment in the stereotactic operating room (focal distance: 4.3 m), yielding undistorted, natural size radiographs. ×1.02–1.05

of brain structures, including the central gray nuclei and the cerebral cortex. The latter is obviously essential for the full definition of the epileptic phenomenon.

This report consists of two parts.

The first is a brief description of "global" stereotactic neuro-radiological localization techniques. In the surgery of epilepsy, their aim is

to localize brain structure in space,

to demonstrate lesions possibly related to the symptoms, and

to allow for intracerebral placement of electrodes within the radiologically localized brain structures (stereo-EEG) [1].

The second is related to the techniques of cortical excision, the extent of which is stereotactically defined by data gathered prior to craniotomy [21].

"Global" Stereotactic Radiological Localization

The patient, under general anaesthesia, is placed in a stereotactic frame first designed in 1949 [11]. Its successive modifications will not be described here. The rectangular frame together with the corresponding radiological equipment allows for *bidirectional, orthogonal* teleradiography giving the three coordinates of brain structures (X, Y on the lateral view, Y, Z on the frontal view). A 5 m focal distance is used and precise centering of X-rays is now achieved by laser beams (Fig. 1 A and B). Thus, all radiographs are practically distortion free and bound by a *common geometry:* enlargement is minimal, and taken into account by a corrected localization grid. A geometrically identical double grid allows for direct intracerebral insertion of electrodes without calculation.

As it is well known, localization of brain structures can be either direct or indirect [14].

A. *The indirect localization* is well known as the classical stereotactic localization method. It is achieved by reference to a base line, usually the bicommissural AC-PC line described in 1952 [12], accepted by most authors and used in most stereotactic atlases of the central gray nuclei [6, 16] (Fig. 2 a).

For indirect localization of telencephalic structures [18], we use a proportional grid system centered on the AC-PC line, taking into account the principal axes of the brain. This method allows for statistical localization of the cortical structures which could not be visualized directly, proportionality compensating in part for difference in brain sizes. By reducing differing cerebral anatomy to a standard common denominator, statistical evaluation of these studies

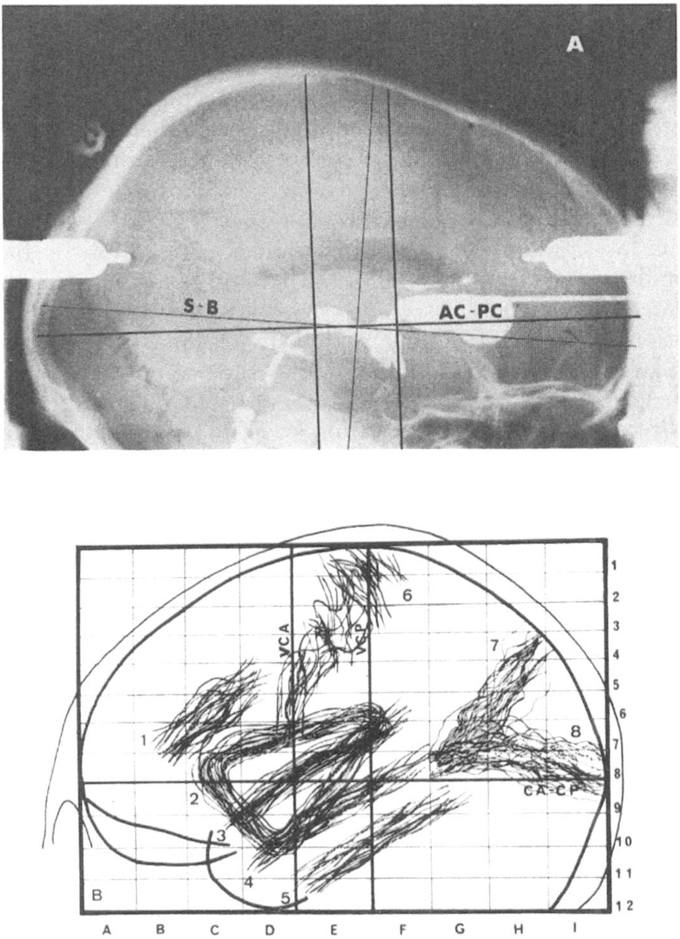

Fig. 2. A. The bicommissural AC-PC line, central reference for indirect localization. In the initial description (Talairach 1949) it follows the hypothalamic sulcus (upper border of AC—lower border of PC). The variant used in the Schaltenbrand-Bailey atlas is indicated as well (S–B). B. The proportional grid localization system based on the bicommissural line, allows for indirect localization of cortical structures (here, outlines of some major sulci: *1* inferior frontal, *2* insula, *3* Sylvian fissure (surface), *4–5* superior and middle temporal, *6* central, *7* parieto-occipital, *8* calcarine; Talairach, Szikla 1967)

is facilitated [18] (Fig. 2 B). This is the fundamental element in the so-called N.A.CRE process of standardization by anamorphosis (Pecker and Scarabin) [4].

Obviously, the most accurate localization of a structure is its *direct localization* in the individual patient. Some structures can be delimited by an adjacent subarachnoidal space, others by characteristic details of the ventriculogram. Gyri and sulci of the cortex can be localized with precision by the tortuous course of arteries running on their surfaces, as has been shown by one of us [7, 8].

This localization by three-dimensional angiography is based on the simultaneous study of lateral and frontal projections and greatly facilitated by stereoscopy [5, 8]. The latter, supplying a three-dimensional image by adding a slightly oblique (6 °) incidence, is particularly helpful to disentangle the superimposed, more or less superficial or deep vessels. In this way, based on the recordings of both *direct and indirect localization*, an accurate stereotactic diagram can be built up, showing the patient's brain with its different anatomical planes. Arteries, veins, subarachnoid spaces, ventricles and possible abnormalities are superimposed on this diagram, on the *AC-PC line*, and on the *proportional grid* [19]. As it will be shown, the diagram can be most useful for cortical excision, as the landmarks of superficial blood vessels may orient the surgeon and allow him to identify the exposed cortical structures.

In *stereo-EEG explorations*, chronic or acute electrodes are placed according to clinical and electrical seizure patterns as described in a preceeding chapter by J. Bancaud. We will leave aside the technique of electrode implantation using twist-drill holes guided through metallic double grids corresponding to the localization grid [11, 17–19]. The method was once considered to be "anti-surgical", but in fact proved to be easier and less traumatic than any other system and with a lower complication rate.

In general, the electrode is orthogonally introduced, in a plane parallel to the frame and thus, parallel or perpendicular to the midline. The advantage of doing this lies in the fact that the electrode follows a plane of known anatomical section which facilitates the localization of its 5, 10, or 15 plots with respect to the explored brain structures. Any other plane of introduction may be used but in that case, only the position of the electrode tip will be known with precision. It is more difficult to appreciate its *anatomical position* accurately in the case of an oblique penetration.

The patient is recorded in the acute or chronic state [19]. The general principles of this type of recording is described in Bancaud's report.

Removal of Epileptogenic Cortex

A plan for surgical excision can be made, if the data furnished by the stereo-EEG investigation indicate an appropriate location of the epileptogenic area, the excision of which should not result in significant deficit. A diagram is prepared to represent the location of the defined epileptogenic area as well as the preferential propagation of electrical discharges in three dimensions [19]. A second drawing based on the first will help to establish the plan of surgical intervention. Individual diagrams are prepared by the surgeon, prior to each operation. Some examples will show the great diversity of epileptogenic areas and of their preferential propagation pathways which are seldom restricted to one lobe (Fig. 3). (The disease process does not take our artificial delimitations into consideration.) They also show that small epileptogenic areas are rather exceptional in our practice. Patients with epilepsy limited to the temporal lobe with 1 or 2 seizures per month, with a 90 per cent surgical success rate and risks lower than those of accidental or suicidal death are quite rare in our department. Limited parietal or frontal epilepsies are also rare. On the other hand, our patient population includes a considerable number of severe cases with large epileptogenic areas and with repeated attacks of status epilepticus. In these cases, surgery is frequently considered as the patient's last chance. The removal will then often be incomplete and could hardly be considered as sufficient, at least theoretically. Nevertheless, as far as long-term results are concerned, even this type of surgery gives sometimes surprisingly good results.

The transfer of gathered data to the surgical field is an essential feature of the method. The main point is to transpose *without deformation* radiological and stereo-electroencephalographic data to the brain itself [10, 20, 21]. At first sight, this approach might seem theoretical. A practical example might be helpful to explain this procedure:

Patient B. G., 27 years.

A. Clinical Data, Stereotactic Localization, Stereo-EEG, Preoperative Diagram

First generalized tonic/clonic seizure at 7 months of age, without hyperthermia. Onset of seizures at the age of 15, with a generalized tonic/clonic seizure. Although under anti-epileptic medical treatment, the patient subsequently presented with "temporal" seizures with the following symptoms: abdominal pain, mastication, nausea, and tachycardy consistently accompanied by sialorrhea, sometimes by dyspraxic activity or by facial twitching and tonic/clonic generalized

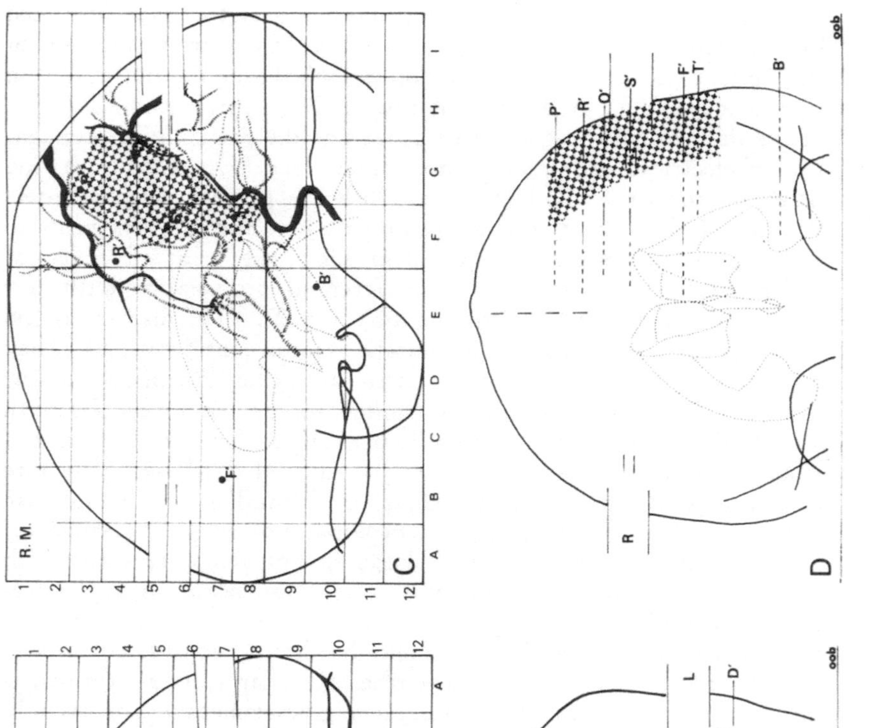
R. E.
A
B
R. M.
C
D
oob

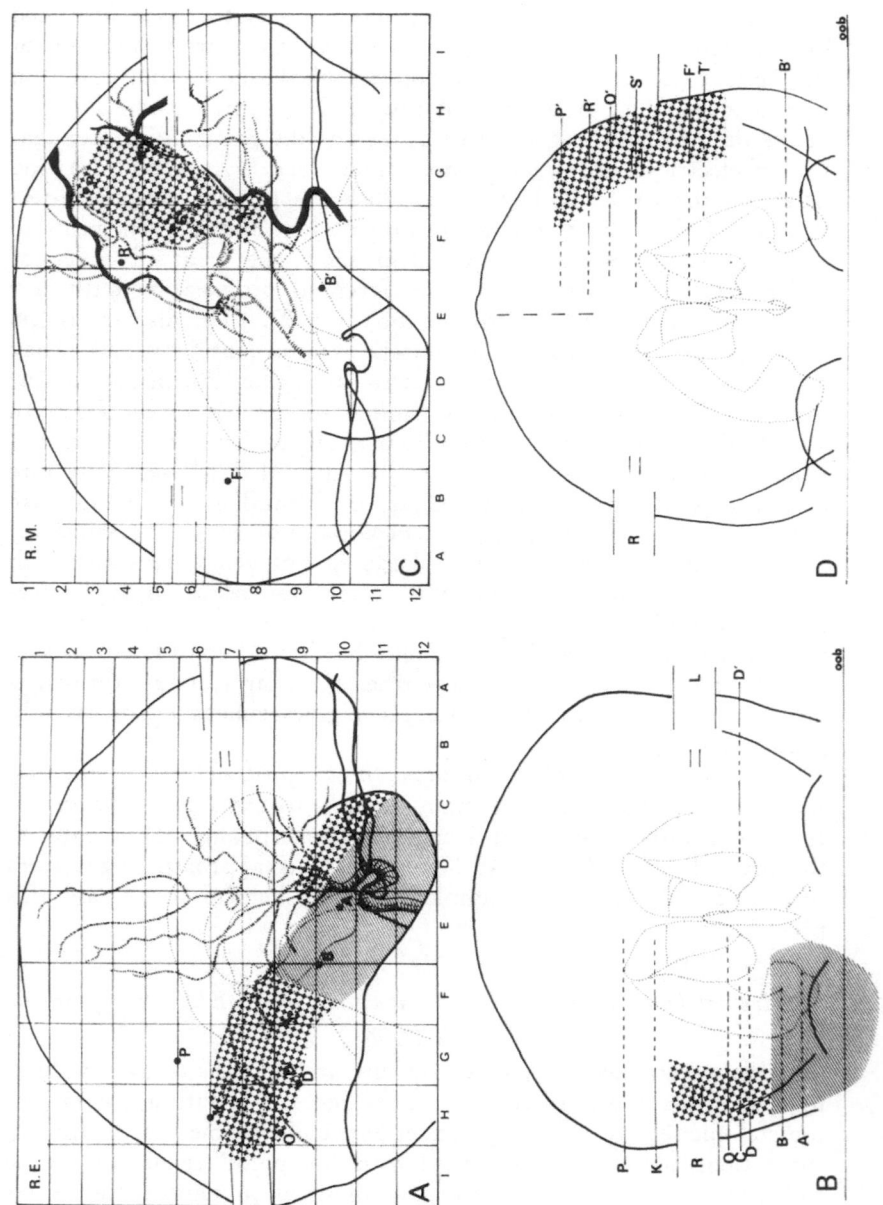

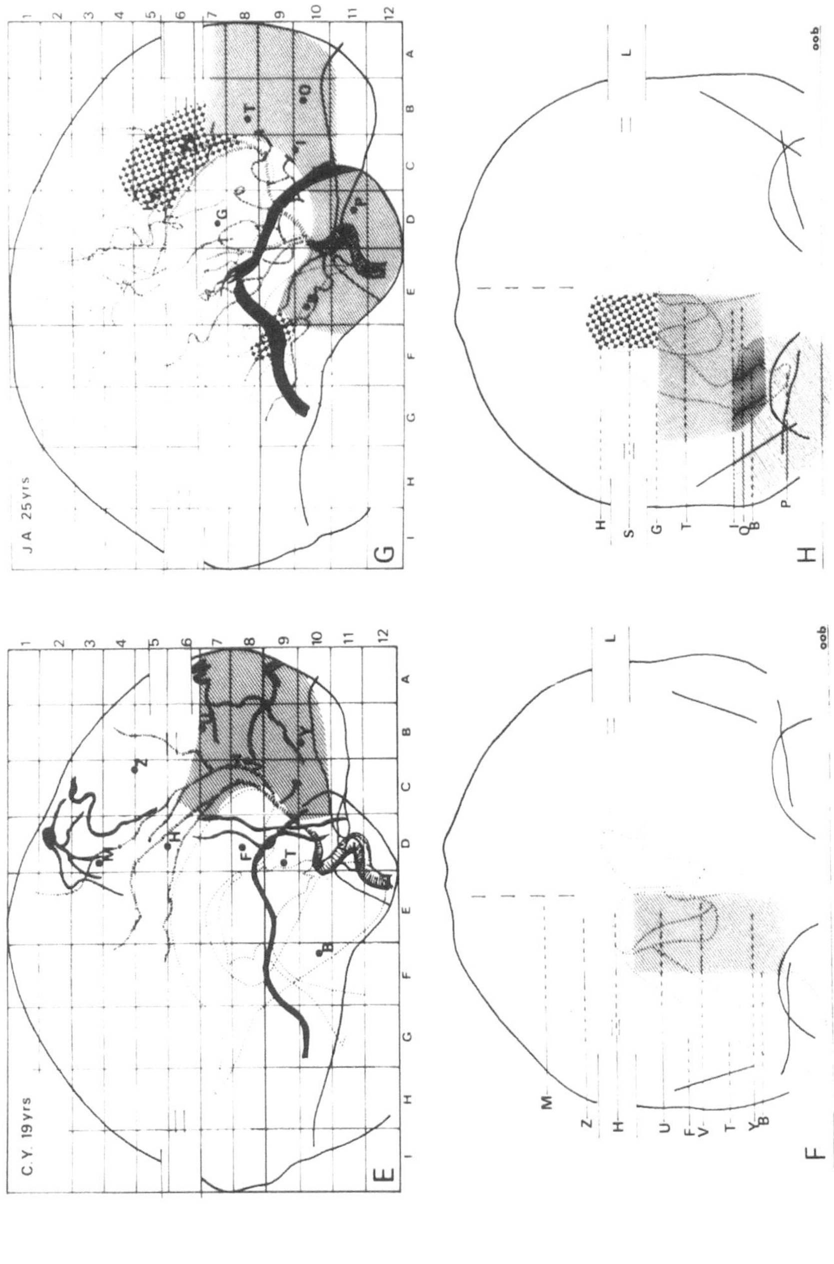

Fig. 3. Preoperative diagrams with plans of cortical excisions according to stereo-EEG and anatomical structures to be spared (ventricular cavities, arteries etc.). Note the diversity of procedures.

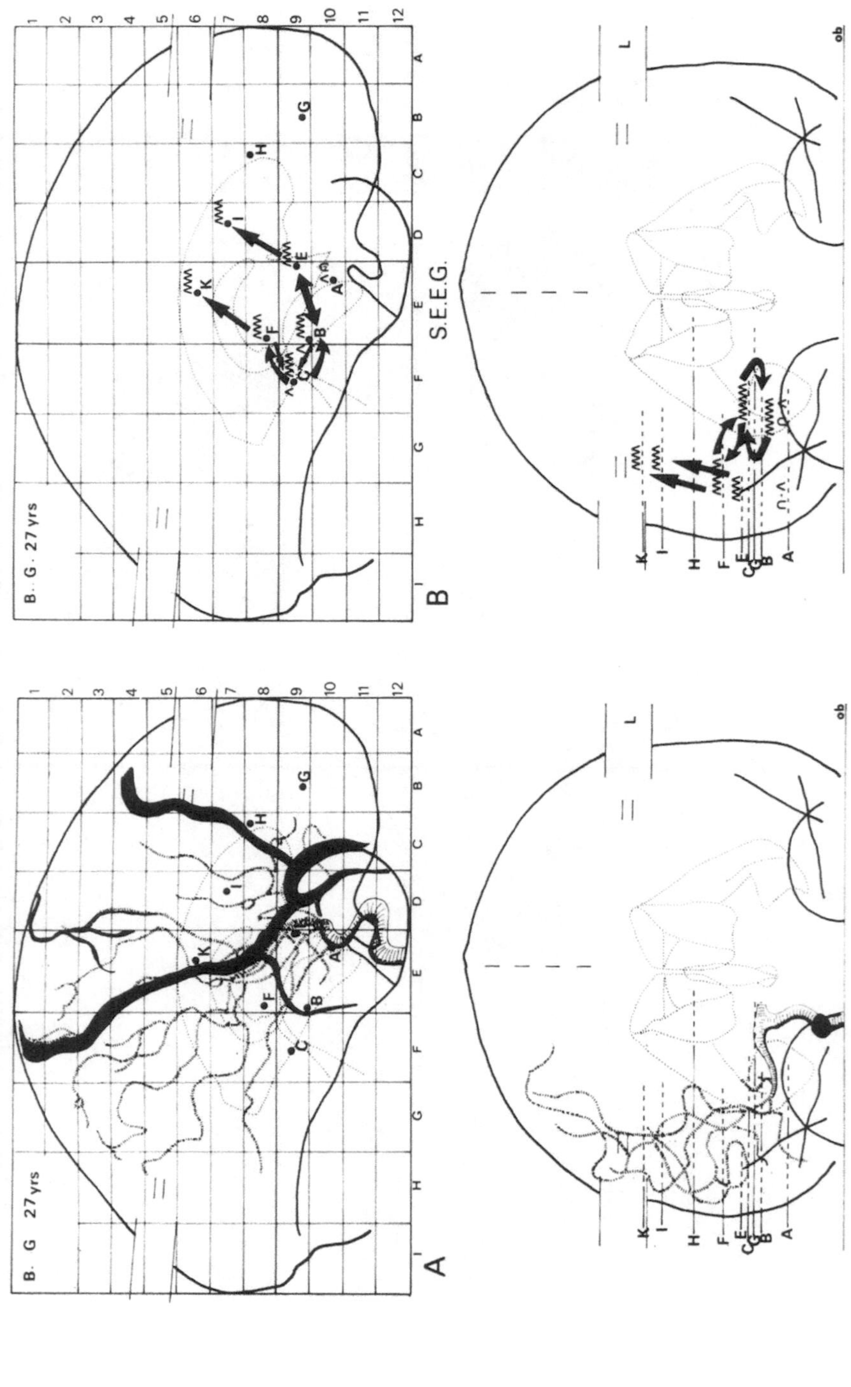
B. G. 27 yrs
A
B. G. 27 yrs
B
S.E.E.G.
L
ob

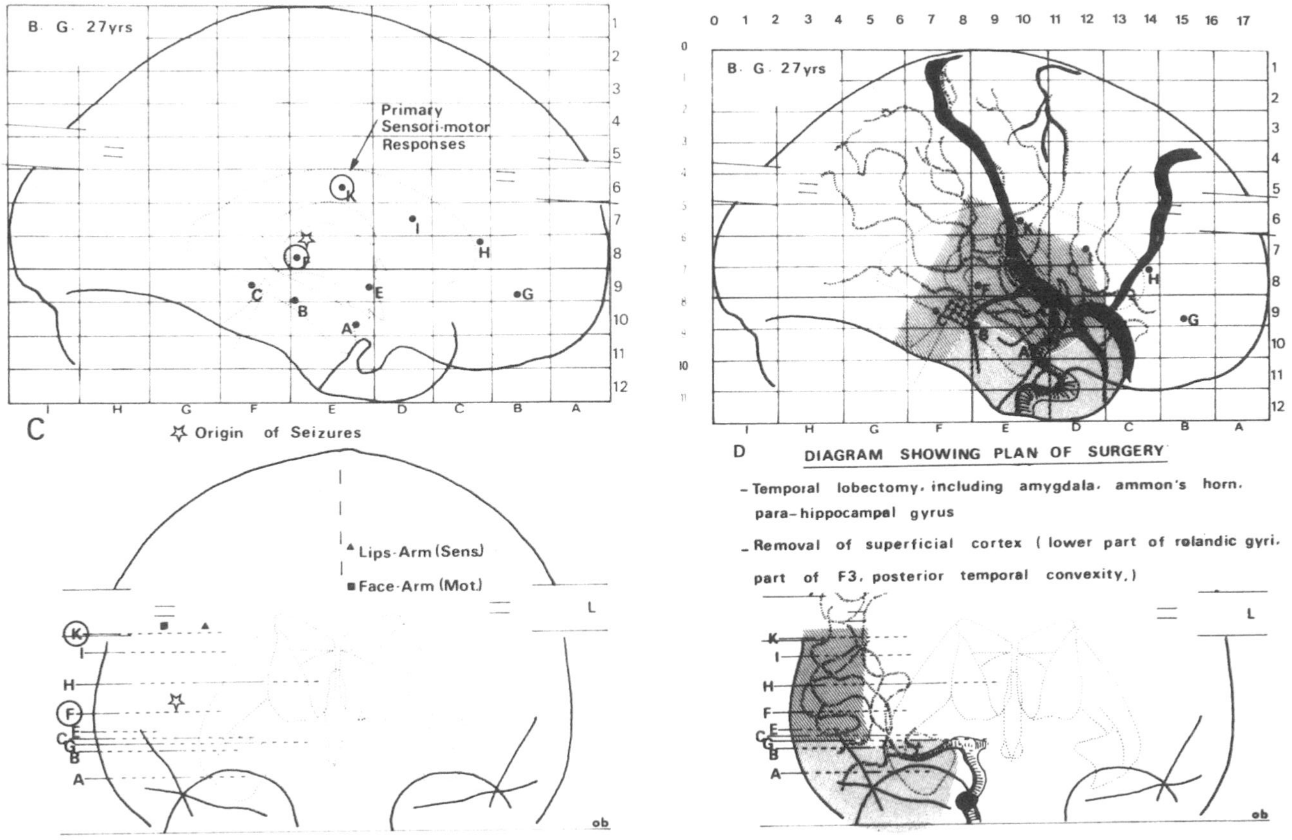

Fig. 4. A. *Anatomical diagram* showing position of arteries, veins and ventricle cavities in relationship to stereotactic base lines. B. *Stereo-EEG diagram* showing the epileptogenic area and its propagation pathways. The arrows indicate the temporal sequence of the seizure. C. *Stereo-EEG: stimulation effects: K* sensitivo-motor phenomena. *F* "Feeling of seizure onset". D. Plan of surgery: dark hatches: lobectomy, clear hatches: external cortical excision, crosses: intraventricular removal of the posterior part of Ammon's horn

fits. Seizures are numerous and often grouped (6 to 10 per day). In this severe atypical temporal lobe epilepsy, the pattern of seizures points to a temporo-periinsular origin. This hypothesis is supported by the findings of the stereo-EEG studies of the temporal lobe as well as of the lower rolandic area above the Sylvian fissure. In fact, in recorded seizures, the SEEG confirms the primordial role of the rhinencephalic structures as well as the immediate involvement of the Rolandic area. It also indicates infra- and supra-Sylvian lesions. Stimulation of electrode K located forward and below the post-central sulcus allows the localization of the Rolandic cortex (exactly corresponding to the arteriographic localization) as well as an area (electrode F) from which the *subjective start of a seizure* is reproduced.

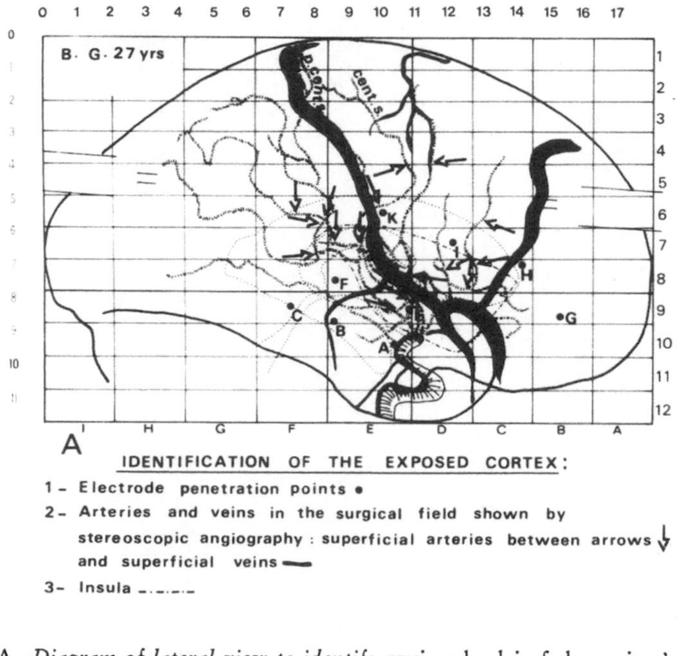

A

Fig. 5. A. *Diagram of lateral view to identify* gyri and sulci of the patient's cortex. B. *Exposed cortex:* identification of sulci (bent arrows) and of "rolandic" parieto-occipital, temporo-occipital arteries (arrows). *A* Electrode implantation points. C. *Exposed cortex:* Transpial and subpial incision (broken lines), respecting the branches of the middle cerebral artery running on the surface of the insula. Localization of the insula underlying the surgical field with the help of the visible landmarks such as superficial veins and arteries, electrode implantation points (dotted line). D. Localization of the temporal horn by the same landmarks

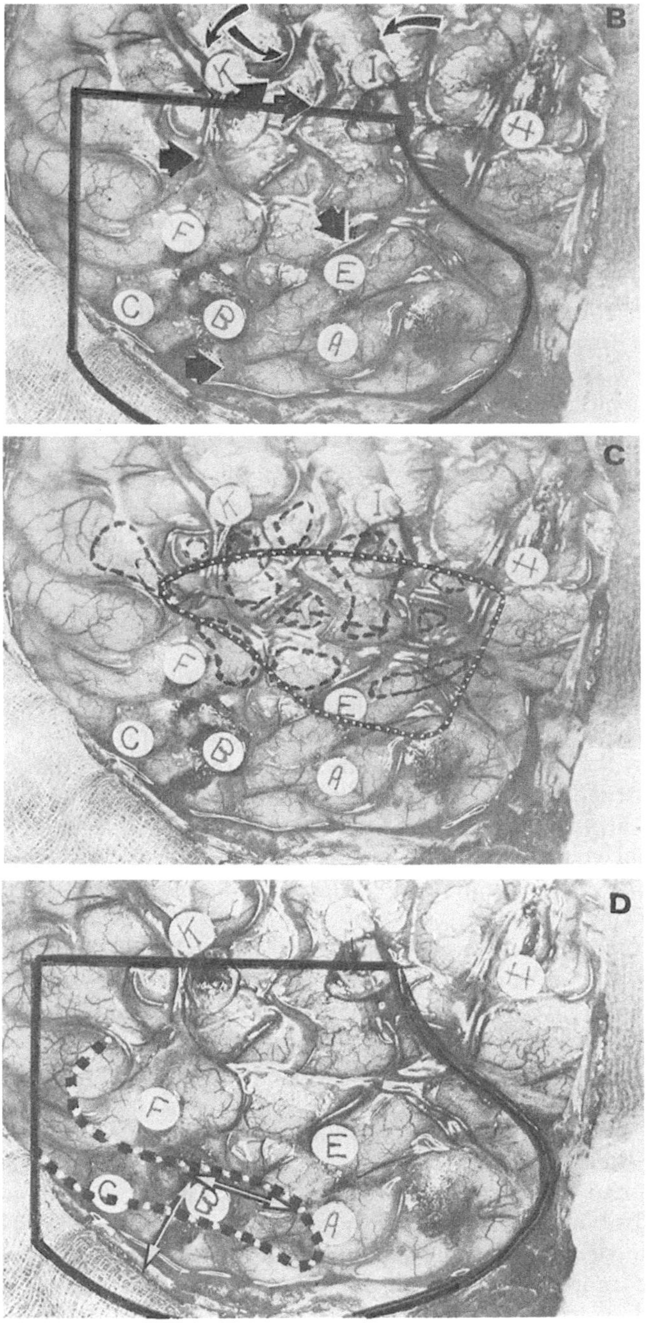

Fig. 5 B, C, D

These data reasonably indicate the need for removal of the temporal lobe with the rhinencephalic structures as well as of the lower part of the central gyri. A preoperative diagram is then prepared on this basis (Fig. 4, A, B, C, D). From then on the surgical problem is related to an accurate identification of the exposed cortex (gyri and sulci) and of the major branches of the middle cerebral artery. If the regional blood flow is to be preserved, surgical destruction should be limited to the removal planned on the diagram. In other words, prior to the surgical procedure, the possible consequences for the patient should be clearly defined. In this particular case, the operation necessarily implies a risk, which should obviously be *controlled as far as possible* so as not to inflict a neurological deficit, which would prove particularly distressing if seizures persist after the procedure.

B. Cortical Removal

The patient is placed on the operating table in an orthogonal position, thus facilitating comparison to the orthogonal radiographs which are undistorted and of approximately natural size. It is often extremely difficult and sometimes impossible to identify cortical structures without such data. In fact it is well known that as far as fissures and sulci are concerned, only the anterior part of the Sylvian fissure can be identified at craniotomy. Also, it is extremely difficult to identify with precision arteries crossing the operative field.

With the important anatomic data reported on the diagram, several structures can be identified on the exposed cortex: the sulci (*e.g.*, precentral, central, postcentral sulci), the superficial arteries, superficial veins, and electrode entry points (Figs. 5, A). These landmarks allow the delimitation of the area of excision according to the diagram (Fig. 5, B, C).

The superficial arteries crossing the exposed cortex and which are to be spared can be clearly recognized. The three main arteries of the sensori-motor area between the vein and penetration point of electrode I, several arteries running to the temporo-parietal convolutions between electrodes K and F, temporo-occipital artery going to the external temporo-occipital junction behind and above electrode E, etc. The underlying insula is also indicated in the diagram (Fig. 5, C). With the help of the electrode penetration points, the location of the *ventricle* can be defined deep to the cortex (Fig. 5, D). Thus it becomes possible to achieve a strictly orthogonal plane of section slightly below the ventricular roof, avoiding penetration into the sublenticular area and more anteriorly the avoidance of injury to the anterior choroidal artery.

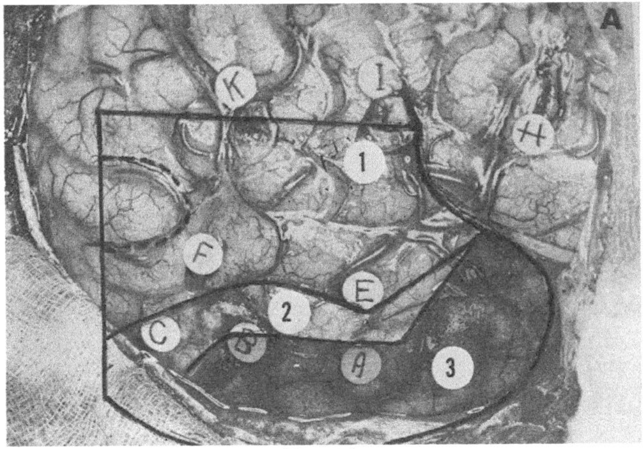

Fig. 6 A

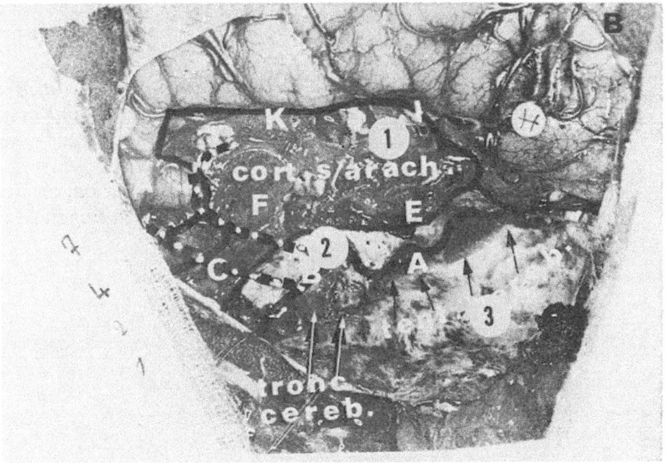

Fig. 6 B

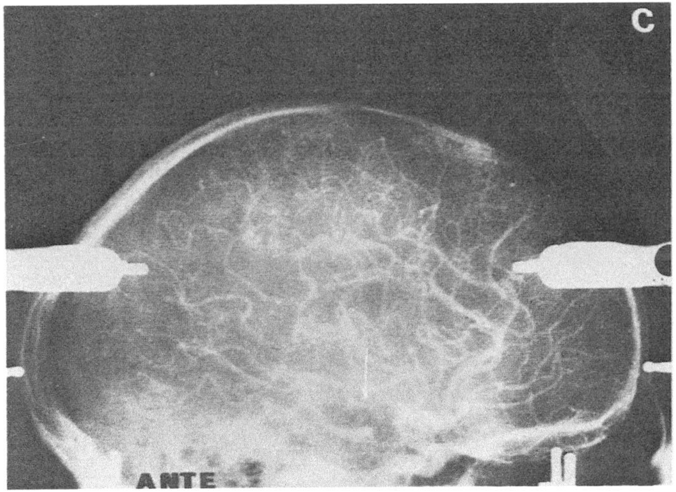

Fig. 6 C

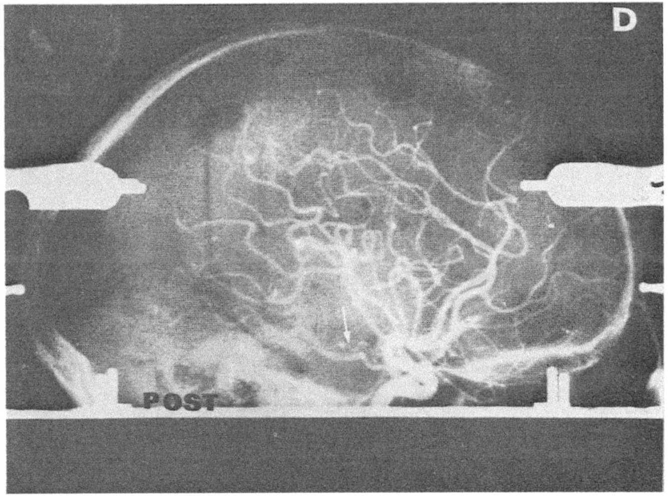

Fig. 6 D

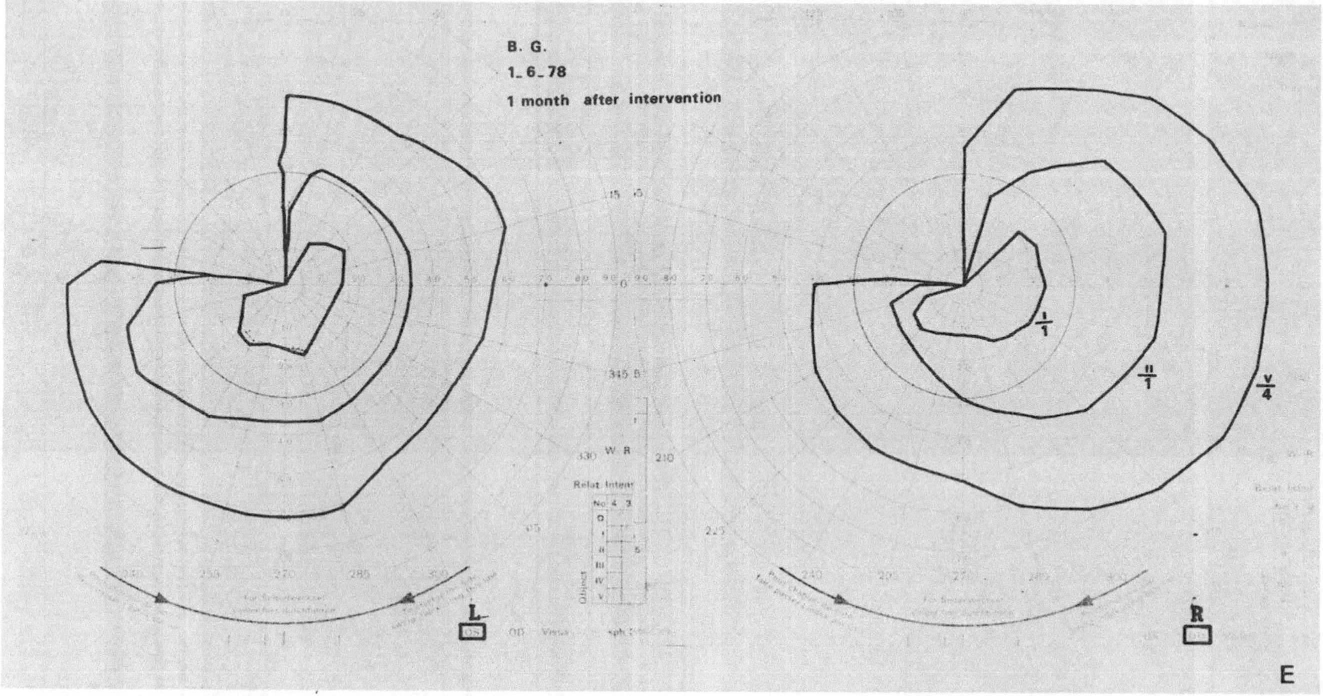

Fig. 6 E

Fig. 6. A. The limits of the *planned excision* are indicated on the exposed cortex corresponding to the preceding informations. *1* Trans- and subsial external cortical excision, *2* simple external cortical excision, *3* complete lobectomy. B. *Photograph* taken at the end of the procedure, showing the execution of the plan. *1* Sub- and transpial excision, *2* external excision, *3* total lobectomy: the brain stem and the tentorium cerebelli are visible. C. and D. *Postoperative angiographic control:* preoperative angiogram; postoperative angiogram performed in the same stereoctaxic projections. All important vessels are patent. Note shifted position of the insula and lowering of the anterior choroidal artery (→). E. *Visual field of patient B:* superior quadranopsia

Precise knowledge of the position of the ventricle allows the limitation of the extent of cortical removal posteriorly so as to spare as much as possible the optic radiation while removing Ammon's horn (5 mm behind electrode B).

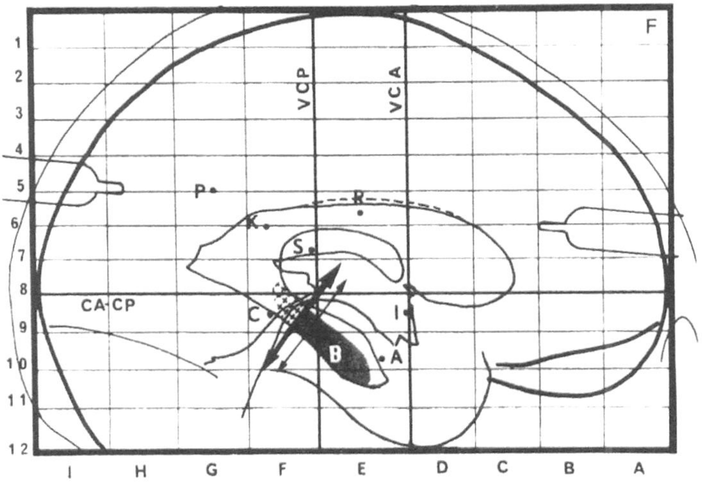

Abb. 6. F. Posterior limit of lobectomy: section level of patient B (thick arrow). Thin arrow indicates a section plane allowing to respect almost completely the visual field in spite of a complete removal of Ammon's horn. The removal (curet) of the whole Ammon's horn is in that case, somewhat more delicate and depends on several factors

Finally, the strategy of the removal can be formulated into an overall plan (Fig. 6, A). In this case, this will be performed in 3 stages firstly *superficial subpial excision* of the suprasylvian Rolandic operculum together with the posterior third of the third frontal gyrus and the posterior three quarters of the superior temporal gyrus. Secondly *superficial removal* of a part of T 1, T 2, T 3 and finally, *total lobectomy* involving part of T 2, T 3, T 4 parahippocampal gyrus, uncus, amygdaloid nucleus and Ammon's horn. The posterior part of the latter will be removed intraventricularly with a curet so as to avoid complete destruction of the optic radiation winding around the temporal horn.

In our opinion the remarkably smooth postoperative course might be related to several facts, namely that the pial membrane on the inner aspect of the temporal lobe is spared, thus closing the cavity of the removal, also after careful haemostasis, the cavity is filled with physiological saline solution and the dura mater hermetically sutured and sealed with an acrylic glue.

C. Postoperative Controls

This is an essential stage of the methodology. A first control is a photograph of the operation field (Fig. 6, B) showing: subpial removal, superficial cortical removal and the extent of lobectomy where the brain stem and the tentorium can be seen. The second is the angiogram which is performed in stereotactic conditions, before the patient is discharged to make sure that vessels are still patent (in particular those crossing the operation field) (Fig. 6, E, D).

The patient had no seizures for 14 months, no neurological deficits apart from a superior quadrant anopsia which he is unaware of, in spite of the extent of the cortical removal (Fig. 6, E).

The following figure illustrates a plane of section 1 cm anterior to the aqueduct, which reduces the visual field deficit to a minimum (Fig. 6, F). This means that Ammon's horn can be completely removed without major destruction of optic radiations, provided surgery is guided by stereotactic data.

Thus it can be seen that operation is not based on intuitive information but on a detailed constructed plan in advance based on the stereotactic method. The precision required by this method transforms each procedure into an actual experiment and success and failure can be more easily assessed and explained. Without doubt this type of planned surgery is more compelling and time consuming but the results bear out its value.

Conclusion

Anatomo-electro-clinical correlations necessary for the localization of an epileptogenic area and of its prefered propagation pathways can be established by pre-operative stereotactic investigations. The same stereotactic methodology may be helpful in performing surgery by the *natural transposition* of three-dimensional radiologic information to the brain itself.

Through successive examinations and controls, this methodology allows for a better evaluation of successes and failures, a better understanding of any postoperative deficit or of its absence. Each new fragment of information will improve the art and science of surgery and our knowledge of brain function.

Finally, we believe that when small brain tumours are diagnosed in seizure patients by the CT scan they require as complete preoperative study and collection of data as in the case of so-called "essential" epilepsy. Thus stereotactic methods will add considerable anatomical precision to the surgical procedure improving thereby its functional result.

References

1. Bancaud, J., Talairach, J., Bonis, A., Schaub, C., Szikla, G., Morel, P., Bordas-Ferrer, M., La stéréo-électroencéphalographie dans l'épilepsie, 1 vol., 321 p. Paris: Masson. 1965.
2. Bancaud, J., Talairach, J., Geier, S., Scarabin, J. M., EEG et SEEG dans les tumeurs cérébrales et l'épilepsie, 1 vol., 351 p. Paris: Edifor eds. 1973.
3. Pecker, J., Scarabin, J. M., Brucher, J. M., Vallee, B., Démarche stéréotaxique en neurochirurgie tumorale, 1 vol., 301 p. Paris: Laboratoire Fabre. 1979.
4. Pecker, J., Simon, J., Scarabin, J. M., Perfectionnement technique dans le repérage stéréotaxique chez l'homme: étude anatomo-radiologique et traitement de l'information. Premiers résultats. Xe Congrès Int. Neurol. (Barcelone) 1973.
5. Rabischong, P., Vignaud, J., Pardo, P., Thurel, R., Yver, J. P., Stereoradiogrammetry and Angiography. In: Advances in Cerebral Angiography, pp. 141—147 (Salamon, G., ed.). Berlin-Heidelberg-New York: Springer. 1975.
6. Schaltenbrand, G., Bailey, P., Introduction to stereotaxis with an atlas of the human brain, 1 vol. New York: Grune and Stratton. 1959.
7. Szikla, G., Bouvier, G., Hori, T., *In vivo* localization of brain sulci by arteriography: a stereotactic anatomoradiological study. Brain Res. *95* (1975), 497—502.
8. Szikla, G., Bouvier, G., Hori, T., Petrov, V., Angiography of the Human Brain Cortex. Atlas of Vascular Patterns and Stereotactic Cortical Localization, 1 vol., p. 273. Berlin-Heidelberg-New York: Springer. 1977.
9. Szikla, G., Peragut, J. C., Irradiation interstitielle des gliomes. Neuro-chir. (Paris) *21* (1975), 187—226.
10. Szikla, G., Stereotactic Neuroradiology and Functional Neurosurgery: Localization of Cortical Structures by Three-Dimensional Angiography. In: Functional Neurosurgery (Rasmussen-Marino, ed.). New York: Raven Press. 1979.
11. Talairach, J., Hecaen, H., David, M., Moussier, M., de Ajuriaguerra, J., Recherches sur la coagulation thérapeutique des structures souscorticales chez l'homme. Rev. Neurol. (Paris) *81* (1949), 4—24.
12. Talairach, J., de Ajuriaguerra, J., David, M., Etudes stéréotaxiques et structures encéphaliques profondes chez l'homme. Presse Méd. (Paris) *28* (1952), 605—609.
13. Talairach, J., Aboulker, J., Ruggiero, G., David, M., Utilisation de la méthode radio-stéréotaxique pour le traitement radioactif in situ de tumeurs cérébrales. Rev. Neurol. (Paris) *90* (1954), 656—657.
14. Talairach, J., Les explorations radiologiques stéréotaxiques. In: Les explorations radiologiques en neurochirurgie cérébrale, pp. 124—152 (David, M., ed.). Paris: Masson. 1954.
15. Talairach, J., Ruggiero, G., David, M., The roentgenologic contribution to stereotaxic investigations of the brain and its practical application in pathologic conditions. Acta Radiol. (Stockholm) *46* (1956), 391—406.
16. Talairach, J., David, M., Tournoux, P., *et al.*, Atlas d'Anatomie stéréotaxique, 1 vol., 294 p. Paris: Masson. 1957.

17. Talairach, J., Tournoux, P., Chirurgie stéréotaxique. In: Traité de Technique Chirurgicale, T3—1, pp. 358—435. Paris: Masson.
18. Talairach, J., Szikla, G., Tournoux, P., Prossalentis, A., Bordas-Ferer, M., Covello, L., Iacob, M., Mempel, E., Atlas d'anatomie stéréotaxique du télé-encéphale—Atlas of stereotactic anatomy of the telencephalon, 1 vol., 323 p. Paris: Masson. 1967.
19. Talairach, J., Bancaud, J., Approche nouvelle de la neurochirurgie de l'épilepsie. Méthodologie stéréotaxique et résultats thérapeutiques. Neurochir. (Paris) *20*, suppl. 1 (1974), 240 p.
20. Talairach, J., Peragut, J. C., Farnarier, Ph., Manrique, M., The Role of the Stereotaxic Radiographic Exploration in the Neurosurgical Intervention. In: Advances in Cerebral Angiography, pp. 215—261 (Salamon, G., ed.). Berlin-Heidelberg-New York: Springer. 1975.
21. Talairach, J., Szikla, G., Stereotactic Neuroradiological Concepts Applied to Surgical Removal of Cortical Epileptogenic Areas. Functional Neurosurgery, pp. 219—242 (Rasmussen-Marino, ed.). New-York: Raven Press. 1979.

Acta Neurochirurgica, Suppl. 30, 55—66 (1980)

Long Term Results of Cortical Excisions Based on Stereotactic Investigations in Severe, Drug Resistant Epilepsies

A. Bonis*

With 16 Figures

This report covers the surgical results of 220 patients (146 of them have been described in detail in 1974, Talairach *et al.*); 74 new cases have since then been operated with a follow-up of at least 18 months.

In order to simplify the study of a great number of amnestic, clinical, electrical, neuroradiologic, stereoelectroencephalographic and anatomo-pathologic data corresponding to 115 parameters, our presentation is identical to that of the study published in 1974.

I. Population

Any study on surgical results in epilepsy requires a study of the *population* involved.

Our population has special characteristics. It includes 133 men and 87 women: this majority of men is not a mere chance but is related to socio-psychologic factors: post-natal skull injuries are more·frequent in men in the relatively small group of this etiology; also men, due to personal and family grounds, tolerate less well than women an exclusion from socio-professional activities.

Fig. 1 gives *the age of the patients* at the time of surgery. The essential point is a considerable predominance of adolescents and young adults: 85% of patients are between 11 and 30 years of age.

Age at onset of seizures (Fig. 2). Seizures generally apeared at an early age. 80% of seizures appear before patients are 16 years

* Service de Neurochirurgie Fonctionnelle de l'Hôpital Sainte-Anne, 1, rue Cabanis, F-75014 Paris, et Unité de Recherches INSERM (U. 97) sur l'Epilepsie, 2ter, rue d'Alésia, F-75014 Paris, France.

0065-1419/80/Suppl. 30/0055/$ 02.40

old and 50% before they are 9 years old (115 patients on 220 patients).

Duration of seizure tendency at the time of surgery (Fig. 3) is 8 to 18 years in more than 80% of patients with a maximum between 11 and 14 years. Patients presented with particularly *frequent* seizures, generally several daily seizures and quite often several seizures per week.

This length of the evolution should be emphasized. We feel that it is a major argument against the existence of secondary independent

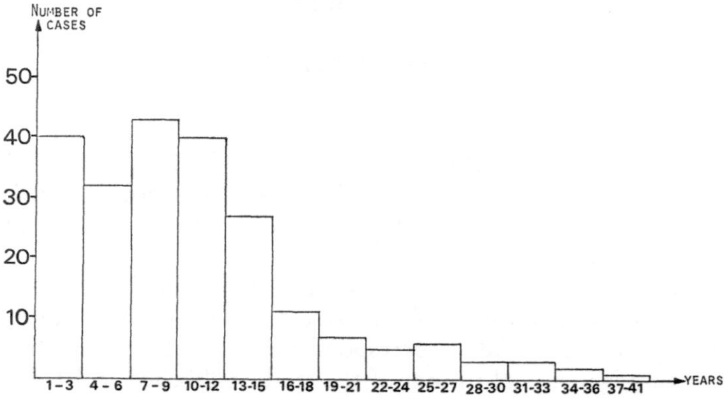

Fig. 1. Age at onset of seizures

pace-maker, more particularly in epilepsies involving the temporal lobe where stereo-EEG shows ictal discharges usually propagating towards contralateral basal limbic structures.

The etiology of the epilepsy (Fig. 4) is known in 60% of our cases and uncertain in 40%. The group of post-traumatic, post-natal epilepsies is clearly less important than groups currently found in statistics on the surgery of epilepsy. In the "miscellaneous" group a distinction should be made between gliomas including 11 astrocytomas and one recurrent operated ependymoma and dysplasic space occupying processes having a possible evolutive potential.

The tumour was discovered accidentally in these patients presenting with a long standing seizure history. No recurrence occurred 5, 8, 10 years or more after surgery not followed by radiotherapy. (These patients recently had tomodensitometric examinations.) These low grade glial tumours in younger subjects might be integrated in the category of surgical epilepsies all the more as they are more frequently discovered by the CT scan.

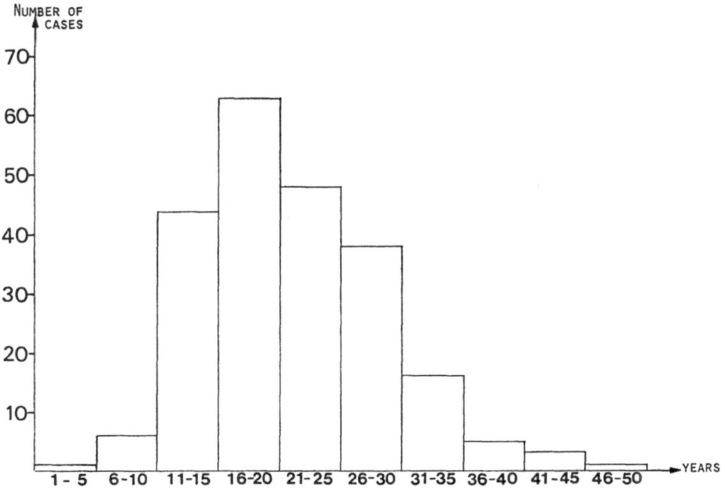

Fig. 2. Age of patients at operation (years)

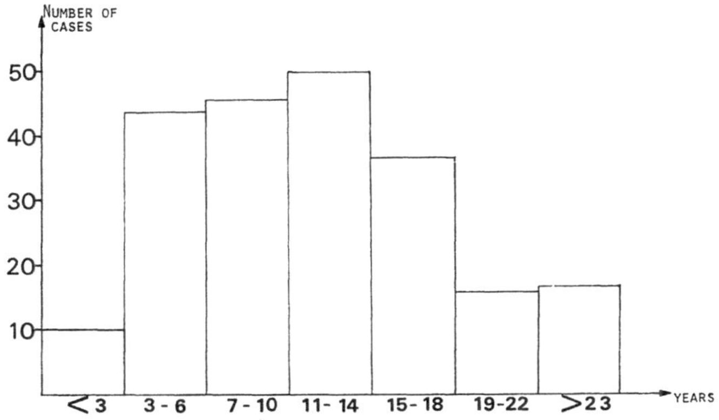

Fig. 3. Duration of epilepsy before operation

Peri-natal	59	
Encephalitis	30	60%
Traumatic	23	
Miscellaneous	20	
Unknown	88	40%

Fig. 4. Etiology

The study of hemispheric dominance is performed through an intracarotid Amytal test, mostly bilateral, in case of uncertainties on speech lateralization (Fig. 5).

We had 34 lefthanded and 5 ambidextrous patients, *i.e.*, 17.1% of patients, 15 with left speech dominance and 24 with right dominance, which might seem paradoxical but can be easily explained by patients important lesions facilitating the transfer of function. Another interesting point is the observation of 3 right hemisphere dominance among 181 right handed patients which might be explained in the same way.

Interictal investigation found neurologic deficits in nearly half of the cases. Paresis was present in nearly 43.1% of the cases, ranging

		Right handed	Left handed	Ambidextrous
Speech dominance	R	3	24	0
	L	178	10	5

Fig. 5

from massive infantile hemiplegia with hypotrophy to slight paretic signs. The other lesions affect in a decreasing order, visual, sensitive and symbolic functions.

The neuroradiologic assessment shows in 68% of the cases more or less important abnormalities.

However, correlated to the location of the epileptogenic area defined by stereo-EEG and to the surgical procedure, these anomalies are directly related to both of these data in only 47% of the cases.

Thus, lesion and epilepsy cannot be confused.

Our population is composed of patients with lesions of the central nervous system. The surgeon's report, stereo-EEG exploration, anatomopathologic investigations respectively show actual lesions in 91% of the cases. However if these criteria are cross-checked, the figures give but 96% of evidenced brain lesions.

The study of neuropsychic conditions is one of the most important factors in considering surgical indications. Out of 220 patients, 43% could be considered as normal at the intellectual and psycho-emotional levels, not taking into consideration a slight intellectual backwardness—often dysharmonious, better explained on poor socio-educational grounds than by a true deficit or moderate and intermittent psychopathic disorders. Both can easily be explained by a frustrating social environment due to this severe and socially handicapping disease. 56.6% of patients present with psycho-emotional problems. The majority have severe personality and behaviour troubles, but 26 subjects are psychotic and 20 could be considered as "pre-psychotic".

As to the actual intellectual level, clinical and psychometric assessment indicates a moderate debility in 77 patients and severe debility in 47 patients corresponding to 56.3% of our cases.

Thus considered as a whole, this population comprises a great number of epileptics with an intellectual deficit and with considerable

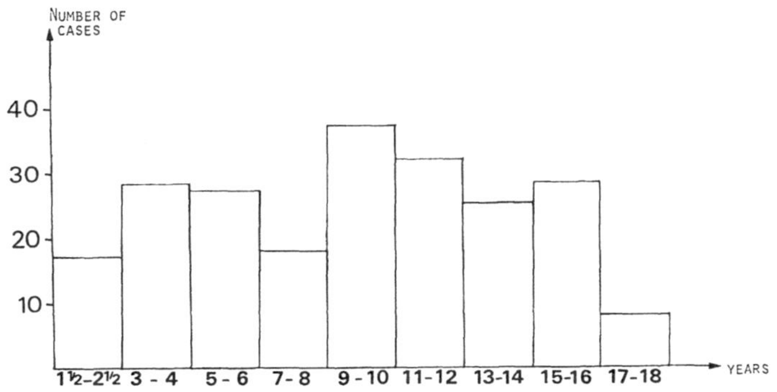

Fig. 6. Follow-up

psychopathologic troubles. Both are probably not directly correlated to epilepsy but rather to the extent of lesions of the central nervous system (severe infantile hemiplegia with severe debility, Kojewnikoff syndrom with diffuse lesions, post-traumatic pathology with important brain damages, bilateral impairment of the brain etc.).

The shortest post-operative period is 18 months (Fig. 6). It is less than 5 years in 45 patients (20% of the cases), over 10 years for 130 patients (*i.e.*, over 59% of the cases). This long follow-up reflects our efforts towards long standing controls of post-surgical evolution.

As far as failures are concerned, the department usually remains a permanent anchoring point where the non-cured patient comes back in order to reach a more satisfactory control of his condition. We ask cured patients to come back every year during the first five postoperative years and afterwards, every 2 to 5 years. We also see them at the occasion of important personal events: marriage, births of children.

The operated hemisphere studied in terms of speech dominance (Fig. 7) shows that most surgical procedures concern the right hemisphere (153 compared to 67 on the left) and procedures are still more predominant on the minor hemisphere (172 compared to 48 on the major hemisphere).

At first sight, this predominance seems easy to explain. However a detailed study on 48 procedures on the major hemisphere including several evolutive tumours leads to the conclusion that sometimes we are overcautious in that respect and that indication of surgical procedures could be taken into consideration more frequently for epilepsies of the dominant hemisphere.

			Speech dominant h.	
			L	R
Side of operation	L	67	45	22
			L	R
	R	153	150	3

Fig. 7. Side of operation—speech dominance

II. Results

Global results on epileptic seizures are clearly favourable (Fig. 8). *Cure* means an absence of epileptic seizures following the immediate postoperative period. It therefore implies the suppression of even minimal seizures and of the signal symptom. 119 patients have no seizures anymore and most of them, no therapy. However, a third of them follow a minimal safety treatment, generally a single evening dose of Phenobarbital for subjects with major lesions (infantile hemiplegia . . .).

42 patients have exceptional seizures, *i.e.*, once or twice a year or less. These seizures often are occasional and bound to various factors (lack of sleep, heavy drinking, infectious syndrom . . .). They generally happen at night. Most of these patients choose to go back to a light safety treatment.

73.3% of our patients can be classified as cured, taking into account both complete suppression of seizures and cases with exceptional seizures.

14.5% of our patients are only improved. This improvement might be quite important to some of them or might be only a reduction in the number of seizures, but, due to a complete maladjustment, their way of life remains the same. This group is in fact quite heterogenous. It include patients with an impressive and important improvement, able to lead a better life than before surgery. This is for instance the case in startle epilepsies with infantile hemiplegia. At the opposite, however, it also includes patients—50%—with less frequent seizures which are still frequent enough to hinder a satisfactory social reintegration.

No seizures	119	54.2%	73.3%
Exceptional s.	42	19.1%	
Marked reduction (> 50%)	32	14.5%	
Unchanged	20	9.1%	26.7%
Mortality	7	3.1%	

Fig. 8. Results: seizures after operation

No seizures	44	59.4%	81%
Exceptional s.	16	21.6%	
Marked amelioration	10	13.5%	
Unchanged	3	4.1%	19%
Mortality	1	1.4%	

Fig. 9. Results 1973–1977. Seizures after operation

9.1% of our patients continue to have identical seizures, thus confirming the failure of our diagnostic and therapeutic approach.

3.1% of patients died. We reported in detail in our 1974 study 6 deaths among 146 patients. Our only death among 74 new patients is a case of frontal epilepsy: one month after cortex excision the patient had a massive pulmonary embolism.

The study of our 1973 to 1977 results (Fig. 9) shows that cured cases reach 81% (suppression of seizures: 59.4% and exceptional seizures: 21.6%). The percentage of improved cases with reduced seizures tendency is 13.5% and that of unchanged seizures falls to 4.1% with 1.4% mortality.

We will briefly recall results published in 1974:

Complete suppression of seizures: 51.8%.

Exceptional seizures: 17.6%.

Complete cure (including both preceeding categories): 69.4%.

Important decrease of seizures: 15%.

Persisting seizures: 11.5%, *i.e.*, failure in 25.6% of cases.

The mortality rate of 4.1% has been analyzed in detail.

This comparison between global results of the 1974 series and global results of the series published here including results on the series of patients operated on from 1973 to the end of 1977 (minimal follow-up of 18 months) shows a clear and continuous progress in results. However, it should not be infered from these facts that there is a gap between the results of procedures up to 1972 (1974 series) and those presented here. In fact, results improved progressively, over the years, experience improving the methodology used in the exploration of our patients and more particularly in stereo-EEG and in making more subtle surgical decisions.

Two additional remarks on these data:

On the one hand, up to 1969, out of 5 patients only one was operated only after a stereo-EEG exploration while since 1973, three patients out of 4 are operated.

On the other hand, taking into consideration the number of seizures recorded before the surgical procedure and more particularly during stereo-EEG exploration, this figure is steadily rising, year after year: 40 to 100%.

The study of results in relation to location of seizures and of surgery will be briefly mentioned:

Frontal removals (35 patients) (Fig. 10) result in over 57% of cures. Success rate in this location is lower as with other locations and particularly with temporal epilepsy. In our opinion this is probably related to the fact that clinical interpretation of frontal seizures is difficult, as well concerning the localizatory value of some signal symptoms as the succession of the observed clinical signs. The extension and the volume of frontal lobes, their close interconnections through the corpus callowum make it more difficult to define the topography and the propagation of the initial ictal discharge.

Central area (27 patients, Fig. 11) results also improved and cures amount to 63% (against 60% in 1974).

Parietal lobe (31 patients, Fig. 12). Three patients have been successfully operated since 1974; these results influence only slightly the statistics: 70.9% of cures against 68% in 1974.

Temporal excisions are by far the most numerous (104 patients, Figs. 13 and 14); it should be recalled that the surgical removal is not necessarily limited to the temporal lobe.

In our whole series, the percentage of cures is 86.5%, including 64.4% of seizure suppression and 22.1% of exceptional seizures against 11.5% where seizure tendency persists.

The number of patients allow for comparing a series of 39 patients operated since 1973 with a global result showing 97.4% of cures against 2.6% of persisting seizures (1 patient).

The inclusion of recent results in overall data from the preceeding series (Figs. 13 and 14) obviously narrows the difference between former surgical results and those obtained since 1973 (in 1974: complete suppression of seizures in 61.7% of cases, exceptional seizures: 19.2% of cases, *i.e.*, a 80.9% success rate; persistence of seizures: 16.2%; two deaths, *i.e.*, 19.1% failure rate).

No seizures	17	48.6%	57.2%
Exceptional s.	3	8.6%	
Unchanged	11	31.4%	42.8%
Mortality	4	11.4%	

Fig. 10. Operation on frontal lobes (35 patients)

No seizures	11	62.9%
Exceptional s.	6	
Unchanged	9	37.1%
Mortality	1	

Fig. 11. Operations in the central area (27 patients)

No seizures	16	51.6%	70.9%
Exceptional s.	6	19.3%	
Unchanged	9	29.1%	29.1%
Mortality	0	0	

Fig. 12. Operations on the parietal lobe (31 patients)

Fig. 15 shows that the success rate increases from frontal (57.2%) to temporal (86.5%) location, with intermediary values in central (62.9%) and parietal (70.9%) excisions.

On our opinion, the improvement of results illustrated by the comparison of the success rate in our 1974 and the present reports is essentially due to a) the experience won in the definition of the epileptogenic area, that is in the field of indication of surgery and b) to the improved utilization of stereotactic data, the last step, that is, the surgical procedure.

Fig. 16. This last table summarizes our corresponding experience. Considering all locations together, an accurate definition of the curative cortical excision obtained by stereoelectroencephalography (157 times) gives 143 successes against 14 failures, *i.e.*, 91.0% of success against 9% of failures. In other words, the diagnostic and therapeutic method lead to success in 9 cases out of 10.

On the opposite, a location thought to be insufficiently defined according to stereo-EEG reports (57 times) gave 19 successes (33.33%) against 38 failures (66.66%).

Taking into consideration 14 procedures ending in failures although the epileptogenic area was supposedly accurately defined,

No seizures	67	64.4%	86.5%
Exceptional s.	23	22.1%	
Unchanged	12	11.5%	13.5%
Mortality	2	1.9%	

Fig. 13. Operation on temporal lobe (104 patients)

No seizures	25	69.4%	97.4%
Exceptional s.	10	28%	
Unchanged	1	2.6%	2.6%
Mortality	0		

Fig. 14. Operation on temporal lobe 1973–1977 (36 patients)

an a posteriori explanation can be found in the evolution of a operative postinfectious disease in 4 patients; in 6 patients failure might be due to an unsufficient number of electrodes (one sees only what one is looking at); this has been in particular the case of certain fronto-temporal or central epilepsies. In 4 patients, the removal was limited because of neighbouring functional structures which had to be spared although the later were included in the epileptogenic area. Thus for these 14 patients where the definition of the cortical removal was estimated accurate, the reason of the surgical failure can be explained in relationship with one or the other step of our progressive diagnostic procedure. We should emphasize that the number of electrodes proved unsufficient in the exploration of 6 patients and recall that the strategy and the efficiency of stereo-EEG exploration must be based on a thorough knowledge of the epilepsy of a given patient and on the validation of hypotheses concerning the initially or secundarily involved cortical areas.

This is for instance the reason of our only failure in the temporal epilepsy group since 1973: persistent seizures after the temporal removal are nearly identical to seizures occurring before the procedure; we regret not to have explored the fronto-orbital and cingular areas as we had done for certain patients.

Concerning those 19 cases where cure was achieved in spite of an unsufficient definition of the epileptogenic area, it appears that

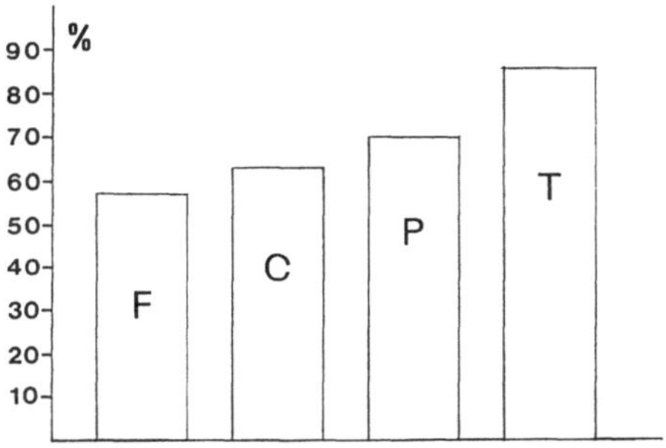

Fig. 15. Success-rate according to site of surgery

Localization estimated correct	143	14	157
Localization estimated inadequat	19	38	57

Fig. 16. Success and failure rate according to accuracy of SEEG localization

9 patients had rare seizures and that no seizures were recorded during the stereo-EEG exploration in 6 patients. Thus, the limits of our methodology are especially related to seizure frequency. In particular some patients with relatively unfrequent but drug resistant seizures could raise difficult problems.

III. Conclusions

These global results lead to brief conclusions. Severe, long standing, drug resistant epilepsies can be cured by surgery, the results of which are predictable according to a global methodology. This global methodology must be multi-disciplinary; clinicians, psychiatrists, neurophysiologists, neurosurgeons, anatomists and neuroradiologists, neuropsychologists play simultaneously and successively their role. The stereotactic methodology seems to be indispensable both at data gathering, and at the final surgical procedure. This method is necessarily bound to semiology, electrophysiopathology, in short, epileptogenic informations; they guide the method which in turn guides them in a continuous and dialectic approach.

Based on this method, complex and extensive surgical procedures can be achieved with a minimum of irreversible sequellae even after a transitory period of neurologic and neuropsychologic or psychopathologic troubles.

In particular, we wish to emphasize the striking tolerance shown by an epileptic undergoing the removal of an extended cortical area involving functional areas perturbed by frequent and repeated disorganizations due to epileptogenic discharges, as was the case for our patients.

We completely agree with the group of Montreal concerning the psychiatric evolution of these patients. An organized dissociated psychosis, severe obsessional or hysterical neurosis remain what they were, just like severe debility will obviously remain unchanged.

However we wish to draw the attention on the difficulties and frequently artificial aspects of psychiatric classifications in severe epilepsies. Quite often it happens that a pessimistic psychiatric diagnosis has to be corrected later on once seizures have completely disappeared.

Reactions due to the seizures themselves and to their psychological influence on the patient lead to interactions with the preferential groups of social integration and in particular with the parental group.

Finally, we feel that surgical procedures should more often be performed or taken into consideration for a greater number of severe epilepsies than it is currently done in France. On the contrary, it can be said without being paradoxical that most severe epilepsies do not pertain to surgery for they often express symptoms due to diffuse lesions in the central nervous system.

Surgery can only be indicated if criteria of a focal origin of seizures are present, though they might be blurred by a fallacious context. In a great number of cases, based on the necessary diagnostic procedures localizing the epileptogenic area, surgery can achieve an efficient therapeutic solution.

References

Talairach, J., Bancaud, J., Szikla, G., Bonis, A., Geier, S., Vedrenne, C., *et al.*, Approche nouvelle de la neurochirurgie de l'épilepsie. Méthodologie stéréotaxique et résultats thérapeutiques. Neurochirurgie, Tome 20, Suppl. 1, 240 p. Paris: Masson. 1974.

Acta Neurochirurgica, Suppl. 30, 67—74 (1980)

Surgical Interruption of the Conduction Pathways for the Control of Intractable Epilepsy

F. J. Gillingham* and D. Campbell*

The definition of the focus of origin and its ablation by open operative surgery of cortical or immediately subcortical lesions has been the foundation stone of surgical endeavour for the control of epilepsy when the disciplined use of drugs has failed. We have just enjoyed an exposition of the classical pioneer work of Penfield and Rasmussen, Talairach and his colleagues, and of the painstaking studies and long-term results from their departments. The success of these procedures, particularly in temporal lobe epilepsy, has been gratifying and moreover they have led to a broad advance in knowledge even beyond that of epilepsy. It would be presumptuous of me to consider for a moment that stereotaxy and the interruption of conduction pathways may have a rival place in this particular field, although no doubt Professor Narabayashi will make a case for it in the next contribution. Indeed, some have claimed that when the pattern of seizures suggests a focal origin which cannot be defined unequivocally by all commonly used methods of investigation, even operative exploration, then a stereotactic lesion in the ipsilateral hemisphere is indicated. This was the basis of the original experimental animal work of Jinnai [1] and his co-workers and the application of this knowledge led to his clinical experience with patients and his well-known lesion in the field of Forel. The results were encouraging and their more recent long term follow-up studies support their findings although they stress the need for accurate placement and size of lesion to avoid side effects and achieve significant reduction of the frequency and severity of seizures [2]. In frequent severe grand mal and minor disabling seizures there is also the difficulty of established secondary foci which may be inaccessible to open operation.

* Department of Surgical Neurology, University of Edinburgh EH3 9YW, Scotland.

0065-1419/80/Suppl. 30/0067/$ 01.60

It is this particular group of patients who are so severely disabled that they are faced with permanent institutional care and especially the young adult which concerns me to-day. In an endeavour to help these poor people surgically, observation and empiricism tended to outstrip our scientific knowledge of the basic mechanisms of the epileptic process. Yet this approach has contributed something of importance to therapy and to our knowledge of the pathways of the epileptic discharge. And over the past few years with the help of small biopsy (25 mg) material from the planned target area and of our neurochemists, there has been a real attempt to understand the interplay of the neurotransmitters involved.

New ideas are seldom new even in stereotactic surgery. Before Jinnai's experimental work Spiegel and Wycis in 1951 [3] had already reported promising results in two patients with petit mal epilepsy from lesions placed in the intralaminar nuclei and later they reported success with pallidotomy and pallido-amygdalotomy leading to the further work on the effects of amygdaloidotomy by Reichert, Narabayashi, Chitonondh and others more recently, notably Hitchcock [4—7]. My own interest was roused in the possibility of the stereotactic control of intractable epilepsy in 1958 from an observation which arose from a stereotactic operation in a man of 55 with postencephalic Parkinsonism. As well as the serious disability of tremor and rigidity he suffered from attacks of compulsive abstract calculation and disturbed consciousness many times a day so that he became almost inaccessible for a good part of it. A stereotactic operation for his Parkinsonism relieved the tremor and rigidity but also reduced the frequency of his compulsive attacks to one or two a week so that he was totally rehabilitated and long term follow-up showed that he remained well [8]. The important point about this is that the lesion made with our standard postero-anterior approach to the basal ganglia, when charted, crossed the posterior limb of the internal capsule bordering on the pallidum. Yet there were no side effects such as paresis or dysarthria. Since those early days others have published encouraging results from lesions at a number of other sites, notably the thalamus and subthalamus [9], the putamen for intractable focal epilepsy [12], internal capsule [13, 14, 29], and the ansa and fasiculis lenticularis [15]. At first sight all these scattered lesions, each with some success, suggests the work of blind men groping desperately in the dark, but as we have seen in our work on the dyskinesias and Parkinsonism, each of these many lesions may lie within a specific pathway and therefore each will modify the propagation of the epileptic discharge in some measure. Most surgeons agree that bilateral lesions are essential for the greatest success in reducing the frequency and severity of seizures but that the second lesion will increase the danger of side effects. This can only be avoided by using meticulous techniques under local anaesthesia with physiological methods for target localization such as depth micro-electrode recording, evoked responses and stimulation. Increasingly the computer is being used to enhance accuracy and this is to be encouraged. But having a human computer in the operating theatre in the form of a speech therapist who monitors speech during the fractionated development of a lesion is the greatest safeguard against an established dysarthria.

Multiple lesions seemed to Mathai [15] and Bouchard [16] to be necessary for the better control of epilepsy. Mathai postulated multiple propagation pathways in the epileptic discharge. This is less certain since the detailed work of Nádvorník [17] with continuous depth recording in the human. He felt that epileptic foci appear to involve a system of anatomical structures, functionally interdependent, which can be plotted on a schematic graph which can be used to plot the location of the proposed lesion. This would suggest a single pathway but the problem remains of the most strategic site for its interruption—the most effective yet with the least side effects.

As one looks at the sites of the various successful lesions used for the relief of epilepsy in recent years one has the curious déja vu phenomenon that we have had this experience before. We have—with the stereotactic management of the dyskinesias and Parkinsonism, the anatomical pathway for epilepsy being similar in part at least to that for the dyskinesias. Perhaps the two neurological disorders share part or the whole of a common pathway and the manifestation of one or the other depends on the origins at cortical or subcortical levels, their nature and the interplay of the specific neurotransmitters involved along intertwined bundles of microscopic pathways. After all, the two disorders of epilepsy and Parkinsonism are closely interrelated clinically by their mutual exclusion. Epilepsy is much less common in Parkinsonism (two in 1,200 Parkinson patients in our series, one in 200 in the normal population). It would therefore suggest that in the future our endeavours with biopsy study will involve micro-biopsy, rather than 25 mgm macrobiopsy and microassay if we are to understand the interplay of the neurotransmitters involved and their significance.

In our own more recent work on the stereotactic amelioration of intractable epilepsy our results have improved as our lesions increasingly involve the globus pallidus adjacent to the internal capsule. The recent and immaculate work of Caveness [18] in studying the pattern of glucose utilization in epileptic monkeys has supported this as an important site for surgical ablation. As the seizures extended from focal to grand mal the utilization of glucose increased greatly in the pallidum, twice that of any other structure studied. He felt that these experiments and data provided fresh insight into the location and extent of increased neuronal activity in focal motor seizures which might provide the location of targets for stereotactic surgery. This may be true for seizures of focal origin as in his experiments but in patients with intractable non-focal epilepsy we may be dealing with a different problem. Obviously the surgical target of the pallidum in the clinical situation has now to be explored more fully but it may yet be too early to be so specific. Stephanova [19] using continuous depth recording concluded that the convulsive component of a seizure may well be associated with discharges along pyramidal and extrapyramidal pathways embracing thalamic, striopallidal, limbic and medio-basal frontal formation including the cortex. This is what she calls the epileptic system with precise foci of discharge within it, the dominant focus being the main trigger in the whole system. She concluded from this work that every patient requiring surgical control of epilepsy needs detailed individual assessment including continuous stereotactic encephalographic recording to determine the dominant focus in each individual case. Thus each patient would require a specific and possibly differently sited lesion or therapeutic focal stimulation on the basis of such recording. Even this is not new for Talairach pointed the way many years ago [20].

The success of treatment would thus depend on the electroencephalographic characteristics and functional structure of the epileptogenic system of each patient. These observations are important and may impose an additional discipline in the stereotactic management of intractable epilepsy, namely stereotactic electroencephalographic recording. A defined pathway there may be but lesions may require to be different to be different for each patient. But the method is not without its dangers—of infection and brain injury from multiple electrode implantation. Such problems have been reported but are being overcome [21, 22].

It would be unfair of me not to include in this survey the open operative approach of the conventional "functional" surgeon in the procedure known as forebrain commissurotomy for intractable seizures. The operation involves division of the corpus callosum, hippocampal commissure, fornix and anterior commissure and its evolution has resulted from the work of Wilson and others who reported encouraging results in a small series [23, 24].

Further experience of this radical operative method by Wilson and others concluded that it could reduce the frequency and severity of the attacks, even in patients in whom epileptic discharges arose from both hemispheres [25]. Indeed a few had no seizures at all with long follow-up even with reduction or withdrawal of anti-epileptic medication. This is at first sight very encouraging but the price of so much gain is the considerable problem of the so-called interhemisphere disconnection syndrome which is not significantly reduced by limiting section of the corpus callosum to its anterior third. The patient is forced to rely upon slower visual and proprioceptive feedback systems, and recent memory, encoding, retrieval and read-out functions are reduced. Lower limb motor function is disturbed because direct interhemispheric interaction is important for the fine regulation of motor function. Prolonged re-education and rehabilitation improved matters only slightly. An additional complication in a number of instances was that of ventriculitis although this seemed to be eliminated by the use of the operating microscope and the preservation of the ependyma of the ventricle during section of the commissures. The overall cost of these complications to the patient and his or her relatives seemed too great even with the benefit of less frequent and severe seizures.

So we turn back to the stereotactic method. A recent personal follow-up study of our own patients, the first of whom was treated in 1967, and a review of the literature in the longer series of other workers, support the effectiveness and relatively low morbidity from stereotactic lesions. For example, twelve out of our fourteen patients have been improved and have remained so. A few have had a 75% reduction in frequency and severity of seizures, the remainder about 50% [25–27]. There is no doubt that patients with a shorter duration of their their epileptic illness have better results than those with a longer duration and that younger patients have better results than the older. In our own relatively small group of patients the lesions associated with the upper, posterior and central part of the pallidum would appear to have been more effective. Any fits remaining in these patients post-operatively are mainly of the "minor" type (not petit mal). The possible greater success of the pallido-capsular lesion is supported by the fact that in three patients unilateral lesions at this site have been sufficient with post-operative medication to control intractable epilepsy. At other sites bilateral operations have always been necessary. The dosage of anti-convulsants could be reduced post-operatively in three patients of the fourteen but it required to be increased in four—but of course with much better control of seizures. In the three with reduced dosage two had lesions at the pallido-capsular junction, one bilateral and one unilateral. Complications have occurred in eight patients with bilateral procedures but were of short duration in five and recovery was complete. Three patients were left with minor degrees of dysarthria, ataxia and intellectual deterioration but tending to improve slowly. Three patients had behaviour problems associated with epilepsy before operation and are now improved. Four patients had intellectual deterioration before operation and one improved. Only one patient worked full time before operation. Following operation seven patients were working with greater or less protection. Two are in full normal work. In five their work potential had not improved. In one patient work capacity deteriorated some years after operation because of a cerebral vascular accident and one died in her bath two years after operation during one of her very infrequent grand mal epileptic attacks, having returned to work. An important aspect of these results in respect of quality of life is that before operation, eight of the fourteen patients were under consideration for total hospital inpatient care. All of these are now enjoying home life and a few are in protected work.

Evidence is now accumulating in the literature that in intractable epilepsy when seizures are severe, frequent and resistant to drug therapy, but without evidence of a focal discharge, stereotactic surgery is the method of choice. Accuracy in placement of lesions is very important and physiological techniques are essential to achieve this. It may also be an essential pre-requisite of definition of the appropriate therapeutic target to use pre-operative continuous electroencephalographic studies to define and ablate the dominant focus of the epileptic system. Whatever is done, there seems little doubt that these studies and operations would be more profitably carried out at a much earlier stage before the epileptic pattern, behavioural changes and intellectual deterioration have become fully established. To do this we have to convince our friends the medical neurologists and the family doctors that we can carry out our surgical procedures safely and with good control of seizures so that our patients have a significantly improved quality of life.

References

1. Jinnai, D., Clinical results and significance of Forel H otomy in epilepsy. Second Int. Symp. on Stereoencephalotomy. Confin. Neurol. (Basel) *27*/1—3 (1966), 1—261.
2. Mukawa, J., Kimura, T., Nagao, I., Forel H otomy for the treatment of intractable epilepsy. Special reference to postoperative EEG changes. Confin. Neurol. (Basel) *37*/1—3 (1975), 302—307.
3. Spiegel, E. A., Wycis, H. T., Thalamic recordings in the mind with special reference to seizure discharges: Electroencephalography and Clinical Neurophysiology, Vol. 2, 1950, pp. 23—27.

4. Riechert, T., Die stereotaktischen Operationen und ihre Anwendung in der Psychochirurgie. Med. Contemp. *72* (1954), 589—599.
5. Narabayashi, H., Uno, M., Longterm results of stereotaxic amygdalotomy for behaviour disorders: Confin. Neurol. (Basel) *27* (1966), 168—171.
6. Gillingham, F. J., Introduction to scientific sessions, third symposium on Parkinson's disease, 1—5. Edinburgh: E & S Livingstone. 1969.
7. Hitchcock, E. R., Observations on the development of an assessment scheme for Amygdalotomy: Surgical Approaches in Psychiatry. Edinburgh: E & S Livingstone. 1973.
8. Gillingham, F. J., Watson, W. S., Donaldson, A. A., Naughton, J. A. L., The surgical treatment of Parkinsonism. Brit. Med. J. *2* (1960), 1395—1402.
9. Mullen, S., Vailati, G., Karasick, J., Mailis, M., Thalamic lesions for the control of epilepsy. Arch. Neurol. (Chic.), *16* (1967), 277—285.
10. Pertuiset, B., Selective stereotaxic thalamotomy in grand mal epilepsy. ICS 193, 72. Amsterdam: Excerpta Medica. 1969.
11. Nittner, K., Combined thalamo/subthalamotomy in the treatment of epilepsy. Confin. Neurol. (Basel) *32*/2—5 (1970), 93—99.
12. Hori, Y., Terada, C., Kanazawa, K., Miyamoto, S., Effect of stereotaxic putamectomy for epileptic seizures. Neurol. Med. Chir. (Tokyo) *10* (1968), 323—324.
13. Kalyanaraman, S., Stereotactic surgery for generalized epilepsy. Inst. Neurol. Madras Proc. *2* (1972), 67—77.
14. Kalyanaraman, S., Stereotaxic surgery for generalised epilepsy. Neurology (Bombay) *18* (1970), 42—45.
15. Mathai, K. V., Taori, G. M., Stereotaxic destruction of ansa and fasciculus lenticularis in the control of seizures. Neurology (Bombay) *20*/2 Suppl. (1972), 169—174.
16. Bouchard, G., Stereotactic operations in generalised forms of epilepsy. Acta Neurochir. Suppl. *21* (1974), 15—24.
17. Nádvorník, P., Sramka, M., Gajdosova, D., Critical remarks on stereotaxic treatment of epilepsy. J. Neurosurg. Sci. *18*/2 (1974), 133—135.
18. Caveness, W. F., Propagation of focal motor seizures in the monkey. Proc. Epilepsy Int. Symp., (1978), 204—205.
19. Stephanova, T. S., Grashev, K. V., Stereoelectro-subcorticography in epilepsy, the focus and epileptogenic system. Acta Neurochir. Suppl. *23* (1976), 27—31.
20. Talairach, J., Bancaud, J., Bonis, A., Tournoux, P., Szikla, G., Morel, P., Stereotactic functional investigations in epilepsy. Rev. Neurol. *105*/2 (1961,) 119—130.
21. Horowitz, M. J., Cohen, F. M., Skolnikoff, A. Z., Saunders, F. A., Psychomotor epilepsy—rehabilitation after surgical treatment. J. Nerv. Ment. Dis. *150* (1970), 273—290.
22. Heath, R. G., John, S. B., Fontana, C. J., Stereotactic implantation of electrodes in the human brain—a method for long term study and treatment. Trans. Biomed. Eng. *23*/4 (1976), 296—304.
23. Wilson, D. H., Culver, C., Waddington, M., Gazzaniga, M., Disconnection of the cerebral hemispheres—an alternative to hemispherectomy for the control of intractable seizures. Neurology (Minneapolis) *25*/12 (1975), 1149—1153.
24. Wilson, D. H., Division of corpus callosum for uncontrollable seizures. Proc. Epilepsy Int. Symp., (1978), 114—115.

25. Gillingham, F. J., Watson, W. S., Donaldson, A. A., Central brain lesions for the control of intractable epilepsy. Epilepsy: Proc. Hans Berger Cent. Symp. (Harris, P., Mawdsley, C., eds.). Churchill Livingstone. 1974.
26. Gillingham, F. J., Watson, W. S., Donaldson, A. A., Cairns, V. M., Stereotactic lesions for the control of intractable epilepsy. Acta Neurochir. Suppl. *23* (1976), 263—269.
27. Gillingham, F. J., Watson, W. S., Central brain lesions for the control of intractable epilepsy. Proc. Epilepsy Int. Symp., 120, 1978.
28. Rossi, G. F., Consideration of the principles of surgical treatment of epilepsy. Brain Res. (Amsterdam) *95*/2—3 (1975), 395—402.
29. Gillingham, F. J., Watson, W. S., Central brain lesions in the control of intractable epilepsy. Proc. Vth European Symp. on Epilepsy. London, July 1972, 91—93.

Acta Neurochirurgica, Suppl. 30, 75—81 (1980)

From Experiences of Medial Amygdalotomy on Epileptics

H. Narabayashi*

Summary

This paper does not present any new cases. From the long-term follow-up study of the cases operated by the stereotaxic medial amygdalotomy, the progressive worsening in clinical pictures of the chronic epileptics, such as changes of pattern of seizures, aggravation of seizure tendency and of emotional and behaviour problems, were found to be parallelly improved. The reason of such beneficial changes is discussed and the possible participation of the limbic structures is suggested.

Keywords: Medial amygdalotomy; pattern of seizures; seizure tendency; behavioral problem; limbic structures.

Introduction

This paper does not intend to report on new cases. Long-term follow-up study of the child cases with amygdaloid surgery was reported in 1976 at the First International Congress of Pediatric Neurology in Toronto [7] and on adult cases in 1977 in Sãọ Paulo Symposium [8]. Both reports include the cases with five to sixteen postoperative years and both were published already. Tables 1 [7] and 2 [8] are the brief summaries of the results in child cases and in adult cases. The detailed analysis of these results and descriptions of neurological, psychological and social status in general and also in each individual case should better be referred to several previous reports by the author [3—8].

Clinical Observations

1. *Indications.* In our observation, the most effectively influenced are the cases presenting severe behavioural and emotional problems together with clear epileptic features in history, seizure problems

* H. Narabayashi, M.D., Professor of Neurology, Juntendo University Hospitals, 2-1-1 Hongo, Bunkyo-ku, Tokyo, Japan.

0065-1419/80/Suppl. 30/0075/$ 01.40

and EEG. No case with either seizure problems only or with behavioural problems only has been included in the series.

From the histories, the etiology of epilepsy in both child and adult group were exogenic, *i.e.*, due to febrile convulsions in childhood, encephalitic or infectious condition, cerebral trauma or in a few cases, birth injury. No case of idiopathic or genuine epilepsy is included. In these cases of acquired epilepsy, epileptic traits usually start with convulsions, sometimes focal and sometimes generalized, immediately, several months or years after the brain damage. After repetition of such seizures in several years course, some of these patients start to present gradual changes in mood and emotional state, often presenting irritableness, unstreadiness in mood, easily excitableness, explosiveness with violence and poor concentration, which result lowering of performances in jobs or in school-results.

In parallel, the convulsive seizure itself also tends to show changes, such as prolongation of postictal dreamy state, or mixture of psychomotor type seizures, as automatism, masticatory movements, visceral or psychic manifestations. These changes may indicate more involvement of the temporal lobe structures. In many instances electrical foci at the temporal area, especially at the anterior temporal area, are added to the original diffuse or localized paroxysmal electrical activity. Such course and gradual changes in clinical pictures of epileptic patients have been well-known and described in the textbook and therefore, the psychological changes in these patients have been accepted as a part of the symptoms of the disease.

2. *Two illustrative cases* from our series, one in children and the other one from the adult cases will be described.

A. *Case 27.* A girl of 27 years of age in 1975 (cited from reference 7)

This patient was epileptic with aggressive and excitable behaviour problems and with very short concentration span. Epileptic fits started 6 months after a mild encephalopathy due to whooping cough infection at 5 years of age. Fits had been continuous until admission for surgery in 1961, occuring two or three times monthly despite anticonvulsant drugs. From around the age of 10, *i.e.*, the third grade at the primary school, a tendency toward emotional change gradually became apparent, with more episodes of excitableness and aggression. Around the age of 13, at the middle school, these changes in mood became more frequent, and she was often violent toward her schoolmates. School achievement became poorer, and she was advised by her teacher not to attend any more. Change of medication did not help at all.

In 1961, at the time of admission for surgery, at the age of 13, the EEG showed bitemporal spikes and left frontal spike activity on the basis of diffuse slowing of about 6–7 c/s. Surgery was performed on June 14, 1961 on the right, and on June 24 on the left medial amygdaloid nucleus. There were no complications acutely and subacutely after surgery, with marked calming effects in the emotional sphere. There were no fits at all after this bilateral surgery, and medication was slowly reduced and finally stopped in 6 months postoperatively. Bilateral temporal spikes disappeared. She again joined the class and graduated from the middle school and the high school with standard academic achievement. After graduation, she worked as a salesgirl in a small department store, and several years later she was married. She is quite social in her new family, is a capable housewife, and is now a mother of two children.

This was one of the most successful cases and we could not find even a single sign of temporal lobe syndrome or any sign of deviation in the intellectual sphere or in personality. On a recent EEG, there was no paroxysmal activity, although medication has not been given for more than 10 years.

B. *Case 125.* An 18-year-old boy (cited from reference 8)

This patient's birth was normal as was his mental and physical development until the age of six. At the age of six he developed tonic seizures with loss of consciousness associated with an episode of high fever, which was presumed to be an encephalitic process of unknown etiology. Convulsive seizures occurred several times a week over the next 10 years, despite trials of various medications.

Around the age of 17, explosiveness, irritableness, and aggressive behaviour began, culminating in a near fatal attack with a baseball bat on his grandfather.

The patient's cooperation was very poor and the EEG had to be done under narcosis. This showed 2.6 cycles per second diffuse slow-wave abnormality with positive spikes. Psychometric tests could not be carried out because of his poor cooperation, but his intellectual capacity did not seem to be low. Bilateral medial amygdalotomy was performed on February 2, 1972.

Postoperatively, this patient's improvement was dramatic, with almost complete calming and with a normalized emotional state. He was not abnormally hypo-emotional, however, and could become angry and unhappy, when other family members, shop mates, or customers treated him badly. To date, no violence has been observed and he is now working in his family's enterprise, management of hotels and shops. There is no spike activity in the EEG but the basic slowing is the same. Medication was stopped about 2 years postoperatively, with no reappearance of seizures afterwards.

Cases like these two cases are experienced the best indication for this type of surgery. Clear exogenic etiology, which indicated the organic brain damage, long-standing grand mal or other types of seizures with slow progressive coloring of temporal lobe involvement and the worsening of abnormal behaviour problems seem to be the essential feature in these cases.

3. *Postoperative changes.* When the medial amygdaloid surgery, unilaterally or bilaterally, was done, almost all of above-described epileptic traits, clinical seizures, EEG paroxysm and psychological and behavioural symptoms, were alleviated. And in about half of the well-improved cases, the patients require no medication afterwards. EEG paroxysm almost completely disappears sustainedly but with no change of basic slow waves and the patient's emotional status and mood are steadier and well-balanced with better concentration, thus producing higher results at school or better work [3].

4. *Medial amygdaloid lesion is important.* In order to obtain such beneficial effects, the small circumscribed coagulation lesion produced through the stereotaxic device has been observed more

effective, when it is placed in the medial part of this big nucleus than in its lateral part, as was reported in Cambridge Meeting [5].

For exactly locating and targetting to the medial amygdale, the following three physiological criteria obtained through the depth electrode, if possible by microelectrode, are essential [4]. These are the recording of injury discharges, which appears when the needle tip reaches and penetrates inside the nucleus and lasts for about twenty seconds, the recording of the spontaneous biphasic spike discharges from the nucleus and of the evoked discharges at the nucleus in response to the olfactory stimulation given to the nose. This olfactory responses are much larger and spiky in the medial subnuclei than in the lateral and therefore, this response often offers the reliable criteria to identify these two subdivisions. Autonomic somatic effects, such as pupillary dilatation or arrest of respiration for several ten seconds in response to high-frequency stimulation of the nucleus are also useful and important.

When all these observations are fulfilled, it is assumed the tip of the needle is exactly located in the medial subnuclei within the amygdala and the small coagulation lesion by controlled hyperthermia is placed.

5. *For temporal lobe seizures.* When the procedure was initiated, the specific effect on the temporal lobe seizures was expected as well as improvement in emotional and behavioural sphere. Seizures of automatism in one case, which also had generalized seizures, have been continuously and successfully alleviated for postoperative eight years until the long-term survey was made [1]. However, our observation indicated that the cases of temporal lobe epilepsy with psychic seizures or with visceral seizures were not influenced in a sustained way. Surgery in three cases with psychic seizures, such as auditory hallucinations or delusions resulted immediate and complete relief of these symptoms, but the seizure similar to the preoperative one recurred within several months or a year in all three cases. Visceral seizures in one case with paroxysmal arrest of respiration at the inhalatory phase and pupillar dilatation, which continued for twenty to forty seconds and then subsided, and abdominal aching had totally disappeared for several months postoperatively but recurred in about six months. The small surgical thermocoagulation lesion confined within the medial part of the amygdaloid nucleus seems not enough for these types of temporal lobe epilepsy. Reoperation to enlarge the surgical lesion was not tried.

6. *Threshold for barbiturates.* Another interesting observation is that in the well-improved cases, the high dosage of intravenous

barbiturates necessary to induce sleep preoperatively becomes much lower, usually to about half, which is almost normal dosage, after the procedure. Chronic epileptic patients are experienced resistant to the barbiturate anaesthesia, requiring higher dosage for sedation than in the normal control. Such study may easily be done because many of these cases require narcosis even for examining routine EEG.

Table 1. *Classification of Improvement in 58 Child Cases*

Classification	No. of cases	
A″	15	68.4%
A′	18	
A	7	
B	13	
C–D	5	

A″ Almost complete normal living. A′ Highly improved in behaviour, staying at special school for handicapped. A Highly improved, but still staying at home. B Moderately improved, mostly staying at home. C Minimum improvement. D No change or slightly worsened.

Table 2. *5 to 17 Years Follow-up Study of 18 Adult Patients*

Classification	No. of cases	
A″	5	11 (61%)
A	6	
B	3	
C	4	

7. *Side-effects.* The possibility of side effects was one of the most serious concern since start of the procedure. Memory loss by this surgery, even after the bilateral procedure, was not detected in clinical observation and also in the memory-test, when it was applicable. Penfield also suggested the nucleus was not related to memory function [9]. Permanent Klüver-Bucy syndrome did not appear in our series of medial amygdalotomy, even after the bilateral procedure. However, we could not dare to enlarge our lesion big enough even to involve the lateral part of the nuclei and therefore, it is not possible to conclude whether the bilateral larger lesion involving most part of the amygdaloid nuclei may cause this syndrome or not.

Discussion

1. The most impressive observation in the long-term follow-up study of the operated cases is that the most benefitted cases in the behavioural and emotional disturbance were also markedly benefitted in other epileptic traits, *i.e.*, in abolition of clinical attacks and EEG paroxysm. As was previously described, the emotional and behavioural problems, mainly for which the indication of surgery was made, were considered as a part of the important basic symptoms in epileptics. But in most of the cases the effects of surgery were seen not only on the behavioural sphere but also parallelly on other symptoms.

2. There will be no doubt that epileptic attacks start by abnormally discharging electrical foci in the gray matter of the brain, which is the classical concept in neurology since Jackson. Surgical procedures aiming to resect the abnormally discharging electrical foci or to cut down their conduction pathway, are based on this understanding. Temporal lobectomy and the stereotaxic fornicotomy were thought of as the methods for the abnormal electrical activity within the temporal lobe.

However, as was explained in the chapter of *clinical observation* in this short paper, there is a group of cases, which show some gradual change in emotional and behavioural aspects or increase in the excitability of neural structures during the years course of repetition of seizures and/or of EEG spikings. Such aggravation of seizure tendency has been suggested by many clinicians, for example, as easier tendency of convulsions. Also with gradual changes in mood and behaviour, the progressive colouring of fits themselves by temporal lobe involvement, such as prolongation of the postictal dreamy state or as mixture of temporal lobe fits is often observable in the natural history of the disease. However, there is no explanation made of such progressive changes, except the neuropathological study on the hippocampal sclerosis in the brains of chronic epileptic patients [10–12].

3. Recent experimental study on the kindling effects in animals seems to offer an important and suggestive key to understand the mechanism of such progressive changes, although the concept of kindling is still somewhat hypothetical [2]. Kindling formation is becoming to be understood generally with more participation of limbic system structures, anatomically, physiologically and pharmacologically. The clinical observation we have learned is that the slowly progressive changes of symptoms, which may possibly be attributable to such progressive functional changes of the central nervous system, can totally be improved by the medial amygdaloid

surgery. In other words, the supposed process of progressive limbic activation would be one of the keys responsible for progressive changes in clinical pictures of epileptic patients and the more experimental studies in animals seem to be needed. It must be remembered that the area removed by temporal lobectomy usually includes the amygdaloid nucleus. The possibility must be investigated that the temporal lobectomy is reducing the level of limbic activation as well as removing the abnormal electrical foci. This paper only suggests the way of possible explanation about the clinical findings obtained through the medial amygdaloid surgery.

References

1. Feindel, W., Penfield, W., Localization of discharge in temporal lobe automatism. A.M.A. Arch. Neurol. Psychiat. *72* (1954), 605—637.
2. Goddard, G. V., McIntyre, D. C., Leech, C. K., A permanent change in brain function resulting from daily electrical stimulation. Exp. Neurol. *25* (1969), 295—330.
3. Narabayashi, H., Mizutani, T., Epileptic seizures and the stereotaxic amygdalotomy. Confin. neurol. *32* (1970), 289—297.
4. Narabayashi, H., Stereotaxic amygdalotomy. In: The neurobiology of the amygdala, pp. 459—483 (Eleftheriou, B. E., ed.). New York: Plenum Publ. Corp. 1972.
5. Narabayashi, H., Shima, F., Which is the better amygdala target, the medial or lateral nuclei? (For behaviour problems and paroxysm in epileptics.) In: Surgical approaches in psychiatry, pp. 130—134 (Laitinen, L. V., *et al.*, eds.). Lancaster: MTP. 1973.
6. Narabayashi, H., The place of amygdalotomy in the treatment of aggressive behavior with epilepsy. In: Current controversies in neurosurgery, pp. 778—781 (Morley, T. P., ed.). Philadelphia-London-Toronto: W. B. Saunders Co. 1976.
7. Narabayashi, H., Stereotaxic amygdalotomy for epileptic hyperactivity—Long-range results in children. In: Topics in child neurology, pp. 319—331 (Blaw, M. E., *et al.*, eds.). New York-London: Spectrum Publ. Inc. 1977.
8. Narabayashi, H., Long-range results of medial amygdalotomy on epileptic traits in adult patients. In: Functional neurosurgery, pp. 243—252 (Rasmussen, T., *et al.*, eds.). New York: Raven Press. 1979.
9. Penfield, W., Mathieson, G., Memory. Arch. Neurol. *31* (1974), 145—154.
10. Sano, K., Malamud, N., Clinical significance of sclerosis of the cornu ammonis. A.M.A. Arch. Neurol. Psychiat. *70* (1953), 40—53.
11. Spielmeyer, W., Die Pathogenese des epileptischen Krampfes. Z. Neurol. Psychiat. *109* (1927), 501—520.
12. Uchimura, I., Zur Pathogenese der örtlich elektiven Ammonshornerkrankung. Z. Neurol. Psychiat. *114* (1928), 567—601.

Acta Neurochirurgica, Suppl. 30, 83—89 (1980)

Neurophysiological Remarks

R. Naquet*

Summary

Certain points in the different reports relating to the stereotaxy of epilepsy are discussed.

The accent is first put on the current superiority of the techniques of stereotaxy used in Man with respect to those currently used in the animal, and especially the Monkey.

In order to appreciate the nature of an epileptogenic lesion in Man, it is then discussed what information one can expect to obtain, given the present state of the techniques, from the data furnished by the positron camera as well as by the enzymatic dosages made on micro samples made in vivo by stereotaxic means.

Based on different examples, the limits of the extrapolation to Man of the different experimental models of epilepsy are considered: particular attention is given to the data furnished by the kindling phenomenon an by status epilepticus obtained by intra-amygdaloid injection of kainic acid. These models allow us to appreciate the differences in symptomatology characterizing epilepsy of amygdaloid origin according to the species. They incite us to be careful in transposing to Man the data found in the animal, if one does not consider the process at the origin of the epileptic discharge on the one hand, and of the species studied on the other.

As a neurophysiologist I would like to make several remarks concerning the different reports which have been presented.

The techniques of stereotaxy such as they have been presented by Talairach and his team have nothing in common with those used in animal experimentation. They are much more complex, certainly very precise and they allow, thanks to the use of stereoangiography, a visualization of the cortical circumvolutions; as far as I know these have never been shown, in vivo, in the animal. According to the classical principles formulated by Horsley-Clarke [8], in most laboratory animals currently used in neurophysiology or in neuroanatomy, and particularly in the cat, the identity of the facial and cranial bone structures for animals of at least equivalent weights, allows a sufficiently precise delineation of the sub-cortical structures. Conversely, in man, these inter-individual differences have made these

* Laboratoire de Physiologie Nerveuse, F-91190 Gif-sur-Yvette, France.

0065-1419/80/Suppl. 30/0083/$ 01.40

principles difficult to transpose without correction, and many neurosurgeons have tried since the 50's to develop radiographic identification techniques which would allow a more precise approach to the subcortical structures [26, 28, 29], and more recently to the telencephalon [30] and the cerebral convolutions [27]. Simultaneously, it was observed in the monkey, that errors could occur [21] if one used only the classical principles. But it is only recently that, in spite of the precision of the stereotaxic atlas [21, 25], and due to studies in the macaca and baboon in which gross errors were found, it has become necessary to establish some corrections based on the neuroradiological data in the macaca [22] as well as in the baboon [13]. Animal experimentation was inspired by techniques used in man, but it remains less developed, especially concerning the visualization of the cortical sulcus. It is true that the goals are not the same and that surgical stereotaxy, at least cortical stereotaxy, is not as important in the animal as it is in man.

I was very interested by the two reports presented by Rasmussen and Gillingham, who emphasized recent neuropharmacological and neurochemical techniques opening new perspectives for a better understanding of the metabolic phenomena which accompany or cause epileptic seizures.

I would like to point out however that the use of the positron camera proposed by Rasmussen seems premature as a better means of locating the exact site of the epileptogenic lesion. The positron camera's definition is still too low to furnish information of this order; as soon as it will have been perfected, I think, with Rasmussen, that we will have an extremely important tool (as is evidenced by the preliminary results obtained with different active substances in the animal as well as in man [5, 6, 10].

Gillingham's enzymatic study made on stereotaxically obtained micro-samples in various subcortical structures supposedly implicated in certain epileptic discharges, is very stimulating. The choice of enzymes is equally interesting, particularly glutamic acid decarboxylase (GAD), the GABA synthesizing enzyme whose role is well known in the control of certain epileptic symptoms. However, I must mention that with this technique, it is necessary to be careful in interpreting the data. The technique of micro-punch on the brain slices, in vitro, has been criticized because it does not permit a perfect dissection of the structures [37]. The use of this technique in vivo is even more doubtful: in this case, by a slight localization error, the sample would cut through two structures or neighboring nuclei having different properties. Enzyme activity and especially that of GAD can vary by as much as a factor of two within the same structure:

for example, in the amygdaloid nucleus, the GAD activity is twice as high as in the central and medial nuclei than in the lateral nuclei [1]. How then can one interpret the variation in the GAD levels in certain epileptogenic lesions without risk of error if one is not sure of the control values or of the subject to subject variation?

The term "so-called kindling process" applied to man by Narabayashi poses a few problems at least from the semantic standpoint. Goddard *et al.* [7] have called "kindling phenomenon" a very particular phenomenon characterized by the setting off of a generalized seizure by repetitive infrathreshold stimulation of a localized cerebral region: the first stimulation has no effect or produces only a brief, practically infraclinical localized after-discharge. During the subsequent stimulations, the after-discharge gets longer, a focal seizure occurs and after a certain number of stimulations (which varies according to the structure stimulated), the focal seizure is followed by a generalized seizure. From this point on, for each stimulation whose intensity is less than that of the first stimulation, the animal can no longer produce a focal seizure alone, each of these being automatically followed by a generalized seizure. The kindling phenomenon is therefore established.

Kindling can only be obtained by stimulation of certain cerebral structures, such as the limbic structures; among these, the amygdaloid nucleus is particularly sensitive since 15 to 20 sequential stimulation are sufficient to induce kindling, whereas 70 sequential stimulation are necessary for the hippocampus. The interval between two stimulation plays a very important role in the setting up of the phenomenon: for maximum efficiency the stimulation must be separated by an adequate time interval, preferably between 12 and 24 hours in the animals used (especially the rat, the cat, and monkey).

It has been shown subsequently that during the induction of kindling it is possible to record interictal discharges of spikes, not only at the level of the stimulated amygdala, but also in different limbic, thalamic and cortical structures on the homolateral side, and for some of these on the contralateral side as well [31, 35]. The appearance of these contralateral interictal discharges is one of the signs of the kindling phenomenon, but is not the kindling itself.

Goddard *et al.* as early as 1969 had already pointed out that in the cat and the rat, the kindling phenomenon could occur within 15 days at a rate of one stimulation of the amygdala per 24 hours; nearly 70 days were necessary in the monkey. More recently, Wada *et al.* [34] have determined that in the rhesus monkey, a true generalized seizure remained an exception, the myoclonus being localized in the contralateral hemibody of the stimulated side.

If one considers the strict definition of the kindling phenomenon, certain authors were perhaps not correct in extending this term to cover only the interictal discharges which could be found at the level of the homotopic contralateral structures. But the fact that these discharges exist in the contralateral side to the stimulation has been of particular interest, because it is analogous to that which have been described in the mirror focus [15, 16], and could allow us to explain the mechanism of the creation of certain of these foci [17, 24]; however, they do not allow us to explain the mechanism of induction of a secondary lesion occurring on the side opposite to the side originally touched, since the kindling is not accompanied by any anatomical lesion whether on the stimulated side or on the contralateral side [3].

The kindling phenomenon obtained by stimulation of the amygdala in the cat and the rat is expressed by a focal seizure of the amygdala type followed by a generalized tonic-clonic seizure. The data furnished by stereotaxic exploration of the amygdala in man has shown that the spontaneous seizures beginning in this structure or the seizures induced by its electrical stimulation do not have the same symptoms. The amygdaloid focal seizure is never followed by a generalized seizure (Bancaud, personal communication). One wonders then if the kindling phenomenon does exist in man. Wada [33] did not hesitate to say that there was no proof that the kindling phenomenon could be provoked by electrical stimulation in man. The data furnished to-day allow us to go even further: if one admits that in man as in the animal, it is amygdaloid stimulation which is the most apt to induce the kindling phenomenon, the possibility that amygdaloid focal seizures should be one day followed by generalized seizures by a mechanism of this type seems improbable. This data could be of some reassurance to stereotactic neurosurgeons who, after the discovery of the kindling phenomenon [24], have been accused of unjustly favouring the induction of epilepsy by repeated stimulation of certain structures during chronic investigation, after implantation of electrodes in the limbic structures.

This discussion of the kindling phenomenon has brought to light the danger of extrapolating without restriction the data furnished by animal experimentation in this domain of epilepsy to man [19]. One must always remember that phylogenesis is the origin of the important differences in epilepsy. Several examples can be quoted.

It has been known for a long time that among the genetic epilepsies, audiogenic epilepsy of the mouse and the white rat [4] does not exist in the cat, the monkey or man; and that inversely, photosensitive epilepsy has to date only been found in man and certain monkeys [9, 18, 36].

Certain species under the effect of various active substances are able to present characteristic epileptic symptoms and some others not: for example, one can quote the epilepsy found in the cat after injection of large doses of penicillin, which is not found in other species and particularly in the baboon [11, 23]. The same is true for the active substances applied directly to the cortex (cobalt, for example, although very epileptogenic in the rat, is much less in the monkey or the cat [20]), or for others injected by systemic or intraventricular ways (opiates which are epileptogenic in the rat [32] are not in the baboon [12].

Finally, the symptoms of seizures induced by electrical stimulation or by the creation of irritative focal lesions are not necessarily the same in the rat, the monkey and man. We have seen how difficult it is to produce generalized seizures from the amygdala during kindling in the monkey [34]. The same is true if one uses other techniques. It has been shown recently that the injection of kainic acid at the level of the amygdala gave rise to true status epilepticus which varied according to the species. In the rat, the status epilepticus begins with focal seizures characteristic of amygdaloid seizures showed by chewing, salivation, facial clonus, but very rapidly generalized tonic-clonic seizures occur, from a clinical as well as electroencephalographic point of view; these seizures are able, by their repetition, to cause the death of the animal [2]. In the baboon, kainic acid set off sustained electrical seizure discharges, affecting not only the amygdala and the hippocampus on the injected side, but also those of the opposite side. The cortex is affected only exceptionally. The clinical symptomatology is minor, apart from some chewing movements sometimes observed at the end of certain seizure discharge [14]. The propagation of an amygdaloid seizure discharge at the level of the neocortex is then much more difficult in the baboon than in the rat. It is highly probable that the same is true in a man with a healthy cortex. Of course it can be different when an epileptogenic scar exists, which modifies the excitability of the damaged structures or those which are nearby. It is logical then to think that the propagation of the epileptic discharge varies with the importance of the type of the epileptogenic lesion and its effect on the neighboring structures. It will thus vary from one subject to another. One can understand the importance of the initial tests (clinical as well as paraclinical) which have been emphasized by Rasmussen and Bancaud and Talairach in the evaluation of the epileptogenic zone and by the excellence of the results obtained these past few years by Talairach's team, who tried, when necessary, to go beyond the classical ablations of the temporal lobe.

References

1. Ben-Ari, Y., Kanazawa, I., Zigmond, R. E., Regional distribution of glutamate decarboxylase and GABA within the amygdaloid complex and stria terminalis system of the rat. J. Neurochem. *26* (1976), 1279—1283.
2. Ben-Ari, Y., Lagowska, J., Action épileptogène induite par des injections intra-amygdaliennes d'acide kainique. C. R. Acad. Sci. (Paris) *287* (1978), 813—816.
3. Brotchi, J., Tanaka, T., Leviel, V., Lack of activated astrocytes in the kindling phenomenon. Exp. Neurol. *58* (1978), 119—125.
4. Collins, R. L., Audiogenic seizures. In: Experimental models of epilepsy, pp. 347—372 (Purpura, D. P., Penry, D. B., Woodbury, D. M., Walter, R. D., eds.). New York: Raven Press. 1972.
5. Comar, D., Maziere, M., Godot, J. M., Berger, G., Soussaline, F., Menini, Ch., Arfel, G., Naquet, R., Visualisation of 11 C-flunitrazepam displacement in the brain of the live baboon. Nature *280* (1979), 329—331.
6. Comar, D., Zarifian, E., Vermas, M., Soussaline, F., Maziere, M., Berger, G., Loo, H., Cuche, H., Kellershohn, C., Deniker, P., Brain distribution and kinetics of "C-chlorpromazine in schizophrenics". Psychiatry Res. juillet 1979, in press.
7. Goddard, G. V., McIntyre, D. C., Leech, C. K., A permanent change in brain function resulting from daily electrical stimulation. Experim. Neurol. *25* (1969), 295—330.
8. Horsley, V., Clarke, R. H., The structure and functions of the cerebellum examined by a new method. Brain *31* (1908), 45—124.
9. Killam, K. F., Killam, E. K., Naquet, R., An animal model of light sensitive epilepsy. Electroenceph. clin. Neurophysiol. *22* (1967), 497—513.
10. Kuhl, D. E., Clinical investigations of local cerebral metabolism and perfusion in stroke and epilepsy using emission computed tomography. Society for Neuroscience, St. Louis, Missouri, Nov. 1978.
11. Meldrum, B. S., Brailowsky, B., Naquet, R., Approche pharmacologique de l'épilepsie photosensible du Papio papio. Actualités pharmacologiques *8* (1978), 81—99.
12. Meldrum, B. S., Menini, Ch., Stutzmann, J. M., Naquet, R., Effects of opiate like-peptides, morphine and naloxone in the photosensitive baboon Papio papio. Brain Res. *179* (1979), 333—348.
13. Menini, Ch., Guillon, R., Leviel, V., Contrôle radiographique simplifié pour l'exploration stéréotaxique du babouin et les injections intracérébroventriculaires chez l'animal chronique. J. Physiol. (Paris) *74* (1978), 15 A.
14. Menini, Ch., Riche, D., Silva-Comte, C., Meldrum, B. S., Naquet, R., Status epilepticus induced by intra-amygdaloid injection of kainic acid in Papio papio. 11th Epilepsy International Symposium, Florence, 1979, in press.
15. Morrell, F., Secondary epileptogenic lesions. Epilepsia *1* (1960), 538—569.
16. Morrell, F., Lasting changes in synaptic organization produced by continuous neuronal bombardment. In: Brain mechanisms and learning. A Symposium, pp. 375—392 (Fessard, A., Gerard, R. W., Konorski, J., eds.). Oxford: Blackwell Scientific Publications. 1961.
17. Morrell, F., Goddard kindling phenomenon: a new model of the "mirror focus". In: Chemical modulation of brain function, pp. 207—223 (Sabelli, H. C., ed.). New York: Raven Press. 1973.
18. Naquet, R., L'épilepsie photosensible. Données humaines et expérimentales. Neurobiol. (Récife) *40* (1977), 145—180.
19. Naquet, R., The limits and perspectives of our knowledge of epilepsy. Progress from research. 10th Epilepsy Symposium, Vancouver, 1978, Raven Press. In press.

20. Naquet, R., Lanoir, J., Essay on antiepileptic drug activity in experimental animals: special tests. In: Anticonvulsivant drugs, pp. 67—122 (Mercier, J., ed.), IEPT Sect. 19, Vol. 1, Oxford: Pergamon Press. 1973.
21. Olszewski, J., The thalamus of Macaca mulatta. An atlas for use with the stereotaxic instruments. Basel, 1952.
22. Percheron, G., Lacourzy, N., Albe-Fessard, D., Lack of precision of thalamic stereotaxy based on cranial landmarks in some species of Macaca. Medical Primatology, pp. 297—304. Basel: Karger. 1972.
23. Prince, D. A., Farrell, D., "Centrencephalic" spike-wave discharges following parenteral penicillin injection in the cat. Neurology (Minneap.) *19* (1969), 309—310.
24. Racine, R., Kindling the first decade. Neurosurgery *3* (1978), 234—252.
25. Riche, D., Christolomme, A., Bert, J., Naquet, R., Atlas stéréotaxique du cerveau de babouin (Papio papio). Editions du C.N.R.S. (Paris), 1968, 207 p.
26. Spiegel, E. A., Wycis, H. T., Stereoencephalotomy (thalamotomy and related procedures). New York: Grune and Stratton. 1952.
27. Szikla, G., Bouvier, G., Hori, T., Petrov, V., Angiography of the human brain cortex. Berlin-Heidelberg-New York: Springer. 1977.
28. Talairach, J., de Ajuriaguerra, J., David, M., Etudes stéréotaxiques et structures encéphaliques profondes chez l'Homme. Presse Méd. *28* (1952), 605—609.
29. Talairach, J., David, M., Tournoux, P., Corredor, H., Kuasina, T., Atlas d'anatomie stéréotaxique des noyaux gris centraux, 283 p. Paris: Masson et Cie. 1957.
30. Talairach, J., Szikla, G., Tournoux, P., Prossalentis, A., Bordas-Ferrer, M., Covello, L., Iacob, M., Mempel, E., Atlas d'anatomie stéréotaxique du télencéphale, 323 p. Paris: Masson et Cie. 1967.
31. Tanaka, T., Lange, H., Naquet, R., Sleep, subcortical stimulation and kindling in the cat. Can. J. Neurol. Sci. Nov. (1975), 447—455.
32. Urca, G., Frenk, H., Liebeskind, J. L., Taylor, A. N., Morphine and enkephalin: analgesic and epileptic properties. Science *197* (1977), 83—86.
33. Wada, J., Kindling as a model of epilepsy. In: Contemporary clin. Neurophysiol., (EEG Suppl. 34), pp. 309—316 (Cobb, W. A., Van Duijn, H., eds.). 1978.
34. Wada, J. A., Mizoguchi, T., Osawa, T., Secondarily generalized convulsive seizures induced by daily amygdaloid stimulation in rhesus monkeys. Neurology *47* (1978), 1026—1036.
35. Wada, J. A., Sato, M., Generalized convulsive seizures induced by daily electrical stimulation of the amygdala in cats. Neurology (Minneap.) *24* (1974), 565—574.
36. Walter, V. J., Walter, W. G., The central effects of rhythmic sensory stimulation. Electroenceph. clin. Neurophysiol. *1* (1949), 57—86.
37. Zigmond, R. E., Ben-Ari, Y., A simple method for the serial sectioning of fresh brain and the removal of identifiable nuclei from stained sections for biochemical analysis. J. Neurochem. *26* (1976), 1285—1287.

Acta Neurochirurgica, Suppl. 30, 91—96 (1980)

C. Communications

Burr-Hole Electrocorticography

J. Broseta*, J. L. Barcia-Salorio, L. Lopez-Gomez, P. Roldan, J. Gonzalez-Darder, and **J. Barberá**

With 1 Figure

Summary

In 17 epileptic patients, most of them with seizures of partial type but with diffuse or focal alternating abnormalities in the electroencephalographic recordings, chronic implantation of subarachnoid electrodes was performed. Through two bicoronal burr-holes and under fluoroscopic control, 13 to 19 insulated monopolar flexible electrodes were introduced in the subarachnoid space, conducting them either to standardized cortical targets, or concentrating them in that area of interest showed by conventional EEG. The electrodes were placed bilaterally and symmetrically, and remained implanted for 10 days. During this period, the activity of multiple foci, the reciprocal dependence between them, its reaction to cortical electric stimulation, barbiturate administration and sleep, were studied. No morbidity was found. Because of the simplicity and safety of this technique, it appears to be a good diagnostic method placed between conventional EEG and stereoelectroencephalography.

Introduction

Nowadays surgical treatment of epilepsy is subject to previous localization of an active focus. The general procedure to this aim is conventional EEG. But this method may give ambiguous results which often disagree with the epileptic clinical picture. Most frequently, this happens when uni- or bilateral synchronous or asynchronous epileptic discharges are recorded. In these cases, Vliegenhart [2] implanted a variable number of cortical electrodes through burr-holes in different cerebral areas to study the electrobiological conditions of the epileptic focus.

* Departments of Neurosurgery and Electroencephalography, Hospital Clínico Universitario, Valencia-10, Spain.

0065-1419/80/Suppl. 30/0091/$ 01.20

Table 1 a. *General Data of the 17 Patients*

Case	Clinical seizure type	Etiology	Neuroradiological findings
1	Temporal lobe seizures	birth anoxia	
2	Temporal lobe seizures	trauma	left temporal horn dilatation
3	Temporal lobe seizures	unknown	left temporal horn dilatation
4	Epileptic absences	trauma	
5	Bilateral epileptic myoclonus	birth anoxia	generalized brain atrophy
6	Somatomotor status epilepticus	birth anoxia	
7	Epileptic absences	birth anoxia	moderate brain atrophy
8	Generalized tonic-clonic seizures	birth anoxia	generalized brain atrophy
9	Myoclonic-astatic seizures	unknown	
10	Temporal lobe seizures	unknown	
11	Epileptic absences	hereditary influence	
12	Generalized tonic-clonic seizures	birth anoxia	generalized brain atrophy
13	Temporal lobe seizures	unknown	
14	Temporal lobe seizures	unknown	
15	Temporal lobe seizures	unknown	
16	Temporal lobe seizures	birth anoxia	moderate brain atrophy
17	Temporal lobe seizures	trauma	

Table 1 b. *General Data of the 17 Patients*

Case	Interictal scalp EEG	Burr-hole ECoG
1	Bilateral epileptiform activity without localization or predominant signs	left anteriotemporal focus
2	Alternating bilateral temporal foci	left temporal focus
3	Bilateral epileptiform activity without localization or predominant signs	left temporal focus
4	Right synchronous discharges	right deep parietal focus
5	Bilateral synchrony	bilateral synchrony
6	Bilateral epileptiform activity without localization or predominant signs	bilateral synchrony
7	Generalized epileptiform discharges without localization	generalized epileptic discharge
8	Generalized epileptiform discharges without localization	generalized epileptic discharge
9	Bilateral synchrony	bilateral synchrony
10	Alternating bilateral temporal foci	left temporal focus
11	Generalized epileptiform activity without localization	generalized epileptic discharge
12	Generalized epileptiform discharges without localization	generalized epileptic discharge
13	Simultaneous bilateral temporal foci	bilateral synchrony
14	Right synchronous discharges	right temporal focus
15	Bilateral epileptiform activity without localization or predominant signs	right midposteriortemporal focus
16	Simultaneous bilateral temporal foci	bilateral synchrony
17	Bilateral synchronous discharges	bilateral synchrony right predominance

Table 1 c. *General Data of the 17 Patients*

Case	Other methods	Treatment	Follow-up	Surgical results
1		left temporal lobectomy	4 years	initial improvement, no change
2	SEEG	left temporal lobectomy	3.5 years	seizure free
3	CS	left temporal lobectomy	3.5 years	seizure free
4		anticonvulsants		
5	PT	anticonvulsants		
6		anticonvulsants		
7		bilateral amygdalectomy	2.5 years	no behavioural disturbances
8		bilateral amygdalectomy	2 years	reduction of behavioural disturbances
9	PT	anticonvulsants		
10	SEEG	fornicotomy	2 years	no behavioural disturbances
11		anticonvulsants		
12		anticonvulsants		
13	PT	anticonvulsants		
14		right temporal lobectomy	1 year	seizure free, anticonvulsants associated
15		right temporal lobectomy	1 year	seizure free, anticonvulsants associated
16	PT	anticonvulsants		
17	PT	right temporal lobectomy *	0.9 years	seizure improvement, anticonvulsants associated

* This patient was operated on because in the electrocorticographic recordings under the penthothal test repeatedly appeared a right secondary synchrony of temporal origin.

Abbreviations: CS cortical stimulation, PT penthothal test.

The purpose of this report is to present the technical details, indications and results obtained on a group of 17 epileptic patients by means of this method of burr-hole electrocorticography.

Method and Clinical Material

A special model of flexible copper wire electrode of high conductivity 0.5 mm diameter and variable length has been designed. It has been insulated with poliamyde esmalt and tipped with a silver sphere of 2 mm diameter. Ethylene oxide sterilized kits of 19 electrodes were normally used in the operation.

Through bicoronal burr-holes performed at 5 cm from the cranial midline, the electrodes were introduced into the subarachnoid space, guiding them fluoroscopically to standardized cortical targets (frontobasal, anterior temporal, basotemporal, posterior temporal, parietotemporal, parietal and occipital regions or concentrating them in that zone of interest showed by the scalp EEG. The electrode derivations were referred to a neutral electrode placed in the cerebral midline at the vertex level (Fig. 1). The electrodes were introduced bilaterally, attempting to reach certain level of symmetry between the homonymous ones. The electrodes were fixed to the burr-hole and passed subcutaneously along to a parallel incision where they were connected to a multiterminal adaptor.

The electrodes remained *in situ* for ten days for electrocorticographic recordings and complementary studies, such as cortical electric stimulation, the penthothal test [1] or sleep.

The selection of patients for burr-hole electrocorticography was always done among epileptic cases who, because of the severity of their epileptic syndrome, were candidates for surgical treatment. In all cases, the scalp EEG did not offer a precise localization. Table 1 summarizes the main data of each of the 17 cases.

Results

The results obtained with burr-hole electrocorticography are discussed according to the four main indications which were considered in the criteria of patient selection.

1. Patients Without Correlation of the Epileptic Clinical Symptomatology and Scalp EEG Findings

Four patients with these characteristics were in the group (cases 1, 3, 6, and 15). The clinical symptoms were those of a focal temporal lobe epilepsy in three cases and of somato-motor epilepsia partialis continua in case 6. Cases 1, 3, and 15 presented as well interictal psychic disorders. However, the scalp EEG recordings repeatedly showed bilateral epileptiform activity without any localizing features. In cases 1, 3, and 15 burr-hole electrocorticography revealed the appearance of a unilateral temporal focus. These three patients were surgically treated by means of a temporal lobectomy; the superficial and deep peroperative open corticography confirmed the focus. After an average follow-up of 2.8 years, cases 3 and 15 are seizure free; case 1 is in the same preoperative condition, although during the first postoperative year he showed significant clinical improvement.

2. Patients in whom EEG Recordings Showed a Uni or Bilateral Synchronous Discharges, Independent of the Epileptic Clinical Picture

In this group cases 4, 5, 9, 14, and 17 illustrated this pattern. They had different types of seizures, but in all cases scalp EEG recordings showed a uni or bilateral synchrony without any localization. Electrocorticography showed the existence of a temporal lobe focus in case 14 only. In the cases with bilateral electrocorticographic synchronous discharges, the penthothal test in subanaesthetic doses was performed. With this technique, case 17 showed a type 2 response with asymmetrical beta recordings, typical of a secondary synchrony with a temporal origin; consequently, this patient was included in the surgical group. After an average postoperative follow-up of 11 months, cases 14 and 17 presented a moderate seizure improvement but they still required drug therapy.

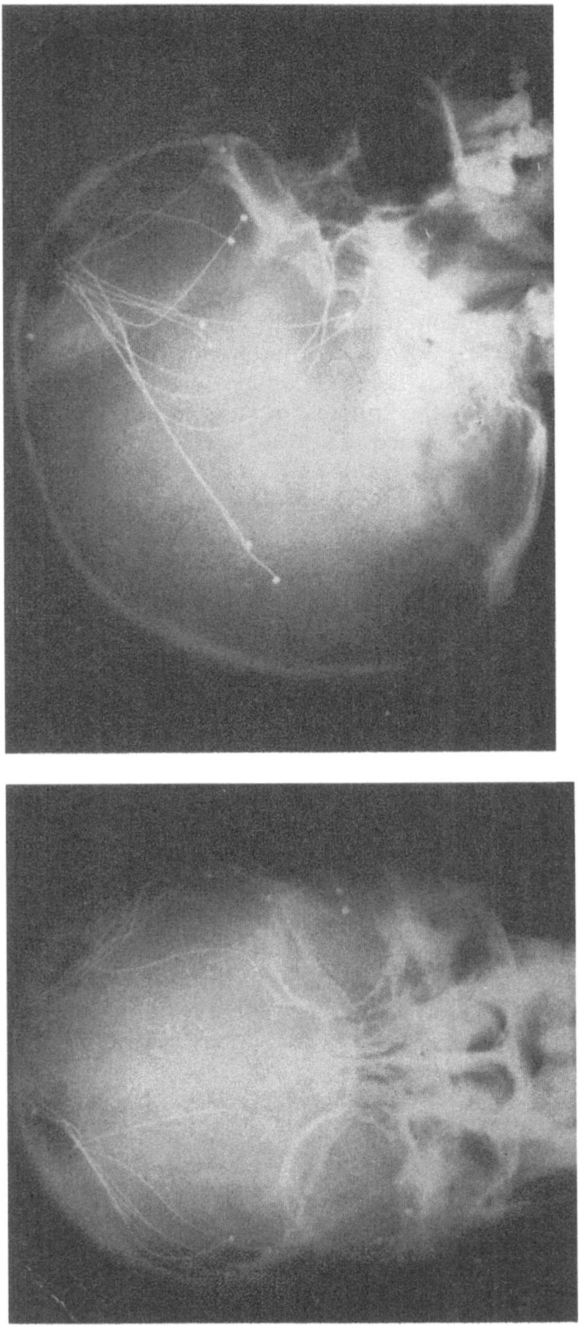

Fig. 1. General distribution of the cortical electrodes on the AP and lateral control radiograms during the attempt to reach basal areas unrecorded by scalp EEG

3. Patients Where the Scalp EEG Showed the Existence of Alternating or Simultaneous Bilateral Temporal Foci

Four patients with these conditions were in this group, all them with a pattern of temporal lobe epilepsy (cases 2, 10, 13, and 16). In addition, all them presented severe psychic disorders. Scalp EEGs repeatedly showed epileptic discharges, sometimes with no localization and others with alternating or simultaneously persisting bilateral temporal foci. Electrocorticography confirmed the presence of a primary unilateral temporal focus in cases 2 and 10, and were therefore regarded as candidates for surgery. Because of the necessity of confirming the epileptic dominant side prior to surgery posterior-anterior transtemporal SEEG with a probe with seven terminals was performed in these two cases. This method also offered the possibility of evaluating the depth of the epileptic focus. In case 2 a left temporal lobectomy was performed while in case 10, because of the predominance of behavioural disturbance over epilepsy, a unilateral stereotactic fornicotomy-anterior commisurotomy was performed.

4. Patients in Whom the Clinical Picture Indicated the Need for Sedative Neurosurgery

The four patients of this group (cases 7, 8, 11, and 12) presented with an aggressive epileptic oligophrenia with differing seizure patterns. The EEG showed only a diffuse deficit of cerebral maturation with bilateral generalized epileptic discharges. In this group burr-hole electrocorticography attempted to show some localization, but failed in all four cases. Despite these results in cases 7 and 8 a bilateral stereotactic amygdalectomy was performed because the severity of psychic symptoms. After an average postoperative follow-up of 27 months, in both patients eretism and aggression remarkedly improved.

Because of the absence of any morbidity, technical simplicity, the low resistence of the electrodes that increases the capability of capturing bioelectrical potentials and, lastly, the facility of chronic implantation that permits deferred studies with auxiliary techniques, burr-hole electrocorticography is in our opinion a simple method that may well fill the gap between conventional scalp EEG and SEEG.

References

1. Lombroso, C. T., Erba, G., Primary and secondary bilateral synchrony in epilepsy. A clinical and electroencephalographic study. Arch. Neurol. *22* (1970), 321—334.
2. Vliegenhart, W. E., Kamp, A., Storm van Leeuwen, W., Van Veelen, C. W., Some experiences with chronic electrocorticography in the localization of an epileptic trigger focus. Paper presented at the Symposium on Stereotactic Treatment of Epilepsy. Bratislava (1975).

Acta Neurochirurgica, Suppl. 30, 97—101 (1980)

Differential Diagnosis Between Temporal and "Perisylvian" Epilepsy in a Surgical Perspective

C. Munari*, J. Talairach**, A. Bonis**, G. Szikla**, and J. Bancaud*

The best operative results with a success rate of 86.5 percent was obtained by our team in temporal epilepsies [4]. We decided to investigate those cases where the relief from seizure tendency was only partially achieved. The purpose of this study is a better understanding and an explanation of the partiality of these results. We tried to figure out, as far as general characteristics are concerned, whether there are any differences between this group of patients and the population of operated patients considered as a whole. It should be recalled that this study has not been computerized.

Material and Methods

The material of this paper includes 23 patients who still present exceptional seizures (not more than two in one year) after surgery for a so-called "temporal" epilepsy.

All these patients were operated on according to procedures previously described by Talairach et Bancaud (1973), Talairach *et al.* (1974), Bancaud *et al.* (1965, 1973), Bancaud (1979), Talairach (1979).

We have especially studied:

1. the general characteristics of this group of patients.
2. the anatomo-electro-clinical organization of the seizures recorded during the stereo-electro-encephalographic (SEEG) exploration (Bancaud *et al.* 1965), with an emphasis on the initial signs characterizing the seizures.
3. the clinical aspects of the persistent, though rare seizures after the cortical removal.

Results

1. General Characteristics

Among the criteria included in the study of our clinical material, most data of this group can obviously be superimposed to the char-

* INSERM — Unité de Recherches sur l'Épilepsie (U. 97), 2ter, rue d'Alésia, F-75014 Paris, France.

** Department of Functional Neurosurgery, Centre Hospitalier Sainte-Anne, 1, rue Cabanis, F-75014 Paris, France.

0065-1419/80/Suppl. 30/0097/$ 01.00

acteristics of the whole population, in particular the duration of the disease and of the post-operative follow-up, the frequency of an epileptic familial background and of neuroradiological alterations (Table 1).

However some differences are present and related, among others, to the following symptoms:

a) Infantile spasm, which preexists in more than fifty percent of cases.

b) Partial motor signs together with a tonic-clonic generalization as a conclusion of partial seizures, in more than half of the cases,

Table 1. *23 Patients. General Characteristics*

Age at the intervention	24	mean (years)
Age at the onset of epilepsy	8	
Duration of the evolution	16	
Post-operative follow-up	6	
Epileptic back-ground	3	no. of patients
Neuroradiological alterations	10	
Insufficient localization by stereo-EEG	3	
Interictal EEG abnormalities (post-operative)	10	

while these phenomena are extremely rare in the whole population who had temporal lobe surgery for epilepsy.

On the other hand, if in three quarters of the cases, a pathological aspect of the cortex has been noted by the surgeon, microscopic examination of surgical samples evidenced minor non-tumoural lesions in only approximately half of the cases.

2. Spontaneous Seizures (During Stereo-EEG)

The recording of spontaneous seizures was impossible for 8 of these patients. The fact that these cases underwent surgery before 1966 has to be mentioned.

Taking into consideration 40 seizures recorded in the remaining 15 patients (Table 2), the initial symptom was, in most cases, either an impairment of consciousness or important neuro-vegetative signs such as pallor, blushing, sweating, tachycardia, varying respiratory frequency etc. ... On the other hand, the so-called "automatic" activities and more particularly oro-alimentary motor activities are extremely rare.

3. Postoperative Seizures

As mentioned before, this group of patients is characterized by persistent though rare seizures (1 or 2 in a year).

A closer investigation of the organization of these seizures (Table 3), evidences the following facts: first, the persistence of an isolated epigastric aura after complete temporal lobectomy as described by Talairach (1979), and this in spite of the fact that these patients present no contralateral temporal epilepsy.

Table 2. *40 Spontaneous Seizures were Recorded (SEEG) in the Other 15 Patients*
The initial symptoms were:

	Seizures	Cases
Impairment of consciousness	11	10
Neurovegetative signs	10	10
Epigastric "aura"	5	4
Visual symptoms	3	3
Auditory symptoms	3	3
"Automatic" dyspraxic activity	3	2
"Automatic" verbal activity	1	1
"Automatic" oro-alimentary motor activity	1	1
Other	3	3

Table 3. *Post-Operative Seizures*

Auditory hallucination		1
Epigastric aura		3
Sialorrhea, dizziness		4
Somatomotor Somatosensitive	lateralized seizures	7
Impairment of consciousness Tonic-clonic generalization		8

Moreover the importance of signs such as sialorrhea or a dizziness has to be taken into consideration together with the existence of partial seizures and their frequently interrelated focal motor or somato-sensory symptoms. Finally the very high percentage of impairment of consciousness and of a secondary tonic-clonic generalization must also be noticed.

Discussion

In our opinion, these data confirm the following:

1. First of all, the importance of an adequate choice of brain structures to be explored by stereo-EEG. Obviously, informations supplied by stereo-EEG depend on the selection of explored brain

structures (Bancaud 1979). A possible extratemporal origin of the seizures must not be underestimated even when they are characterized by an apparently early temporal semiology with the persistence of the following symptoms: epigastric "aura", sialorrhea and/or deglutition, lateralized somatomotor activity, tonic-clonic generalization.

2. On the other hand, the importance in our methodology of the recording of spontaneous seizures in view of stereo-EEG localization of epileptogenic areas should be recalled. I wish to mention once more that in one third of these patients no spontaneous seizure could be recorded by stereo-EEG.

Some hypotheses on the origin of the exceptional seizures presented by these patients might be defined:

1. The persistance of an epigastric aura after removal of the temporal lobe leads to the conclusion that at least in certain cases, this aura is related to functional troubles in other structures, for instance the insula or supra-Sylvian areas (Penfields and Rasmussen 1950).

2. Phenomena such as sialorrhea, deglutition, are, in our experience, related to the involvement of the Rolandic operculum; also localized motor seizures are related to the central area, the tonic-clonic generalization implying the participation of frontal structures.

The symptoms we mentioned suggest the necessity to take into consideration the exploration of extratemporal structures.

Definition of the extent of the cortical excision is a second and different problem: if it is true that the removal of the Rolandic and/or parietal operculum increases the probalility of complete recovery, it is also true that this additional removal, increases the functional risk of surgery. Even though stereotactic investigations reduce to a considerable extent the probability of these risks, we think that for these patients, the decision on the extent of cortectomy should be discussed with the patient, who alone can decide whether the risks of a motor deficit are preferable to the risk of persisting seizures, even if the frequency of the latter is to remain exceptional.

References

1. Bancaud, J., Surgery of epilepsy based on stereotactic investigations: the plan of the SEEG investigation. Fourth Meeting of the European Society for Stereotactic and Functional Neurosurgery. Paris 1979, July 12–14.
2. Bancaud, J., Talairach, J., Schaub, C., Szikla, G., Morel, G., Bordas-Ferer, M., La stéréo-électro-encéphalographie dans l'épilepsie, 321 pp. Paris: Masson et Cie. 1965.
3. Bancaud, J., Talairach, J., Geier, S., Scarabin, J. M., EEG et SEEG dans les tumeurs cérébrales et l'épilepsie, 351 pp. Paris: Edifor. 1973.

4. Bonis, A., Surgery of epilepsy based on stereotactic investigations: long-term results. Fourth Meeting of the European Society for Stereotactic and Functional Neurosurgery. Paris 1979, July 12–14.
5. Penfield, W., Rasmussen, T., The cerebral cortex of man, 248 pp. New York: Macmillan. 1950.
6. Talairach, J., Three dimensional investigation of the brain. Utilization of stereotactic data in open surgery. Fourth Meeting of the European Society for Stereotactic and Functional Neurosurgery. Paris 1979, July 12–14.
7. Talairach, J., Bancaud, J., Stereotaxic approach to epilepsy. Methodology of Anatomo-Functional Stereotaxic Investigations. Progr. Neurol. Surg. *5* (1973), 297—354.
8. Talairach, J., Bancaud, J., Szikla, G., Bonis, A., Geier, S., Vedrenne, C., Approche nouvelle de la neurochirurgie de l'épilepsie. Méthodologie stéréotaxique et résultats thérapeutiques. Neurochirurgie *20* Suppl. 1 (1974), 1-240-1.

Acta Neurochirurgica, Suppl. 30, 103—112 (1980)

Clinical and Chronotopographic Psychomotor Seizure Patterns

(SEEG Study with Reference to Postoperative Results)

H. G. Wieser*, H. P. Meles, C. Bernoulli, and **J. Siegfried**

With 8 Figures

Summary

In 29 selected patients who underwent stereo-electroencephalographic exploration because of uncontrolled psychomotor epilepsy, 213 seizures were recorded. These seizures were analyzed in 10-second-intervals with respect to the sequence of clinical signs and the electrical chronotopographic patterns. By the aid of a computerized cluster analysis four comparatively distinct localization-patterns were found: a) opercular, b) frontobasal-cingular, c) temporobasal-limbic and d) posterior temporal neocortical.

The lowest trend for propagation to the opposite hemisphere is found in a) followed by d). Fairly strong tendency for contralateral propagation is seen in c). Strategically important structures for contralateral propagation are: 1. amygdala and hippocampus, and to a lesser degree 2. the frontal cortex. Seizures propagating to the parietal cortex very often involve the frontal area of the same side before affecting the opposite hemisphere.

For each of these "epileptic clusters" the characteristic clinical signs are pointed out. Special emphasis was put on the primictal symptom-sequence.

By this and a similar study with Bancaud *et al.* we show that significantly better postoperative results are found, when strategy for surgery was based on the evidence of several SEEG recorded spontaneous seizures. In some patients belonging to the "temporobasal-limbic" cluster stereotactic procedures proved successful.

Keywords: SEEG; Electro-clinical correlation; psychomotor epilepsy.

29 patients with a drug resistant psychomotor epilepsy and therefore potential candidates for a neurosurgical intervention were in-

* Departments of Electroencephalography and Neurosurgery, University Hospital, CH-8091 Zürich, Switzerland.

0065-1419/80/Suppl. 30/0103/$ 02.00

vestigated by stereo-electroencephalography [11]. Their selection was based on the following criteria:

primarily psychomotor seizures; no other types except rare secondary generalization;

several spontaneous seizures in every patient stereo-electro-encephalographically recorded; a minimum of 2, averaging 7.6 per patient;

optimal conditions: patient awake and cooperative; there were no complications, unusual frequency of seizures or decompensation;

recording of electro-clinical manifestations with surface and depth electrodes, polygraphy, videosystem with synchronized moving pictures of patient and EEG as well as a magnetic tape for off-line analysis.

Methods

213 spontaneous seizures were recorded and analyzed in intervals of 10 seconds. For every interval clinical symptoms, localization of ictal activity and its bioelectrical pattern were defined. The clinical analysis comprehends 80 symptoms, the topographical 40 points on each side. The EEG rating of the ictal discharge was graded by the following scale: 0 = no ictal change, 1 = questionable including flattening, 2 = rhythmic respectively superimposed ictal discharge, 3 = clonic discharge, 4 = tonic discharge. The analysis of long lasting seizures was interrupted as soon as a steady state of clinical and/or EEG phenomena was reached. In this way 563 10-second-intervals were found and studied by cluster analysis (Fig. 1). The correlation matrix included 80 or 160 variables. Distances were calculated from absolute correlations and clusters were formed using the single-linkage algorithm [4]. At first symptoms and localizations of all the intervals were examined separately, then both together and finally the weights of the different ictal patterns were optimised. The homolateral propagation of the ictal discharge was analyzed for every seizure. If there was a contralateral projection, the electrotopographic constellation both before and afterwards was examined.

Results

1. The ictally active parts interdepend much more than that of the clinical symptoms. Only a few symptoms depend strongly on specific localizations. Thereby most symptoms can be caused by epileptic discharges of different origin and accordingly are not reliable for topographic diagnosis.

2. At least 4 EEG clusters can be delimited and graded as follows:

a) The opercular cluster is the most distinct. It remains confined to the temporal, frontal and parietal opercula without crossing over the superior temporal sulcus. There is no contralateral projection. If the cluster increases homolaterally, the frontal propagation is more intense than the parietal. It correlates strongly with the symptoms auditory hallucinations, constriction and sensory aphasia (Fig. 2).

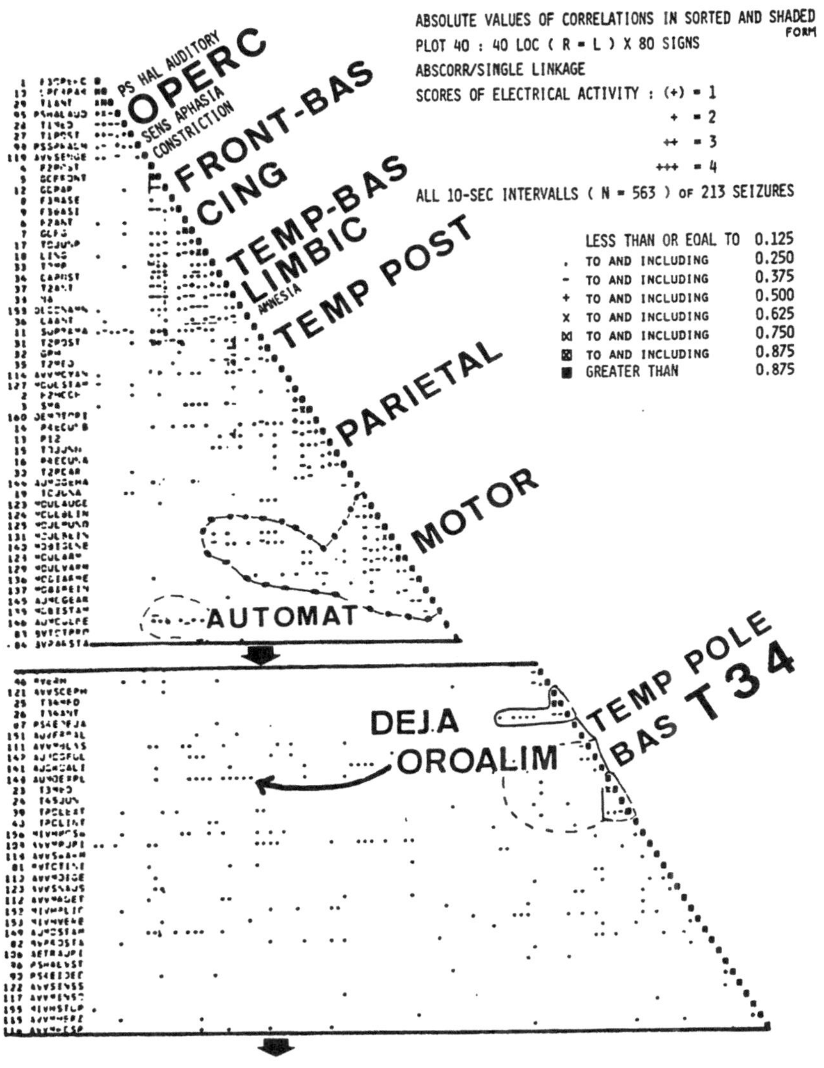

Fig. 1. Example of a cluster analysis with reduced variables demonstrating the topographic clusters and their varying coherence with single symptoms

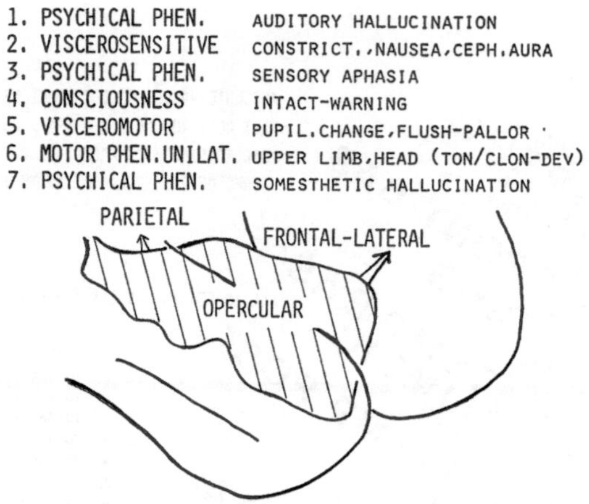

Fig. 2. Opercular cluster with symptoms

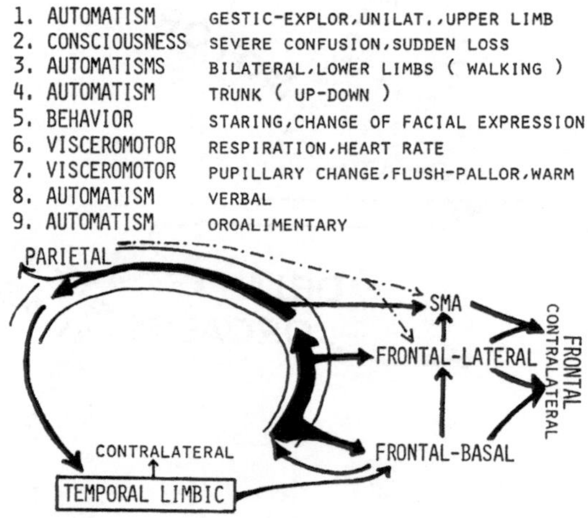

Fig. 3. Frontobasal-cingular cluster with symptoms

b) The frontobasal-cingular cluster is very compact by itself, but has close relations to the temporobasal-limbic. It correlates in a high degree with automatisms [2] (Fig. 3).

c) The temporobasal-limbic cluster coheres well but has multidirectional connections [8] (Fig. 4). One can isolate a "subcluster" consisting of the temporal pole and the anterior T 3 + 4, which correlates with visceromotor symptoms, progressive loss of consciousness,

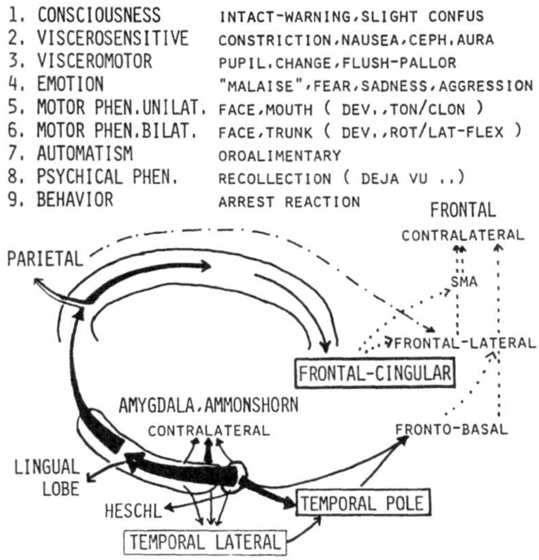

Fig. 4. Unilateral temporobasal-limbic cluster with symptoms

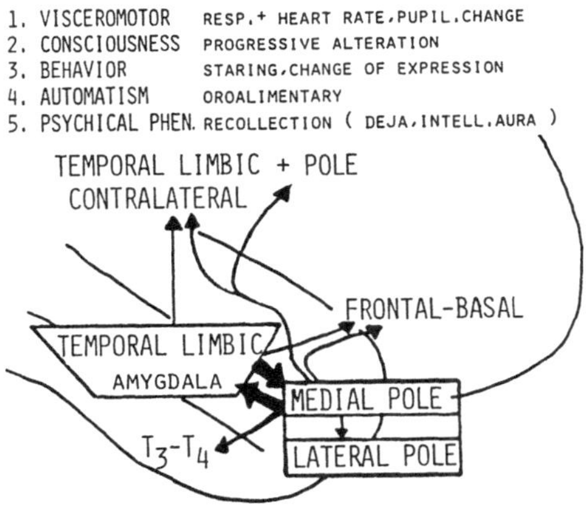

Fig. 5. Subcluster of temporal pole and anterior T 3 + 4 with symptoms

déjà-experiences and oroalimentary automatism (Fig. 5). The whole temporobasal-limbic cluster is markedly linked both homolaterally to the frontobasal-cingular, and contralaterally to the limbic cluster. It is characterized by intact consciousness, viscerosensitive and -motor phenomena and emotion [1].

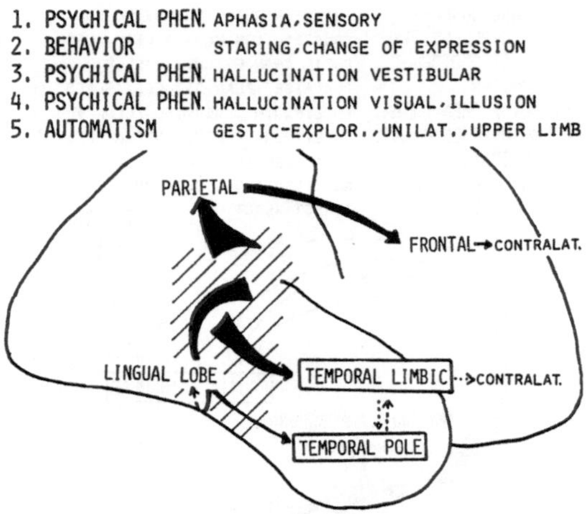

Fig. 6. Temporal posterior cluster (except Heschl) with symptoms

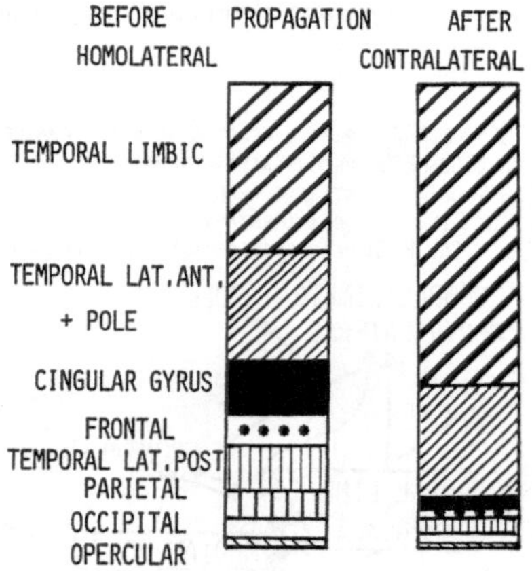

Fig. 7. Quantitative diagram of the electrotopographic constellations before and after contralateral propagation of the ictal discharge

d) The posterior temporal neocortical cluster is still recognizable as being distinct. It is connected to the frontobasal-cingular by the homolateral parietal lobe [10]. The typical symptoms are psychic phenomena, especially sensory aphasia and peculiar behaviour (Fig. 6).

3. If the analysis is restricted to the first 10-second-interval the topographic clusters remain essentially the same. Only the frontobasal-cingular becomes less distinct and therefore plays a minor role

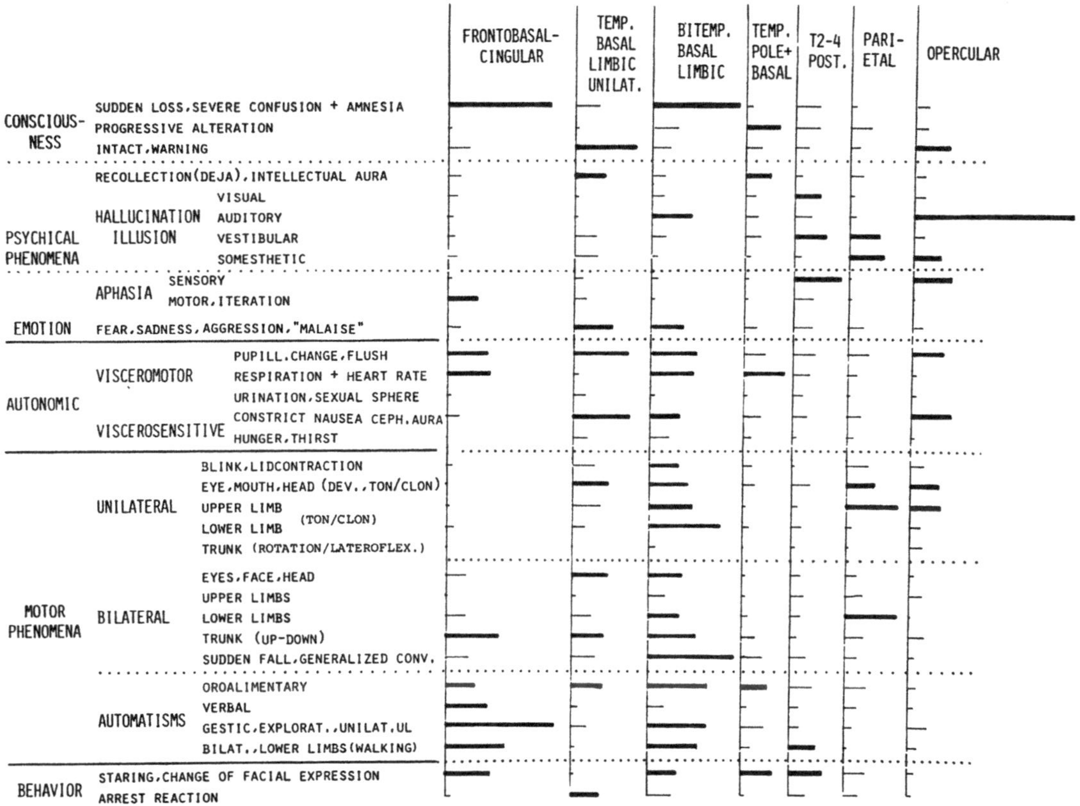

Fig. 8. Synopsis of the epileptic clusters with symptoms using the correlation coefficients of all 563 10-second-intervals. The length of the bars represents the incidence of a symptom related to the topographic cluster

as the primary locus. With respect to the symptoms of the first 10-second-interval the following findings are remarkable: The opercular cluster is also correlated with auditory hallucinations, mimic changes and visceral sensations. The frontobasal-cingular cluster has less automatism but (mostly contralateral) deviation, warning, nausea and changes of respiration (mostly arrest). The temporobasal-limbic cluster including temporal pole and anterior T 3 + 4 consists of arrest reaction, psychic phenomena and viscero-sensitive symptoms. Within the posterior temporal cluster visual and auditory hallucinations or illusions as well as déjà-experiences are enhanced [9].

4. The analysis of the contralateral propagation (Table 1) deals only with unequivocal ictal activity (*i.e.*, grades 3 + 4). 44% of the seizures are propagated contralaterally, consisting of those 60% in the first and 24% in the second 10 seconds. Prior to the projection the ictal activity shows the following topographic distribution: 1/3 temporobasal-limbic, 1/4 temporal lateral anterior + pole, with less frequency gyrus cinguli and frontal regions as well as temporal lateral posterior. 2/3 of the involved contralateral structures are temporo-basal-limbic, 1/5 is temporal lateral anterior + pole (Fig. 7). It looks as if the contralateral temporal limbic structures had a magnetic effect on the discharges. Both anterior and hippocampal commissures are very probably the anatomical substrate of this propagation.

Discussion

The findings are discussed mainly in view of their surgical implications. The clinical semiology alone does not suffice for the precise definition of the epileptogenic area. The interdependency of the symptoms is too vague and their localizing reliability is usually ambiguous (Fig. 8). On the other hand the electrotopographic clusters are accurately differentiated and highly coherent. The interpretation of this discrepancy is rather difficult. The clinical manifestations could represent mostly "distant effects" or could be caused by the epileptic dysfunction of one or several systems. The situation is complicated by the intricacy of excitatory and inhibitory mechanisms and of perturbations. Nevertheless some reliable symptoms exist: Auditory hallucinations, elementary visual phenomena and motor or sensory aphasia (Fig. 8). The automatisms, despite their correlation with the fronto-cingular cluster, are less reliable since they as well as the cluster are underrepresented in the initial ictal stage. As far as the electrotopographic clusters can be identified with the epileptogenic area their dimensions might be inconvenient to a precise diagnostic evaluation. Consequently a stereo-electroencephalographic exploration of a patient with psychomotor seizures cannot be limited to the temporal lobe but has to include both the frontobasal-cingular regions and the contralateral limbic structures.

From the methodological point of view one has to emphasize the importance of recording spontaneous seizures which are the most relevant information allowing the neurosurgeon to operate successfully. We could demonstrate together with Bancaud [12] that interictal activity and induced seizures are less reliable. Correspondence concerning the lateralization only is found between spontaneous respectively electrically and chemically induced seizures in 77% respectively 62%. This difference can partially be explained by the marked tendency of the temporobasal-limbic cluster to contralateral projection.

Table 1

Seizures total		213
With contralateral propagation		94 (44%)
Right → left		64
Left → right		30
Propagation within	0–10 seconds	56 (60%)
	10–20 seconds	23 (24%)
	20–30 seconds	7 (7.5%)
	30–40 seconds	8 (8.5%)
	Later than 40 seconds	0

Under these conditions the surgical results in temporal lobe epilepsy are satisfactory. 72% of the patients can be cured by conventional resection of the epileptogenic area. The stereotactic procedures are less effective. They cannot be applied in the opercular or temporal-posterior types but could be useful in cases with temporobasal-limbic as well as frontobasal-cingular localizations. In the former case we obtained good results by amygdalotomy or selective hippocampectomy. Fornicotomy in the latter case is often unsuccessful [3] because it interrupts only a projectional pathway but does not destroy the original point of the seizure. Its combination with an anterior commissurotomy has been recommended by different authors [7]. For similar reasons Ganglberger [5] completes the amygdalotomy by an interruption of the amygdalo-thalamic fibre tract described by Klingler and Gloor [6].

References

1. Bancaud, J., Talairach, J., Bresson, M., Morel, P., Accès épileptiques induits par stimulation du noyau amygdalien et de la corne d'Ammon (Intérêt de la stimulation dans la détermination des épilepsies temporales chez l'homme). Rev. Neurol. *118* (1968), 527—532.
2. Bancaud, J., Talairach, J., Geier, S., Bonis, A., Trottier, S., Manrique, M., Manifestations comportementales induites par la stimulation électrique du gyrus cingulaire antérieur chez l'homme. Rev. Neurol. *132* (1976), 705—724.
3. Barcia-Salorio, J. L., Broseta, J., Stereotactic Fornicotomy in Temporal Epilepsy: Indications and Long-Term Results. In: Stereotactic Treatment of Epilepsy, pp. 167—175 (Gillingham, F. J., Hitchcock, E. R., Nádvorník, P., eds.) Acta Neurochirurgica, Suppl. 23. Wien-New York: Springer. 1976.
4. Dixon, W. J., Brown, M. B., BMDP-77 Biomedical Computer Programs. Berkeley: Univ. of California Press. 1977.
5. Ganglberger, J. A., New Possibilities of Stereotactic Treatment of Temporal Lobe Epilepsy (TLE). In: Stereotactic Treatment of Epilepsy, pp. 211—214 (Gillingham, F. J., Hitchcock, E. R., Nádvorník, P., eds.). Acta Neurochirurgica, Suppl. 23. Wien-New York: Springer. 1976.
6. Klingler, J., Gloor, P., The Connections of the Amygdala and the Anterior Temporal Cortex in the Human Brain. J. Comp. Neurol. *115* (1960), 333—369.
7. Mundinger, F., Becker, P., Groebner, E., Bachschmid, G., Late Results of Stereotactic Surgery of Epilepsy Predominantly Temporal Lobe Type. In: Stereotactic Treatment of Epilepsy, pp. 177—182 (Gillingham, F. J., Hitchcock, E. R., Nádvorník, P., eds.). Acta Neurochirurgica, Suppl. 23. Wien-New York: Springer. 1976.
8. Nauta, W. J. H., Connections of the Frontal Lobe with the Limbic System. In: Surgical Approaches in Psychiatry, pp. 303—314 (Laitinen, L. V., Livingston, K. E., eds.). Lancaster: MTP. 1973.
9. Penfield, W., Jasper, H., Epilepsy and the Functional Anatomy of the Human Brain. Boston: Little, Brown. 1954.
10. Powell, T. P. S., Sensory Convergence in the Cerebral Cortex. In: Surgical Approaches in Psychiatry, pp. 266—281 (Laitinen, L. V., Livingston, K. E., eds.). Lancaster: MTP. 1973.
11. Talairach, J., Bancaud, J., Szikla, G., Bonis, A., Geier, S., Vedrenne, C., Approche nouvelle de la neurochirurgie de l'épilepsie. Neuro-Chirurgie *20*, Suppl. 1 (1974), 1—240.
12. Wieser, H. G., Bancaud, J., Talairach, J., Bonis, A., Szikla, G., Comparative Value of Spontaneous and Chemically and Electrically Induced Seizures in Establishing the Lateralization of Temporal Lobe Seizures. Epilepsia *20* (1979), 47—59.

Acta Neurochirurgica, Suppl. 30, 113—116 (1980)

Stereo-EEG and Surgery in Partial Epilepsy with Temporo-Parieto-Occipital Foci

F. Marossero*, G. P. Cabrini, G. Ettorre, L. Ravagnati, V. A. Sironi, G. Miserocchi, and **E. D. F. Motti**

With 2 Figures

Summary

Six cases of partial epilepsy operated on for lesions at the temporo-parieto-occipital junction are presented. Three cases had signs of enlargement of one lateral ventricle at the temporo-parieto-occipital carrefour, three had a lateral homonymous hemianopsia and all showed lateralizing interictal EEG abnormalities. The manifold features of the seizures could not be related to the involvement of one or more definite cortical areas.

Since clinical, radiological, scalp EEG investigations provided no sufficient data to map the epileptogenic lesion to be excided, stereo-EEG studies with chronic depth electrodes were performed. Besides permitting the exact delimitation of the epileptogenic lesion, depth EEG gave the clue for interpreting physiopathological mechanisms underlying the electroclinical seizures in each case.

Keywords: Surgery for epilepsy; depth EEG.

Introduction

Preoperative identification of the epileptogenic lesion in cases of partial epilepsy with complex and elementary symptomatology and scalp EEG abnomalities on a large temporo-parieto-occipital area is often difficult without stereo-EEG studies.

Stereo-EEG recordings of the ictal electrical phenomena, besides giving operative informations, allow the interpretation of the ictal clinical phenomena, which are often due to an early secondary involvement of functional systems distant from the primary epileptogenic lesion [1—5].

This paper presents six cases of partial epilepsy with epileptogenic lesion located at the temporo-parieto-occipital junction, operated on according to the data of chronic stereo-EEG investigations.

* Istituto di Neurochirurgia, Ospedale Policlinico, via F. Sforza, 35, I-20122 Milano, Italy.

0065-1419/80/Suppl. 30/0113/$ 01.00

Material and Method

From 1959 to 1977, 160 patients have been surgically treated at our institution for partial epilepsy unresponsive to pharmacological treatment.

Scalp EEG in forteen of them showed interictal spike foci on large temporo-parieto-occipital areas. This paper deals with 6 patients of this group (4 females and 2 males, aged from 18 to 25 years), who underwent surgical ablation of the epileptogenic lesion after chronic stereo-EEG studies.

Talairach's apparatus was used for stereotactic placement of chronic multi-leads stainless steel electrodes. Daily recordings for 2 to 4 weeks were made on a 16-channel EEG recorder.

Results

In all six cases (Fig. 1) ictal symptoms included haemianopsic scotomata or elementary hallucinations, subjective phenomena hardly fitting any one category (loke bodily sensations, "growing heart", "feeling of flying", "suffocation", etc.), motor automatisms varying in pattern and complexity. Five cases presented adversive phenomena associated on occasion to tonic postures. Four cases presented brief spells of loss of consciousness. Somatomotor and somatosensory phenomena were seldom observed. A single case had complex hallucinations. The only interictal abnormalities observed at neurological examination were lateral homonymous quadrantopsy in three cases; in two other cases post-ictal haemianopsy was present.

At neuroradiological study the ipsilateral lateral ventricle was uniformly dilated in three patients. History was non-contributive for any specif etiology in all cases.

Scalp EEG study evidenced mostly lateralized paroxysms often prevailing over a wide temporo-parieto-occipital area. Some recordings showed independent temporal spikes on the same side. Bifrontal paroxysmal bursts of spikes and slow waves were often observed.

Electroclinical seizures mostly followed a stereotyped pattern: a brief phase of low voltage fast activity followed by rhythmic activity diffused to the whole hemisphere site of interictal abnormalities, along with early controlateral propagation. On occasion the electrical seizure seemed bilateral at onset. In effect, while scalp EEG study afforded a secure lateralization (mainly based on interictal abnormalities), it did not allow a more precise focalization.

It was then decided to submit our patients to intracerebral recording with chronic stereotactically implanted electrodes (stereo-EEG).

Stereo-EEG in all six cases demonstrated a well delimited epileptogenic lesion, enabling us to perform a cortical ablation. Depth recording in all six cases evidenced that interictal paroxysmal abnormalities clearly predominated on temporo-parieto-occipital region where a slowing of background activity was also present. Independent temporal abnormalities were also present in 5 cases (Fig. 2).

Electroclinical seizures in all cases originated in the area of maximal interictal abnormalities (Fig. 2). Early and intense secondary

Hemianopsic scotomata	■ ■ ■ ■ ■ ■	Bodily sensations	■ ■ ■ ■ ■ ■
Adversive phenomena	■ ■ ■ ■ ■	Automatisms	■ ■ ■ ■ ■ ■
Somatotopic sensorimotor phenomena	■ ■ ■	Pseudo-absence	■ ■ ■ ■
Arrest (of speech, motor activity)	■ ■ ■	Hallucinations	■
Drop attacks	■	Cognitive-dysmnesic phenomena	■

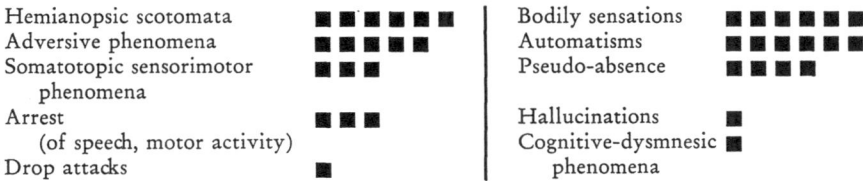

Fig. 1. Partial epilepsies with parieto-occipital focus. Ictal symptoms in the six patients

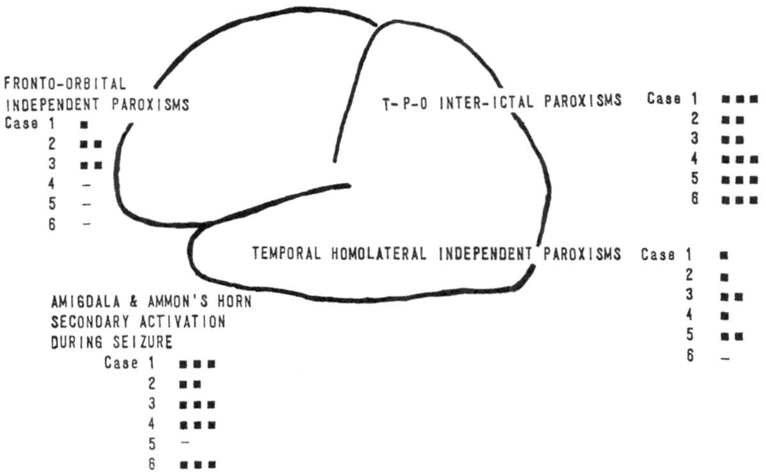

Fig. 2. Depth-EEG patterns in temporo-parieto-occipital epilepsy

activation of temporo-rhinencephalic structures was present in 5 cases. Ictal and/or interictal fronto-orbital paroxysms were present in 3 cases clearly of secondary nature (Fig. 2).

Corticography routinely performed during surgery sometimes helped in definition on the limits of the epileptogenic area.

Follow-up ranged from 3 to 7 years after surgical ablation of the epileptogenic lesion defined by stereo-EEG. Three patients are seizure free and two had a worth-while reduction of seizure frequency. One patient, who had only a limited excision of her left occipital epileptogenic lesion, showed no improvement.

Discussion

Partial epilepsy with temporo-parieto-occipital epileptogenic lesions often present diagnostic preoperative difficulties. Stereo-EEG represents in these cases the primary investigation for recognition of the exact location and extent of the epileptogenic lesion to be surgically treated.

Stereo-EEG study of the temporo-spatial evolution of the electro-clinical seizures arising in the temporo-parietal convexity allows also the correct interpretation of the manifold symptomatology on these partial epilepsies. Early secondary involvement of the rhinencephalic structures can explain the complex symptomatology which often characterizes the spontaneous seizures of the patients with occipital epileptogenic lesion [1, 2].

References

1. Bancaud, J., Bonis, A., Morel, P., Talairach, J., Szikla, G., Tournoux, P., Epilepsie occipitale à expression "rhinencéphalique" prévalente (Corrélations électrocliniques à la lumière des investigations fonctionnelles stéréotaxiques). Rev. Neurol. *105* (1961), 219—225.
2. Bancaud, J., Les crises épileptiques d'origine occipitale (étude stéreo-électro-encéphalographique). Rev. Oto-Neuro-Ophtal. *6* (1969), 299—314.
3. Huott, A. D., Madison, D. S., Niedermayer, E., Occipital lobe epilepsy. A clinical and electroencephalographic study. Europ. Neurol. *11* (1974), 325—339.
4. Ludwig, J. I., Ajmone Marsan, C., Clinical ictal patterns in epileptic patients with occipital electroencephalographic foci. Neurology *25* (1975), 463—471.
5. Tokeda, A., Bancaud, J., Talairach, J., Bonis, A., Bordas-Ferrer, M., A propos des accès épileptiques d'origine occipitale. Rev. Neurol. *121* (1969), 306—315.

Acta Neurochirurgica, Suppl. 30, 117—120 (1980)

Relationship Between the Location and Delimitation of the Epileptogenic Zone and Surgical Results. A Report of 24 Patients Operated on Using the Technique Described by J. Talairach *et al.*

R. Garcia Sola*, **J. Miravet**, **J. Brasa**, **L. Nombela**, and **G. Bravo**

Summary

The authors present the surgical results of the first 20 out of 24 medically uncontrollable epileptic patients operated on using the technique described by Talairach *et al.* The minimum postoperative follow-up period was 6 months and the mean 19.6 months. 12 patients became seizure free. Three patients have had a significant decrease in the number of seizures and 5 have had the frequency of attacks reduced to 20–50% of the preoperative level. In 11 of the 20 patients, the epileptogenic zone lay in the frontal lobe.

Of the 12 patients in whom the delimitation of the epileptogenic zone was correct, only one has seizures, and these occur only 20% as frequently as during the preoperative period. Five patients with frontal epilepsy showed obviously bilateral foci in the SEEG study. In these cases it was decided to resect the more severely affected side and overall results have been poor.

It is apparent that the correct location and delimitation of the epileptogenic zone and achievement of optimal surgical results is more difficult in frontal lobe epilepsy and in epilepsy of the temporo-parieto-occipital area.

Introduction

This paper is a preliminary report of the surgical results in the first 20 medically uncontrollable epileptic patients operated on in the last 2.5 years using the technique described by Talairach and Bancaud [2].

Material and Methods

This procedure involves the following steps [3, 4].

1. A study of the EEG recorded during interictal periods and an accurate electroclinical study of the seizures, paying great attention to the pattern of the seizures themselves, recording them simultaneously on videotape and EEG. Using the collected data, we are able to advance an hypothesis about the anatomical functional localization of the origin of the seizures and the most probable pathways of propagation.

* Services of Neurosurgery, Clinic Neurophysiology and Neuroradiology, Clinica Puerta de Hierro, Universidad Autonoma de Madrid, S. Martin de Porres 4, Madrid-35, Spain.

0065-1419/80/Suppl. 30/0117/$ 01.00

2. A stereoencephalographic (SEG) study using bilateral carotid angiograms, ventriculography and pneumoencephalography is performed under stereotactic conditions. The CT scan findings are integrated with the SEG findings.

3. Using the anatomical information obtained by SEG, and the data from the Talairach's stereotactic atlas [4], depth electrodes are placed in the regions previously selected. With the patient fully conscious, a stereoelectroencephalographic (SEEG) study of both spontaneous and electrically induced seizures is performed in order to delimitate exactly the epileptogenic, lesional and irritative zones, the pathways of propagation of the seizure activity and the correlating functions of the explored brain regions.

4. Finally, the patients have the epileptogenic and lesional zones removed by surgery.

In the 20 patients considered, the postoperative follow-up ranged from 6 to 31 months, with a mean of 19.6 months. Three patients with a follow-up under 6 months have been excluded, as has a patient who died during the immediate postoperative period from massive pulmonary embolism.

Results

The mean age of patients at operation was 18.9 years (the youngest was 7 and the oldest was 28 years old). The mean time elapsed from commencement of seizures to surgery was 12.25 years (3 to 24 years).

As far as etiology is concerned, in 4 patients there was clear evidence of birth trauma or anoxia, and in 3 there was known postnatal trauma. There were 5 cerebral gliomas of grade I–II (Kernohan's classification). In 2 patients, we found postinflammatory brain scarring and in another 2 there were cerebral vascular malformations (Sturge-Weber and cavernous angioma). In 10 patients the etiology is unknown.

Localization of the epileptogenic zone and surgical results are reported in Table 1. We should emphasize the high incidence of frontal lobe epilepsy (present in 11 out of 20 patients). Of the 4 cases of post-surgical exceptional seizures, one suffered from one seizure during the radiotherapy for a grade II astrocytoma of the temporal region, and the other 3 presented with auras in the early postoperative period. All of them became eventually seizure free.

When considering the relationship between the delimitation of the epileptogenic zone (EZ) and surgical results (Table 2), we found that, out of 12 patients in whom the localization was correct, 11 were classified as successes (7 total remission, 4 exceptional seizures). One patient with temporal epilepsy was considered to have been unsuccessful; only an 80% reduction in the number of preoperative seizures was obtained. This patient was reexplored and reoperated two months ago and she has since followed a very good postoperative course both clinically and EEGcally.

Of the three patients with inadequate definition of the epileptogenic zone (for instance due to widespread cerebral lesion), one with frontal epilepsy has experienced a significant decrease of seizures; the other two patients suffered from temporo-parieto-occipital area epilepsy.

Table 1. *Localization of the Epileptogenous Zone and Surgical Results*

Localiz. E.Z.	N.	T.R.	E.S.	M.R.	P.S.
Frontal	11	4	1	2	4
Temporal	4	1	2	1	0
Occipital	2	1	1	0	0
T.-P.-O. area	2	1	0	0	1
Parietal	1	1	0	0	0
Total	20	8	4	3	5

T.R. total remission, E.S. exceptional seizures, M.R. marked reduction, P.S. persistent seizures.

Table 2. *Delimitation of the Epileptogenous Zone and Surgical Results*

SEEG	N.	T.R.	E.S.	M.R.	P.S.
Correct delimitation of the E.Z.	12	7	4	1	0
Insufficient delimitation of the E.Z.	3	1	0	1	1
Bilaterality	5	0	0	1	4

The five patients in whom there was a bilateral epileptogenic involvement are considered separately because of this. These patients had frontal epilepsy and the epileptogenic zone which seemed to be predominant was removed. Only one of the patients had a significant decrease of seizures.

Discussion

Although the number of cases considered is to small to allow statistically significant conclusions, it is clear that the correct delimitation of the epileptogenic zone and the achievement of optimal surgical results is more difficult to obtain in frontal epilepsies and in epilepsies of the temporo-parieto-occipital region. These difficulties are attributed [1, 3] to the following reasons: A. The hypothetical localization of the epileptogenic zone on the basis of the electroclinical studies is more difficult to achieve when dealing with focal epilepsies from these areas than when dealing with temporal or parietal or occipital epilepsies. B. If this localization is not correct, the subsequent SEEG of these areas may fail to provide sufficient information on the localization of the epileptogenic zone, particularly if a limited number of depth electrodes is used. C. In addition, there is a great incidence of bilateral epileptogenic zones in frontal lobe epilepsy.

The patients with bilateral epileptogenicity must be analyzed in more detail. In our five cases, we found that: there was a focal predominance on the scalp EEG; such a predominance (concerning both lesional and irritative activities) was confirmed in the SEEG; the threshold of the electrical brain stimulation provoking the seizure was markedly lower on the predominant side. Our decision to operate was favoured by the pressure of the patients and of their relatives because of the highly disabling consequences of the epileptic syndrome. Nevertheless, we always stressed that, in our opinion, the results of surgery were highly unlikely to be satisfactory. We have obtained a decrease in the frequency of seizures, ranging from 20 to 50% of preoperative frequency.

Conclusion

In conclusion, preoperative localization of the epileptogenic zone must be as precise as possible. Future results will rest upon the degree of precision achieved. Operation is therefore only performed in those patients in whom there is exact definition of the epileptogenic zone.

Only when the patient's situation is unendurable because of the intensity and frequency of medically uncontrollable seizures, may the decision be taken to operate without precise definition of the epileptogenic zone. This is frequently due to multiple diffuse lesions. Corticoectomy is as conservative as possible, consistent with palliation, and operation is undertaken not for cure, but in an attempt to make the seizures more amenable to medical therapy.

References

1. Bancaud, J., Talairach, J., Bonis, A., Scaub, C., Szikla, G., Morel, P., Bordas-Ferrer, M., La Stéréo-électroencéphalographie dans l'épilepsie. Paris: Masson. 1965.
2. Talairach, J., Bancaud, J., Stereotaxic exploration and therapy in epilepsy. In: Handbook of Clinical Neurology. Vol. 15, pp. 758—782 (Vinken, P. J., Bruyn, G. W., eds.). Amsterdam: North-Holland Publ. Co. 1974.
3. Talairach, J., Bancaud, J., Szikla, G., Bonis, A., Geier, S., Vedrenne, C., Approche nouvelle de la Neurochirurgie de l'épilepsie. Méthodologie stéréotaxique et résultats thérapeutiques. Neurochirurgie *20* Suppl. 1 1974.
4. Talairach, J., Szikla, G., Tournoux, P., Prossalentis, A., Bordas-Ferrer, M., Covello, L., Jacob, M., Mempel, A., with the col. of Buser, P., and Bancaud, J., Atlas d'Anatomie Stéréotaxique du Télencéphale. Paris: Masson. 1967.

Acta Neurochirurgica, Suppl. 30, 121—126 (1980)

Medically Intractable Epilepsies of Tumoural Aetiology. Report of 4 Cases Treated According to the Method Described by J. Talairach *et al.*

R. Garcia Sola*, J. Miravet, C. Parera, and **G. Bravo**

With 4 Figures

Summary

The authors present 4 patients with medically uncontrollable epilepsy of tumoural aetiology (grade I–II gliomas). In two of them, CT scan showed probable neoplastic lesions, located deeply in the left frontal and right temporal lobes respectively, reflected in the SEG studies only in the second case. The other two were patients with left frontal gliomas in whom seizures did not disappear after removal of the tumour. After SEEG studies defined the epileptogenic zone and the lesion and these were removed, complete suppression of the seizures was achieved in two patients and the other two only unfrequently suffered seizures.

We emphasize the importance of SEEG studies for success in treating patients with gliomata previously diagnosed by CT scan, and who have seizures uncontrolled by anticonvulsants as the only symptom.

Introduction

In the 2.5 years, we have operated on 24 medically uncontrollable epileptic patients [2] according to the method described by Talairach and Bancaud [3, 4]. We present the procedures carried out in 4 out of 5 patients with epilepsy due to tumour who have been followed up for more than 6 months.

Cases Reports

Case 1

M. Z. B., a 15-year-old male patient, suffering 2–3 seizures per month from the age of 12. There were clinical signs of intoxication by his antiepileptic medication. On the CT scan there was a small hypodense area (Fig. 1), deep in the left fron-

* Services of Neurosurgery, Clinic Neurophysiology and Neuroradiology, Clinica Puerta de Hierro, Universidad Autonoma de Madrid, S. Martin de Porres 4, Madrid-35, Spain.

0065-1419/80/Suppl. 30/0121/$ 01.20

tal lobe. The stereoencephalographic study (SEG) was normal. After stereo-electroencephalography (SEEG) the lesion and epileptogenic focus were delineated and surgically resected. The histopathological diagnosis was grade I Astrocytoma. The patient has been free of seizures (19 months follow-up).

Case 2

M. S. S., a 16-year-old male patient, reported 4–5 seizures daily since the age of 3, and had been referred to our Service with the diagnosis of uncontrollable epilepsy. The CT scan revealed a deep temporal hypodense image with invasion of mesencephalic structures. The SEG ventriculogram showed a stenosis of the mid-portion of the right temporal horn (Fig. 2). After SEEG a right temporal lobectomy and partial resection of the tumour were performed. The histopathological diagnosis was grade I–II Astrocytoma. The patient suffered one seizure during radiotherapy, but has been seizure-free for the first 10 months of post-operative follow-up.

Case 3

M. R. A., a 9-year-old girl with generalized seizures since the age of 6. At the age of 7 a surgical resection of a left frontal grade II cystic Astrocytoma had been performed. Two months later she was reoperated on due to recollection of the cyst, followed by postoperative radiotherapy. Up to five seizures daily ocurred for the next 15 months in spite of medication. The CT scan showed a porencephalic cyst secondary to operation, with no signs of tumour recurrence. After SEEG, the lesion in the antero-external border of the scar was resected (tumour recurrence) and the epileptogenic focus in the Supplementary Motor Area was also resected (Fig. 3). In the 9 months since surgery, she has suffered only one seizure due to failure to take antiepileptic medication. In the EEG the preoperative paroxysmal discharges have disappeared.

Case 4

M. L. G., a 13-year-old girl with epilepsy from age of 5. At age 8, resection of a left frontal oligodendroglioma with postoperative radiotherapy was performed. Two years after surgery she still suffered more than 2–3 seizures daily. The CT scan showed a porencephalic cyst secondary to surgery, and calcification. At this time she was again operated on with resection of the surgical scar and of the calcifications. The histopathological study showed no evidence of recurrence of tumour. As the seizures persisted, a SEEG was performed, followed by resection of the lesional area (with no evidence of tumour recurrence) and of the epileptogenic focus located in the Supplementary Motor Area and Cingulum (Fig. 4). She has had no seizures in the six months following surgery, and the paroxysmal discharges seen prior to the operation have disappeared from the EEG.

Discussion

In the two first cases a suspected tumour was demonstrated by CT study. In the two last cases a standard excision of tumour was not enough to eliminate the epileptogenic focus.

Although the number of cases reported is small, we believe that they demonstrate the importance of SEEG exploration in cases of epilepsy refractory to medical treatment even if a benign glioma is suspected. This exploration [1] will yield precise data for the deline-

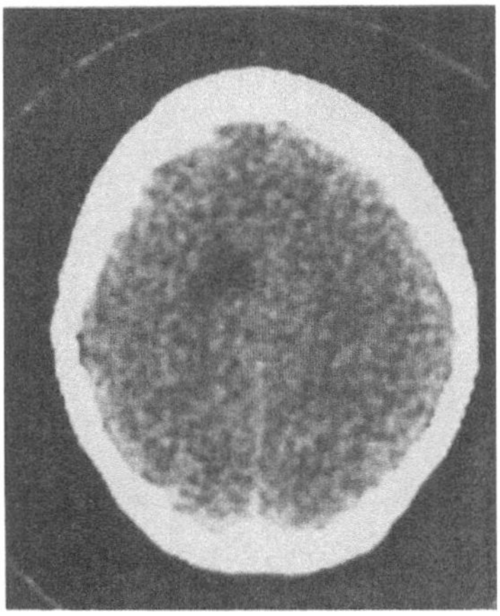

Fig. 1. M. Z. B. The small hypodense area without contrast enhancement

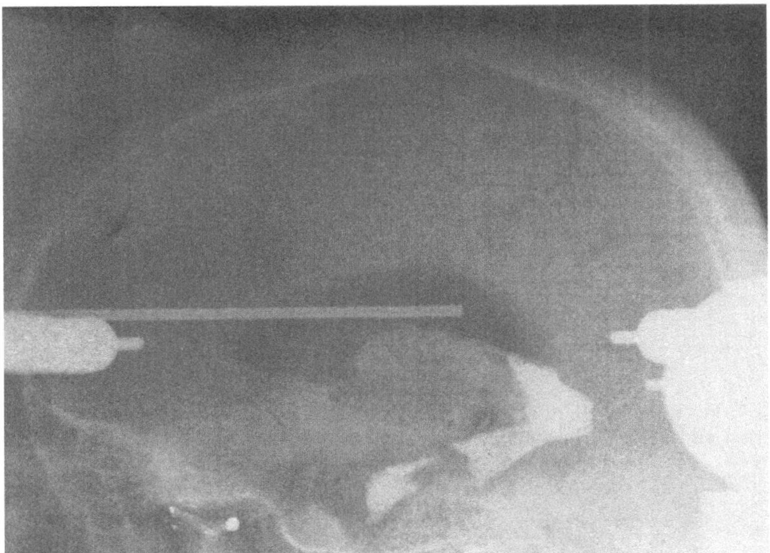

Fig. 2. M. S. S. Stereotactic pantopaque ventriculography: stenosis of the mid-portion of the right temporal horn

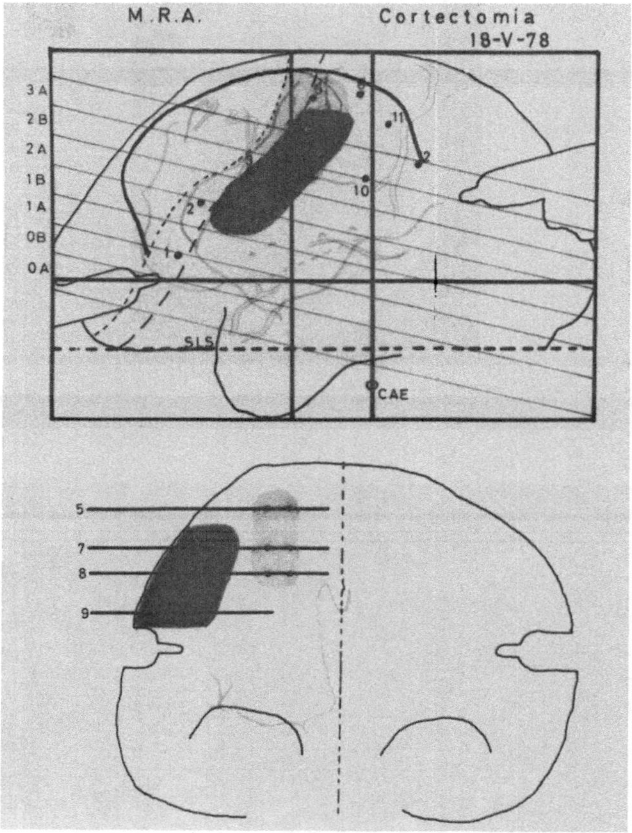

Fig. 3. M. R. A. *0 A . . . 3 A:* planes of the CT scan. Dotted lines: the postero-internal and external borders of the porencephalic cyst. The lesion (in dark gray) and the epileptogenic zone (in clear gray) were resected

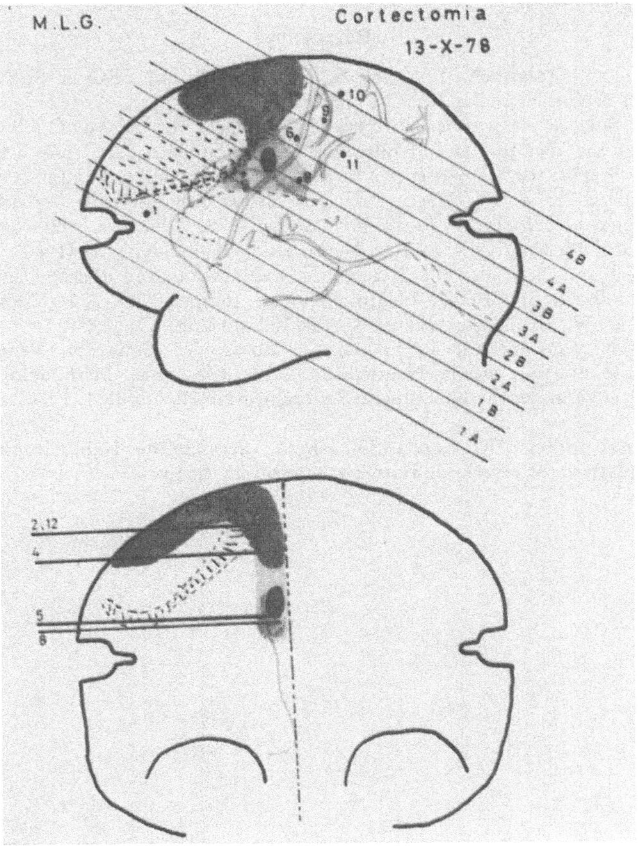

Fig. 4. M. L. G. *1 A . . . 4 B:* planes of the CT scan. The lesional area (in dark gray) corresponded to the border of the porencephalic cyst (electrodes 2, 4, 12). The epileptogenic zone (in clear gray) was surrounding a residual calcification (in dark)

ation and later resection not only of the lesion, but also of the epileptogenic zone responsible for the seizures which are the symptoms causing the patient to seek medical treatment.

References

1. Bancaud, J., Talairach, J., Geier, S., Scarabin, J. M., EEG et SEEG dans le tumeurs cérébrales et l'épilepsie. Paris: Edifor. 1973.
2. Garcia Sola, R., Miravet, J., Brasa, J., Nombela, L., Bravo, G., Relationship between the location and delineation of the epileptogenic zone and surgical results. Report of 24 patients operated on using the technique described by J. Talairach *et al.* IV. Meeting of the European Society for Stereotactic and Functional Neurosurgery, Paris, July 12–14, 1979. Advances in Stereotactic and Functional Neurosurgery 4. Acta Neurochir. (Wien) Suppl. *30* (1980), 117—120.
3. Talairach, J., Bancaud, J., Stereotactic exploration and therapy in epilepsy. In: Handbook of Clinical Neurology, Vol. 15, pp. 758—782 (Vinken, P. J., Bruyn, G. W., eds.). Amsterdam: North-Holland Publ. Co. 1974.
4. Talairach, J., Bancaud, J., Szikla, G., Bonis, A., Geier, S., Vedrenne, C., Approche nouvelle de la Neurochirurgie de l'épilepsie. Méthodologie stéréotaxique et résultats thérapeutiques. Neurochirurgie *20*, Suppl. 1. 1974.

Authors' address: R. Garcia Sola, M.D., Servicio de Neurocirugia, Clinica Puerta de Hierro, S. Martin de Porres 4, Madrid 35, Spain.

Acta Neurochirurgica, Suppl. 30, 127—135 (1980)

Anterior Callosotomy in Epileptics with Multiform Seizures and Bilateral Synchronous Spike and Wave EEG Pattern

F. R. Huck*, J. Radvany, J. O. Avila, C. H. Pires de Camargo, R. Marino jr., P. C. Ragazzo, D. Riva, and **P. Arlant**

With 3 Figures

Summary

Cerebral commissurotomy is a well established procedure in the treatment of epileptics refractory to drug therapy. Breeching of the ventricles in complete commissurotomy carries a certain morbidity. This has led others to perform operations in which the entire corpus callosum or only its anterior portion with or without the anterior commissure were sectioned. Sectioning of the anterior corpus callosum alone is justified by: a) frequent appearance in patients of seizures attributable to a frontal focus, b) clinical and experimental evidence that frontal discharges spread accross the corpus callosum leading to subsequent generalized its, c) the attempt to understand the mechanisms involved in generalized seizures, d) even further reduced surgical morbidity and neuropsychological disability.

Five epileptics were submitted to anterior callosotomy. The seizures in all of them suggested a frontal focus and consisted of absences, adversive, tonic, atonic, and tonic-clonic attacks. All patients were incapacitated by the frequency of seizures. Their EEGs showed paroxysms of bilateral synchronous slow spike and wave with uni-, or multiple (including bilateral symmetrical) focal accentuation. In two patients there were additional independent temporal lobe discharges. Neuropsychological evaluation showed cognitive deficits caused by inattention paroxysms and absences. After anterior callosotomy there was marked reduction in frequency of all types of seizures, the greatest improvement being in the reduction of frequency of absences. There was a marked decrease in physical, social and neuropsychological disabilities.

Keywords: Epilepsy; commissurotomy; corpus callosum.

Introduction

Spread of the epileptic discharge from one hemisphere to the other through the corpus callosum has been recognized since 1940 [2].

* Divisão de Neurocirurgia Funcional, Hospital das Clínicas, Universidade de São Paulo, C.P. 8091, 01000 S. Paulo, SP., Brazil.

0065-1419/80/Suppl. 30/0127/$ 01.80

Based on the improvement in epileptics suffering from tumours or infarcts of the corpus callosum, Van Wagenen and Herren [10] started to section various combinations of interhemispheric connections. Bogen and Vogel [1] demonstrated unequivocal improvement after the section of the entire corpus callosum, anterior commissure and massa intermedia. Their patients became the subject of classical studies on disconnection of the two hemispheres [3, 4].

Marcus [6, 7] studied the interaction of acute large bilateral epileptogenic foci in homologous areas of cerebral cortex in cats. This interaction often resulted in rapid production of persistent synchronous and symmetrical patterns of bilateral discharges including spike and slow wave complexes. Synchrony of bilateral discharges failed to occur after total section of the corpus callosum. The synchronous patterns of bilateral discharges occurred also in preparations in which large bilateral blocks of cerebral cortex had been isolated from subcortical structures but remained connected by the corpus callosum.

Marcus [8], in studies of the monkey cerebral cortex, concluded that recurrent bilateral synchronous and symmetrical patterns of discharge were established most easily following the production of bilateral frontal foci.

Wilson *et al.* [11, 12] analyzing the literature and their own experience concluded that section of the entire corpus callosum, without breeching the ventricles, was the procedure with least morbidity and greatest benefit.

In view of all experimental and clinical evidence discussed above we decided to restrict our surgical target to the anterior portion of the corpus callosum thus further decreasing morbidity. The area sectioned included all the interfrontal transcallosal fibres [9].

Material and Methods

Patient selection fulfilled the following criteria: 1. Uncontrolled epilepsy in spite of good therapeutic serum levels of commercially available anticonvulsants (phenytoin, carbamazepine, primidone, phenobarbital, clonazepam, nitrazepam, ethosuximide); 2. Seizures occurring weekly or more frequently; 3. Duration of epilepsy of at least four years; 4. Incapacity due to epilepsy and not to coexisting organic lesion; 5. Multiform seizures, some suggestive of frontal focus; 6. No severe mental retardation, as long as this could be distinguished from recurrent clinical and subclinical absences; 7. EEG including sphenoidal leads showing bilateral synchrony of spike-slow wave paroxysms with the demonstration, whenever possible, of uni-, or bihemispheric foci. The attempt to demonstrate this often required temporary reduction of anticonvulsant dosage; 8. Supportive family environment.

All patients were assessed for two to three months in hospital paying special attention to observation and description of seizures, administration of various anticonvulsant combinations, with simultaneous serum anticonvulsant level determi-

Table 1. *Clinical Manifestations: Types and Frequency of Seizures*

			Before frontal callosotomy									After frontal callosotomy							
Name	Age	Age of onset	Absences	Absences + automatisms	Atonic seizures	Adversive seizures	Tonic seizures	Tonic clonic seizures	Myoclonic seizures	Decreased attention	Date of operation	Absences	Absences + automatisms	Atonic seizures	Adversive seizures	Tonic seizures	Tonic clonic seizures	Myoclonic seizures	Decreased attention
WS	24	9	20/d	1/wk	1/wk	1/d	—	1/yr	—	2+	02/78	2/mo	—	—	6/yr	—	1/yr	—	0
PRN	23	10	20/d	—	3/wk	1/mo	—	2/yr	—	2+	05/78	1/mo	—	—	—	—	—	—	0
LLF	20	2	ctls	—	3/d	3/yr	—	1/yr	—	3+	06/78	5/d	—	1/mo	3/yr	—	—	—	1+
HF	28	2	ctls	1/mo	5/d	4/d	5/d	1/yr	—	4+	06/78	2/wk	—	1/wk	1/wk	4/yr	1/yr	—	1+
DL	42	20	ctls	4/d	2/wk	6/d	—	2/yr	—	4+	09/78	10/d	1/wk	2/mo	1/wk	—	2/yr	—	2+

ctls = countless, d = day, wk = week, mo = month, yr = year.

nations, neuropsychological investigations, psychiatric interviews, sequential EEGs, air encephalogram and arteriography.

None of the patients had abnormal clinical neurological signs.

Table 2. *Pre- and Post-operative Electroencephalograms*

PT	Pre-operative EEGs	Post-operative EEGs
WS	Generalized bisynchronous spike-slow-wave or polyspike-slow-wave (sleep) maximal right or left fronto-central. Trains of multiple spikes, maximal left central.	Short trains of multiple spikes or spike-slow-wave, restricted to one hemisphere: right or left
PRN	Generalized bisynchronous spike-slow-wave or polyspike-slow-wave (sleep), no focal accentuation.	Spike-slow-wave restricted to one hemisphere: right or left. Short trains of multiple spikes, restricted to right.
LLF	Generalized bisynchronous spike-slow-wave, maximal right central and right temporal.	Repetitive generalized synchronous polyspike-slow-wave (sleep). Irregular spike-slow-wave, restricted to right fronto-central and right fronto-temporal.
HF	Repetitive bilaterally synchronous spike-slow-wave or polyspike-slow-wave (sleep) maximal right or left fronto-central.	Short repetitive spike-slow-wave or polyspike-slow-wave over left hemisphere or bilaterally synchronous.
DL	Generalized synchronous spike-slow-wave, maximal right or left fronto-central. Independent left temporal spikes.	Spike-slow-wave mostly restricted to one hemisphere: right or left, less often bilaterally synchronous. Independent left temporal spikes.

The surgical procedure consisted of a two-inch trephine frontal parasagittal craniotomy. The dura was opened in a semicircular fashion and the bridging veins coagulated with bipolar forceps. The mesial aspect of the frontal lobe was then retracted with a self-retaining spatula and the branches of the anterior cerebral artery were exposed and dissected away from the midportion of the anterior corpus callosum. The callosal fibres were then divided using careful suction under the microscope. The section was commenced at the more inferior rostrum and extended 6–7 cm upwards sparing the thin wall of the ventricle. A radiopaque thread marker was left in place.

Re-evaluation is being carried out at 1, 6, 12, and 24 months after the operations and less frequently subsequently.

Results

The clinical and EEG changes after surgery are summarized on Tables 1 and 2. Anticonvulsants were maintained unaltered for all patients. In the first two or three days after surgery all the patients had transient decrease in spontaneous speech initiation and movement

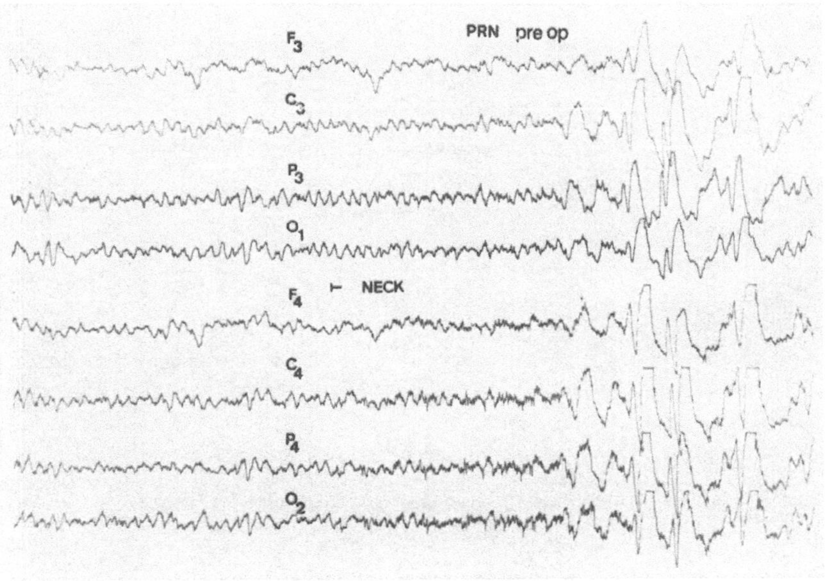

Fig. 1. Patient 2, pre-operative EEG, patient awake. Generalized bilateral synchronous slow spike and wave discharge

of the left arm. All types of seizures decreased in frequency. The most remarkable improvement was in the frequency of absences and in the level of consciousness reflected even on the patients' facies. There was a change in the phenomenology of the remaining fits in three patients: in patient W. S. the motor phenomena that usually accompanied absences (staring and blinking) continued without the subjective sensation of being "switched-off"; in patient H. F. the abrupt tonic fits with a fall became a slow leaning backwards; the global atonic fits in H. F. and L. L. F. were transformed into brief head nodding.

The most impressive EEG change after surgery was disruption of the generalized bilateral synchronous slow spike and wave discharges (Fig. 1). This disruption was complete in two patients, partial in two, and in one, bisynchrony continued only during sleep. After the operation, the slow spike and wave or polyspike and slow wave discharges became confined to part or whole of one hemisphere alone or were randomly and independently seen in one or the other hemisphere (Figs. 2 and 3).

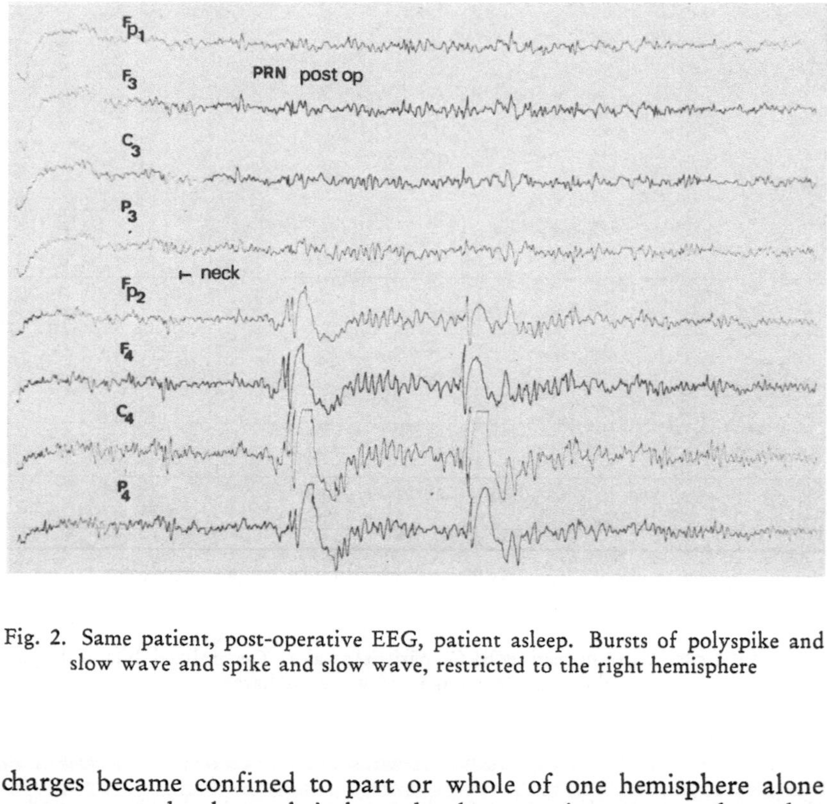

Fig. 2. Same patient, post-operative EEG, patient asleep. Bursts of polyspike and slow wave and spike and slow wave, restricted to the right hemisphere

In three patients neuropsychological evaluation before the operation showed global impairment of cognitive functions by an almost continuous disturbance of attention. In the remaining two patients the inattention was sufficiently intermittent to allow the diagnostic isolation of a premotor syndrome. Six months after surgery the attention of all five patients had improved considerably and both a premotor and a mild prefrontal syndrome became apparent in all of them. By 12 months in the two patients so far tested the premotor syndrome had disappeared. There was marked improvement in the patients' general physical and social capacity: two patients stopped wearing helmets, one abandoned his wheelchair and two returned to school. Before surgery the psychiatric evaluation revealed flatness of affect, disorganized and impoverished thought as well as decreased

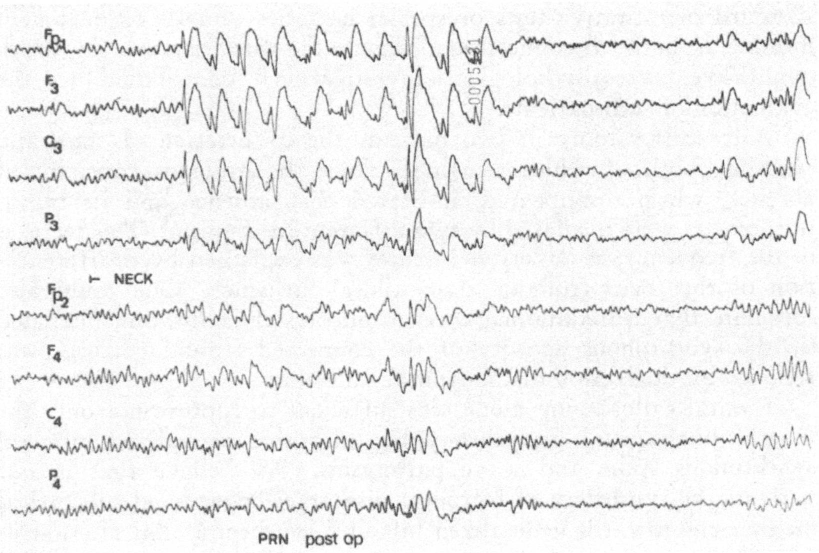

Fig. 3. Same patient as before, post-operative EEG, asleep. Spike and slow wave discharge, restricted to the left hemisphere

pragmatism, initiative and will, all of which varied greatly from patient to patient and from time to time in each patient. All these improved remarkably.

Discussion

The improvement in absences and attention, the rupture of bilateral synchronous spike and slow wave discharges were both associated with heightened level of consciousness. The premotor syndrome, most probably due to almost continuous transcallosal electrical abnormalities in both frontal lobes, disappeared by 12 months in two patients, probably due to reorganization of skilled motor acts with greater participation of subcortical structures. The appearance of a mild prefrontal syndrome in two patients is attributable to the section of the frontal callosum per se because, in spite of the marked impairment of attention before the operation, these patients were tested and did not exhibit such signs. The ease with which a mild prefrontal syndrome could have been overlooked in the face of the remarkable and global improvement in part justifies why this has not been pointed out previously in the literature. Psychological studies of commissurotomized epileptics have so far consisted of standard quantitative tests or special batteries of tests to document interhemispheric disconnection. This is the first instance in which qualitative neuropsychological investigation[5] contributed to the evaluation of such patients.

After callosotomy in two patients the dissociation of stare and blinking, both of which remained, from the previous concomitant absence, which disappeared, indicated that absence and its motor phenomena were mediated by two different mechanisms. The decrease in the frequency of adversive seizures was explained by deafferentation of the focus from its transcallosal influence. One could also speculate that a maintained cortico-subcortical facilitation mediated by the synchronous activity of the connected frontal cortices, was relieved by the section of the frontal callosum.

Frontal callosotomy alone was sufficient to rupture not only the frontal parasagittal bisynchrony but also the generalized bilateral synchronous spike and wave paroxysms. We believe that in our patients the synchrony of bifrontal discharges engendered subcortical mechanisms towards generalized bilateral synchrony. An alternative hypothesis would be to suppose spread of discharges from the bifrontal transcallosal synchrony posteriorly in each hemisphere. These discharges in the posterior part of the hemispheres would in turn become secondarily bisynchronous across the posterior callosum. In either circumstance section of the frontal corpus callosum arrests generalization of the seizure.

References

1. Bogen, J. E., Vogel, P. J., Neurologic status in the long term following complete cerebral commissurotomy. In: Les syndromes de disconnexion calleuse chez l'homme, p. 227 (Michel, F., Schott, B., eds.). Lyon Hop. Neurol. 1975.
2. Erickson, T. C., Spread of the epileptic discharge. Arch. Neurol. Psychiat. *32* (1940), 429.
3. Gazzaniga, M. S., Bogen, J. E., Sperry, R. W., Some functional effects of sectioning the cerebral commissures in man. Proc. Natl. Acad. Sci. U.S.A. *48* (1962), 1765.
4. Gazzaniga, M. S., Risse, G. L., Springer, S. P., *et al.*, Psychologic and neurologic consequences of partial and complete cerebral commissurotomy. Neurology *25* (1975), 10.

5. Luria, A. R., Higher cortical functions in man. New York: Basic Books Inc. Publishers. 1966.
6. Marcus, E. M., Watson, C. W., Bilateral "epileptogenic" foci in cat cerebral cortex: mechanisms of interaction in the intact, the bilateral cortical callosal and adiencephalic preparation. Electroencephal. Clin. Neurophysiol. *17* (1964), 454.
7. Marcus, E. M., Watson, C. W., Bilateral synchronous spike wave electroencephalographic patterns in the cat: interaction of bilateral cortical foci in the intact, the bilateral cortical callosal and the adiencephalic preparations. Arch. Neurol. *14* (1966), 601—610.
8. Marcus, E. M., Watson, C. W., Symmetrical epileptogenic foci in monkey cerebral cortex. Mechanisms of interaction and regional variations in capacity for synchronous discharges. Arch. Neurol. *19* (1968), 99—116.
9. Pandya, D. N., Karol, E. A., Heilbronn, D., The topographical distribution of interhemispheric projections in the corpus callosum of the rhesus monkey. Brain Res. *32* (1971), 31.
10. Van Wagenen, W. P., Herren, R. Y., Surgical division of commissural pathways in the corpus callosum. Arch. Neurol. Psychiat. *44* (1940), 740—759.
11. Wilson, D. H., Reeves, A., Gazzaniga, M., Culver, C., Cerebral commissurotomy for control of intractable seizures. Neurology *27* (1977), 708—715.
12. Wilson, D. H., Reeves, A., Gazzaniga, M., Division of the corpus callosum for uncontrollable epilepsy. Neurology *28* (1978), 649—653.

Acta Neurochirurgica, Suppl. 30, 137—143 (1980)

Anterior Callosotomy as a Substitute for Hemispherectomy

J. O. Avila*, J. Radvany, F. R. Huck, C. H. Pires de Camargo, R. Marino jr., P. C. Ragazzo, and D. Riva

With 4 Figures

Summary

Two patients with epilepsy and large hemispheric lesions underwent section of the frontal fibres of the corpus callosum for the treatment of seizures refractory to medical treatment. A severely retarded girl of 18 had encephalotrigeminal angiomatosis (Sturge-Weber syndrome) with multiple daily absences, tonic-clonic, myoclonic, atonic and adversive seizures since infancy. All types of fits—with the exception of adversive seizures and rare tonic-clonic fits—disappeared after anterior callosotomy. Another moderately retarded girl of 18 had an old cystic lesion over the entire territory of the left middle cerebral artery. She had had right hemiplegia since infancy and frequent brief absences and massive myoclonus triggered by unexpected sensory stimuli since the age of six years. Following anterior callosotomy there was an almost complete disappearance of the absences and a marked reduction of her startle myoclonus.

Frontal callosotomy is a useful procedure in epileptics with large hemispheric lesions and carries less risk than hemispherectomy or total commissurotomy.

Keywords: Epilepsy; commissurotomy; hemispherectomy; corpus callosum.

Introduction

Serious, even fatal early and late complications of cerebral hemispherectomy have been extensively documented [3, 5, 7, 9]. Laine [7] and Griffith [5] suggested, and Luessenhop [8] and Wilson [12] carried out, commissurotomies in epileptics with large hemispheric lesions which were refractory to drug management. The operation consisted of section of the anterioı commissure, the entire corpus callosum and, in some cases, of one of the fornices. Complications due to breaching of the ventricles in these and other cases of commissurotomy [13, 14] led to a more limited number and extent of the commissural sections. Indeed, once it is accepted that the seizure discharge spreads from

* Divisão de Neurocirurgia Funcional, Hospital das Clínicas, Universidade de São Paulo, C.P. 8091, 01000 S. Paulo, SP., Brazil.

0065-1419/80/Suppl. 30/0137/$ 01.40

the cortical focus through the corpus callosum to the contralateral homologous cortex [2], it seems justifiable to section only the part of the corpus callosum which connects the involved cortex with its homologous counterpart as long as the cortical focus is well defined by clinical and electroencephalographic manifestations of the seizure.

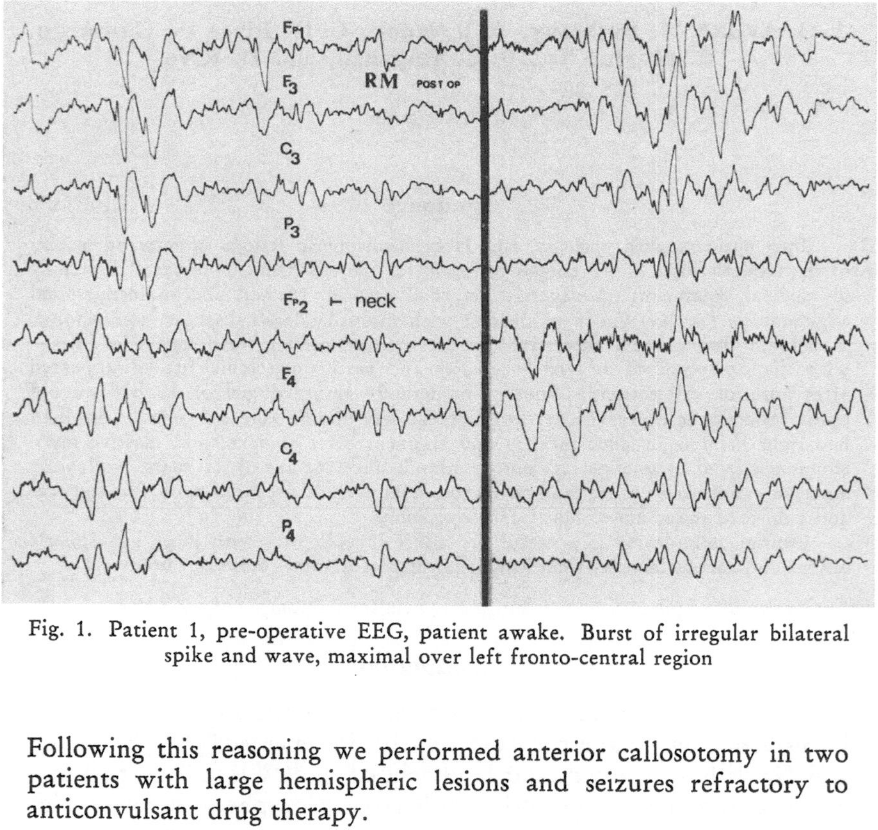

Fig. 1. Patient 1, pre-operative EEG, patient awake. Burst of irregular bilateral spike and wave, maximal over left fronto-central region

Following this reasoning we performed anterior callosotomy in two patients with large hemispheric lesions and seizures refractory to anticonvulsant drug therapy.

Materials and Methods

These two cases are part of a larger series of patients undergoing similar surgical procedures; the remaining cases are discussed elsewhere [6]. Though there are no basic physiopathological differences between the groups, the fact that these two patients had large hemispheric lesions led us to stress some particular aspects of the results obtained, especially when compared to patients submitted to larger commissurotomies or hemispherectomies. The protocol for preoperative investigation is described elsewhere [6].

Patient 1 (R. M.). This 18-year-old girl had a right nevus flammeus over the right frontal and periorbital regions. Deviation of her eyes to the right was noticed in the first month of life. Her fits began at three months and increased in frequency with age up to 30 convulsions a day—generalized tonic-clonic fits, head

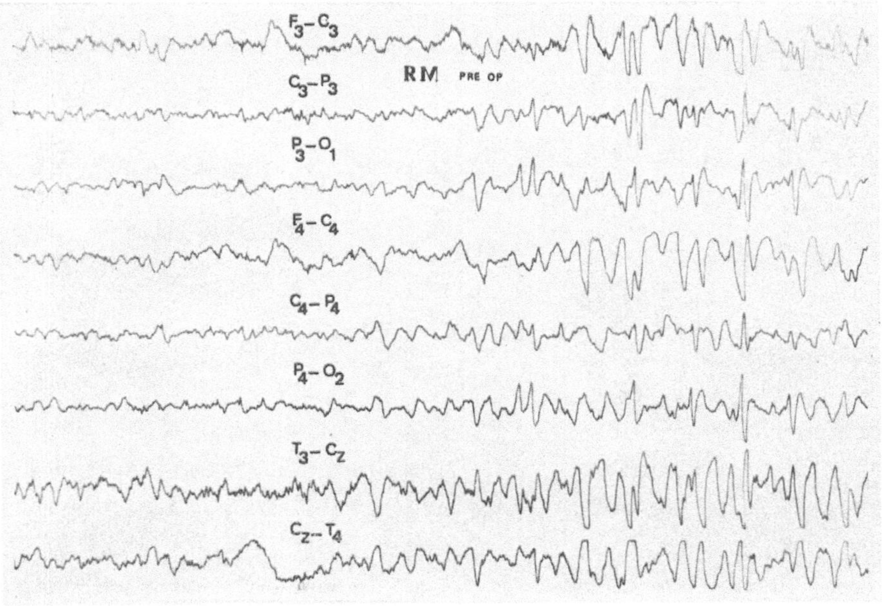

Fig. 2. Patient 1, post-operative EEG, patient asleep. Left: burst of spike and slow wave, restricted to the left hemisphere. Right: irregular spike and wave burst over the left frontal region. Slow wave predominance over the right anterior quadrant

and eye deviation to either side with homolateral arm raising, myoclonic jerks of the upper extremities and very frequent absences with or without falling. She was treated with various combinations of anticonvulsants, which were only transiently effective in spite of maintained adequate serum levels. These included phenytoin, phenobarbital, primidone, carbamazepine, clonazepam and nitrazepam. She was severely mentally retarded. Her admission was necessitated by unmanageable aggressive behaviour at home. Examination revealed no elementary gross motor disfunction. The EEG showed generalized multiple spike and slow wave complexes, and spike and slow wave activity maximal over fronto-central leads (Fig. 1). An air encephalogram revealed marked right hemisphere atrophy with a dilated right ventricle and characteristic occipital calcification. A bilateral carotid angiography showed no abnormalities on the left, but abnormal venous drainage of the whole right hemisphere with no discernible cortical veins and grossly dilated and distorted internal veins on the right.

A right fronto-parietal craniotomy was performed and the anterior 6 cm of the corpus callosum were divided down to but sparing the ventricular wall by means of a small sucter, and preserving all the bridging vessels over the corpus callosum. There was a marked decrease in the frequency of absences, atonic spells and—most of all—tonic-clonic seizures after surgery; these now occur about once

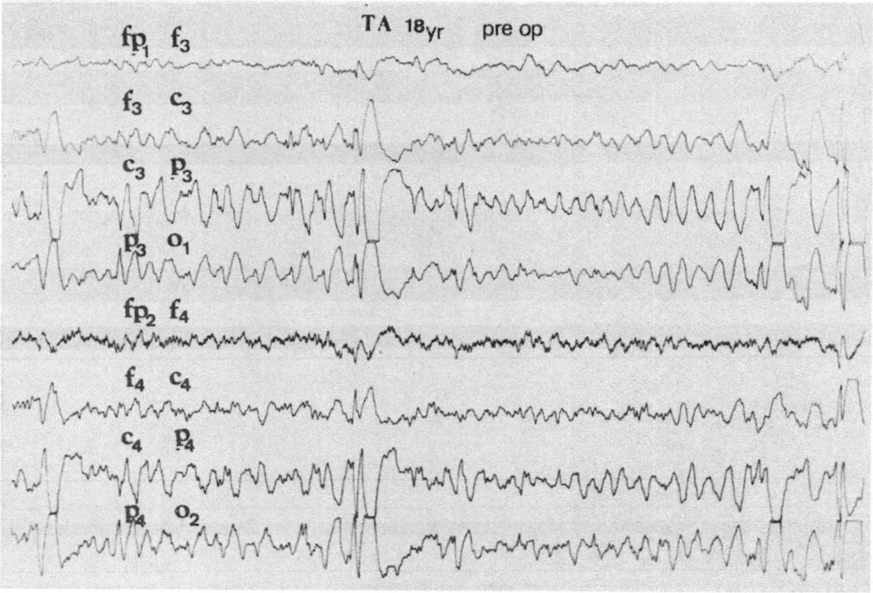

Fig. 3. Patient 2, pre-operative EEG, patient awake. Irregular bilateral spike and slow wave burst, maximal at centro-parietal regions

every two months. The drug regimen was unaltered. The adversive fits did not show any change in frequency. There was a marked improvement in her behaviour and for the first time she was able to be placed in a nursery school. EEG findings after 11 months are displayed on Fig. 2.

Patient 2 (T. A.). This 18-year-old girl, the elder of twins, was delivered at term by caesarian section, weighed 3,200 g and was in good condition immediately after birth.

The patient had a respiratory arrest of unknown length while her sister was being resuscitated. She was discharged from hospital after ten days in good condition. Her motor development was abnormal from the first month. She could not open her right hand at four months, sat without support at nine months and began to walk unassisted after 18 months, with a very evident right-sided hemiparesis. There was hypoplastic development of right face and limbs; she was moderately retarded and often incontinent of urine. The patient began to have very frequent fits at eight, consisting of sudden massive myoclonus predominant on the right side, ten or more times per day, almost always triggered by unexpected sensory stimuli such as sudden noises, lights or touch. She had also countless absences accompanied by a slight deviation of her gaze towards the right. By the time she was referred to us the patient had already been treated with clonazepam, nitrazepam, ethosuximide, phenytoin and carbamazepine in various

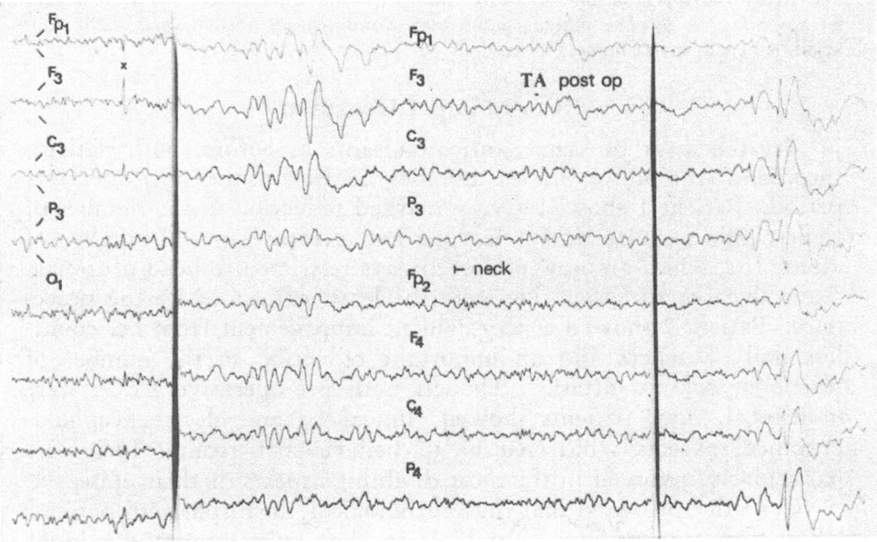

Fig. 4. Patient 2, post-operative EEG taken after six months. Patient awake. Left: Left frontal isolated spike discharge. Middle: Sharp-slow wave burst over the left fronto-central region. Right: Bilateral spike-slow wave discharge, maximal over posterior regions (common reference recording to the neck)

combinations which had to be changed frequently due to loss of control on seizures, in spite of adequate serum levels. EEG studies showed frequent paroxysms of slow spike and wave complexes, pseudo-periodic and more marked over the parasagittal area (Fig. 3). An air encephalogram showed a huge pseudo-porencephalic cyst involving predominantly the left parietal lobe. The left ventricle was grossly distorted from the frontal horn to the atrium. The right hemisphere was normal. The left carotid angiogram showed very poor perfusion over the middle cerebral artery territory with small irregular arteries and hypoplastic cortical veins over the left frontal and parietal lobes. Amobarbital injection did not result in change in language function.

The patient underwent a left fronto-parietal craniotomy which revealed a huge cyst involving the frontal, parietal and upper temporal lobes and deepened in a cone-shaped fashion towards the intact wall of the left lateral ventricle. Electrocorticography with the aid of auditory stimuli revealed spike activity over the frontal border of the cyst and an independent focus over the posterior parietal lobe. The same technique described for patient 1 was used to section the anterior 4 cm of the corpus callosum.

There was a marked decrease in the number of absences down to four or five daily from the first post-operative day. This observation parallelled a much better performance in neuropsychological tests involving persistent attention compared with the pre-operative results. The frequency of startle myoclonus did not change until clonazepam was given again in doses of 8–10 mg daily. Similar doses had had no appreciable effect before the operation. EEG evolution after surgery is shown in Fig. 4. The patient shows now a much more normal social behaviour and is independent at home.

Results and Discussion

Treated with the same anticonvulsants as before, both patients showed a diminution in the number of fits in the post-operative period. Patient 1 showed a very marked reduction in the number of tonic-clonic seizures and a less marked decrease in the number of atonic fits, which are now almost always restricted to head dropping. Adversive fits to either side were the least influenced by the procedure. Patient 2 showed a very evident improvement from her countless daily absences and an important reduction in the number of startle myoclonus attacks. Though both pre-operative EEGs were multifocal, these patients showed clinical [1, 4] and electroencephalographical aspects which led us to believe that frontal foci were particularly involved in the most disabling aspects of their epilepsy.[1]

Griffith [5] proposed that the "pathological" hemisphere of patients whose fits render them candidates for hemispherectomy should be functionally isolated by a total commissurotomy plus a capsulotomy. Wilson *et al.* [14] described a patient who was temporarily freed from his adversive and tonic-clonic fits after section of the anterior corpus callosum. The return of seizures was attributed to a new pathway through the intact posterior corpus callosum, as the patient became almost seizure-free after section of the remaining portion. The activation of the contralateral cortex by way of the corpus callosum may play an important role in the involvement of the contralateral subcortical grey matter (thalamic nuclei, MRF, and possibly lower reticular structures) thus mediating an important step in the propagation of a seizure [2, 10, 11]. The persistence of some generalized fits could be explained either by propagation through the remaining posterior callosal fibres or by random "synchronization" of bilateral independ foci which would be enough to initiate the subcortical mechanisms involved in propagation. The use of serial procedures in more patients would help to clarify this aspect. Once sophisticated

EEG recordings can define where the most prominent epileptic activity occurs, around large lesions, it would appear reasonable to attempt an isolation of this area alone as a first step towards disconnection of this cortex from its homologous counterpart, especially in patients showing secondary generalized epilepsy with multifocal accentuation and probable secondary bilateral synchrony. It is simpler and carries less risk than hemispherectomy or total commissurotomy.

References

1. Bancaud, J., Talairach, J., Hypothèses neurophysiopathologiques sur la épilepsie-sursaut chez l'homme. Rev. Neurol. *131* (1975), 559—571.
2. Collins, R. C., Kennedy, C., Sokoloff, L., Plum, F., Metabolic anatomy of focal motor seizures. Arch. Neurol. *33* (1976), 536—542.
3. Falconer, M. A., Wilson, P. J. E., Complications related to delayed haemorrhage after hemispherectomy. J. Neurosurg. *30* (1969), 413—426.
4. Geier, S., Bancaud, J., Talairach, J., Bonis, A., Szikla, G., Enjelvi, M., The seizures of frontal lobe epilepsy. Neurology *27* (1977), 951—958.
5. Griffith, H. B., Cerebral hemispherectomy for infantile hemiplegia in the light of the late results. Ann. R. Coll. Surg. *41* (1967), 183—201.
6. Huck, F. R., Radvany, J., Avila, J. O., Pires de Camargo, C. H., Marino, R., jr., Ragazzo, P. C., Riva, D., Arlant, P., Anterior callosotomy in epileptics with multiform seizures and bilateral synchronous spike and wave EEG pattern. Acta Neurochir. (Wien), Suppl. 30 (1980), 127—135.
7. Laine, E., Pruvot, P., Osson, D., Résultats éloignés de l'hémisphérectomie dans les cas d'hémiatrophie cérébrale infantile génératrice d'épilepsie. Neuro-Chirurgie *10* (1964), 507—522.
8. Luessenhop, A. J., dela Cruz, T., Fenichel, G. M., Surgical disconnection of the cerebral hemispheres in intractable seizures (Results in infancy and childhood). JAMA *213* (1970), 1630—1636.
9. Oppenheimer, D. R., Griffith, H. B., Persistent intracranial bleeding as a complication of hemispherectomy. J. Neurol. Neurosurg. Psychiat. *29* (1966), 229—240.
10. Wada, J. A., Sato, M., The generalized convulsive state induced by daily electrical stimulation of the amygdala in split-brain cats. Epilepsia *16* (1975), 417—430.
11. Williams, D., The thalamus and epilepsy. Brain *88* (1965), 539—556.
12. Wilson, D. H., Culver, C., Waddington, M., Gazzaniga, M., Disconnection of the cerebral hemispheres. An alternative to hemispherectomy for the control of intractable seizures. Neurology *25* (1975), 1149—1153.
13. Wilson, D. H., Reeves, A., Gazzaniga, M., Culver, C., Cerebral commissurotomy for the control of intractable seizures. Neurology 27 (1977), 708—715.
14. Wilson, D. H., Reeves, A., Gazzaniga, M., Division of the corpus callosum for uncontrollable epilepsy. Neurology *28* (1978), 649—653.

Acta Neurochirurgica, Suppl. 30, 145—149 (1980)

Late Results of Stereotactic Radiofrequency Lesions in Epilepsy

F. Marossero*, L. Ravagnati, V. A. Sironi, G. Miserocchi, A. Franzini, G. Ettorre, and **G. P. Cabrini**

Summary

Thirty-five patients with partial complex seizures and two patients with generalized epilepsy were treated by stereotactic radiofrequency lesions. Follow-up from 2 to 13 years was available in 30 patients. The stereotactic targets in patients with partial complex seizures were: a) Amygdala; b) Ammon's horn; c) parahippocampal gyrus; d) Fornix. Depending on scalp EEG and depth electrode studies, each patient had one or more target coagulated, unilaterally or bilaterally. In the 2 cases of generalized epilepsy, bilateral Forel field lesions were performed. Late surgical results are discussed in relation to the depth EEG studies and the number and site of stereotactic lesions.

Keywords: Surgery for epilepsy; late results; depth EEG; radiofrequency (r.f.) lesions.

Stereotactic coagulation of the epileptogenic lesion and interruption of the pathways of seizure propagation have been widely used in the past 20 years for the treatment of medically intractable epilepsy [3, 1].

The recent review of the literature by Ojemann and Ward [3] shows, however, that there are not as yet generally accepted indications and target areas for stereotactic procedures in epilepsy.

This paper presents the late results of stereotactic surgery in a series of 30 patients, in relation to the preoperative clinical, EEG and depth EEG studies, and to the number and site of stereotactic lesions.

Material and Method

At the neurosurgical Institute of the University of Milan, 160 patients have been treated for non tumoural epilepsy over the past 20 years. Stereotactic radiofrequency lesions were performed in 37 patients. This report is based on the study

* Institute of Neurosurgery, University of Milan, via F. Sforza, 35, I-20122 Milano, Italy.

0065-1419/80/Suppl. 30/0145/$ 01.00

of a group of 30 patients with an available follow-up from 2 to 13 years from the stereotactic procedures.

There were 22 males and 8 females, ranging in age between 11 and 50 years. Twenty-eight patients had psychomotor seizures, occasionally with secondary generalization, and scalp EEG signs of temporal lobe involvement, and two presented primary generalized seizures. The neuroradiological investigations were normal.

Table 1. *Targets of Stereotactic Radiofrequency Lesions in 30 Patients*

Targets	Unilateral	Bilateral
Amygdala	22	5
Ammon's horn	10	—
Hippocampal gyrus	2	—
Fornix	8	4
Fasciculus uncinatus	6	2
Fields of forel	—	2
Fusiform gyrus	2	—

Table 2. *Late Results in Patients with Partial and Generalized Epilepsy.* Outcome groups A, B, C: refer to the text

	Outcome			
	Group A	Group B	Group C	Total
Partial epilepsies	6	7	15	28
Generalized epilepsies	—	—	2	2
Total	6	7	17	30

Preoperative depth EEG studies, either acute or chronic, were performed in 23 cases, for the exact identification of the epileptogenic lesion. The Talairach apparatus and technique were used for stereotactic identification of the structures to be studied, and of the targets to be coagulated [4]. A series of neurophysiological tests were performed in all patients for the exact localization of the surgical targets [2]. Wyss radiofrequency lesion generator and Wyss electrodes were used to perform the stereotactic lesions.

The lesions were placed in the following structures: Amygdala, Ammon's horn, hippocampal gyrus, fasciculus uncinatus, fusiform gyrus, fornix, and the fields of Forel (Table 1).

Results

General Results

The patients have been divided into 3 outcome groups, according to the effect of the r.f. lesions on seizure frequency (Table 2).

Table 3. *Late Results in Patients Divided According to the Preoperative EEG Studies.* Outcome groups A, B, C: refer to the text

Patients		Outcome		
		Group A	Group B	Group C
Without depth EEG study	5	—	1	4
With bilateral temporal depth EEG focus	10	1	5	4
With unilateral temporal depth EEG focus	7	3	1	3
With rhinencephalic focus	2	2	—	—
With also extratemporal foci	4	—	—	4

Table 4. *Late Results of 10 Patients with Bitemporal EEG Foci After Unilateral and Bilateral Radiofrequency Lesions.* Outcome groups A, B, C: refer to the text

Lesion		Outcome		
		Group A	Group B	Group C
Unilateral	(5)	1	3	1
Bilateral	(5)	—	2	3

Group A includes 6 patients with no seizure recurrence, or with only occasional seizures (less than twice per year).

Group B includes 7 patients who presented a worth-while reduction of seizure tendency (from daily seizures, to free intervals of at least one month).

Group C includes 17 patients who had no significant improvement after surgery. The 2 patients with primary generalized seizures, treated by bilateral Forel campotomy, ended in this group.

Results of Rhinencephalic r.f. Lesions

The group of 28 patients with partial complex epilepsy and EEG signs of temporal lobe involvement were treated by rhinencephalic coagulation, to destroy the epileptogenic lesion or to interrupt functional pathways. Table 3 shows the correlation between surgical outcome and preoperative EEG studies.

Results in patients who had been operated on, using only the data of clinical and scalp EEG, without depth EEG studies, have not been satisfactory.

In a group of 10 patients with bitemporal scalp EEG foci, a primary epileptogenic lesion could not be identified even by depth EEG. Different rhinencephalic structures were then coagulated, according to depth EEG data in individual patients (amygdala, Ammon's horn, parahippocampal gyrus, fornix, fasciculus uncinatus), either unilaterally or bilaterally. Surgical results appear not to be different from those obtained by unilateral temporal lobectomy, in a similar group of our patients. The outcome in bilateral r.f. lesions was not different from unilateral ones (Table 4).

In a group of 7 patients, depth EEG studies confirmed the presence of a unilateral epileptogenic lesion. Unilateral stereotactic coagulations of rhinencephalic structures were performed, even if there was a definite indication for an anterior temporal lobectomy, with rather encouraging results (Table 3).

In 2 cases, depth EEG studies revealed a very discrete epileptogenic lesion, with spontaneous seizures originating and developing in the amygdala and anterior Ammon's horn, and r.f. lesions of these regions have given excellent results.

In a last group of 4 patients, in whom r.f. rhinencephalic coagulations were performed as functional procedures in order to interrupt anatomical pathways involved in the development of the seizures, the results have been disappointing (Table 3).

Discussion

Our results suggest that stereotactic surgery is a useful surgical procedure in the treatment of temporal lobe epilepsy diagnosed by depth EEG investigations.

Patients with unilateral epileptogenic lesions can benefit from unilateral coagulation of the structures involved in the seizures, as determined by depth EEG. This procedure is often successful in abolishing the seizures completely, especially when they are shown to originate unilaterally in discrete portions of the rhinencephalic formation, by depth EEG investigations. On the other hand, this approach does not exclude the subsequent excision of the temporal lobe, in the event of failure.

The results in cases of bitemporal epileptogenic lesions are not as good as in the unilateral ones, but do not appear to be worse than those obtained by unilateral temporal lobectomy, in our experience.

Rhinencephalic coagulations appear to be unsuccessful in preventing seizure recurrence in cases where the epileptogenic lesion is extratemporal and the rhinencephalic structures are only secondarily involved.

References

1. Gillingham, F. J., Hitchcock, E. R., Nádvorník, P. (eds.), Stereotactic treatment of epilepsy. Acta Neurochir. Supplementum 23. Wien-New York: Springer. 1976.
2. Maspes, P. E., Marossero, F., Cabrini, G. P., Neurophysiological tests for stereotactic identification of rhinencephalic "targets". Schweizer Archiv Neurol. Neurochir. Psychiat. *111* (1972), 331—340.
3. Ojemann, G. A., Ward, A. A., Jr., Stereotactic and other procedures for epilepsy. In: Advances in neurology, Vol. 8, pp. 241—263 (Purpura, D. P., Penry, J. K., Walter, R. D., eds.). New York: Raven Press. 1975.
4. Talairach, J., Bancaud, J., Szikla, G., Bonis, A., Geier, S., Vendrenne, C., Approche nouvelle de la neurochirurgie de l'épilepsie. Méthodologique stéréotaxique et résultats thérapeutique. Neurochirurgie *20*, Suppl. (1974), 1—240.

Acta Neurochirurgica, Suppl. 30, 151—159 (1980)

Stereotactic Lesions in Primary Epilepsy of the Limbic System

G. Bouvier[1], **J. M. Saint-Hilaire**[2], **R. Maltais**[3], **R. Bélique**[4], and **P. Desrochers**[5]

With 7 Figures

Summary

Chronic depth electrodes have proven useful in diagnosing primary epilepsy of the limbic system. Five patients had small lesions in the amygdala and hippocampus. There was a 50% reduction of the seizures frequency. No complication were observed and patients were ambulant the day following surgery. It is felt that stereotactic lesions larger than produced by the leucotome used should be performed provided we have proofs that the epileptogenic focus is in a restricted area. Stereotactic lesions may also have a role in interrupting pathways clearly proven as participating in the epileptic discharge. Only under these conditions, will it be possible to say that stereotactic lesions are effective in specific type of epilepsy.

Keywords: Chronic depth electrodes; stereotactic lesions; primary epilepsy of the limbic system.

Stereoencephalography and stereoangiography have permitted a three-dimensional study of the telencephalic structures and this has been abundantly illustrated by Talairach *et al.* [8] and by Szikla *et al.* [6]. Stereoelectroencephalography, as introduced by Bancaud *et al.* [1], has improved our understanding of epilepsy; our surgical results support this technique.

This method appears quite sophisticated and prompt the question: "if such great efforts are made to define the epileptogenic zone, the irritative zone and the lesional zone, then why perform standard craniotomies and remove large pieces of cerebral cortex?".

[1] Service de neurochirurgie, Hôpital Notre-Dame, Montréal, Canada, H2L 1M4.
[2] Service de neurologie, Hôpital Notre-Dame, Montréal, Canada.
[3] Departement de radiologie, Hôpital Notre-Dame, Montréal, Canada.
[4] Département de physique bio-médical, Hôpital Notre-Dame, Montréal, Canada.
[5] Département de génie mécanique, Université Laval, Ste-Foy, Québec, Canada.

0065-1419/80/Suppl. 30/0151/$ 01.80

First of all, a craniotomy with cortectomy is not a standard operation. The surgical move is "guided" by the stereoencephalography and stereoelectroencephalography exploration (Fig. 1). Thus, the neurosurgeon knows exactly where he is and what has to be removed.

In other cases, such as those which we now report, it is felt that a more functional approach is indicated, that is, "selective lesions of accurately identified brain structures".

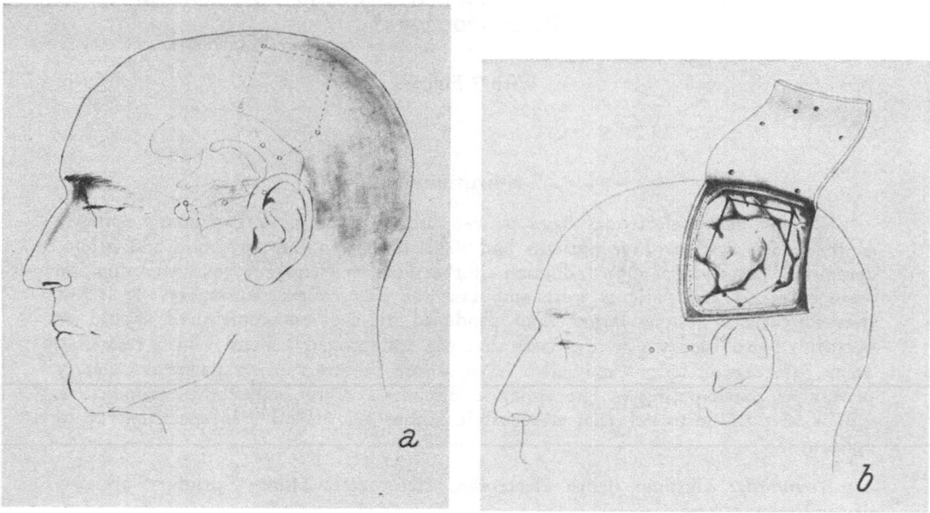

Fig. 1 a, b. After proper definition of the epileptogenic focus by stereoelectroencephalography, it is easy to do a pre-operative planning. Each surgical step has been predicted from skin marks to cortex. It is thus possible to remove exactly what has to be removed and not more, sparing important vessels or important brain areas

Of the sixty patients explored by stereoelectroencephalography at Hôpital Notre-Dame since 1975, 15 were found to have a primary focus in the limbic structures of the temporal lobe. Five of these were treated by stereotactic lesions.

Many authors have reported different stereotactic procedures for epilepsy [3] with the aim of interrupting conducting pathways: some procedures were reported as effective, whilst other procedures have given poor results. Some approaches appear logical but are not always supported by objective electrophysiological investigations. Talairach *et al.* [7] have created stereotactic lesions in the limbic system

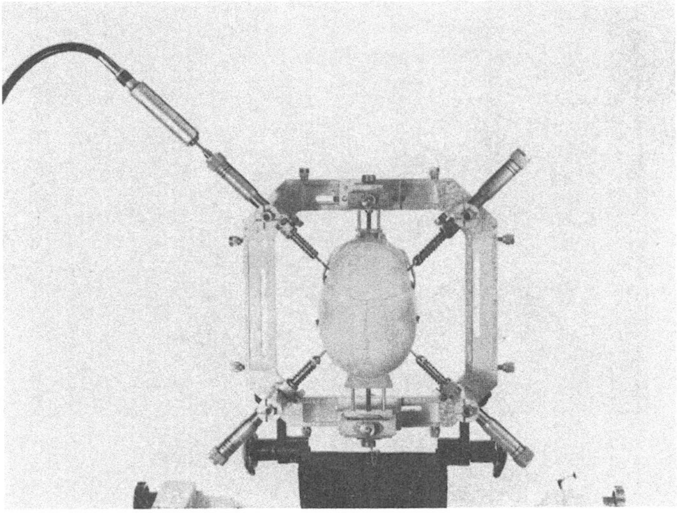

Fig. 2. This is the Talairach stereotactic frame as modified by Bouvier *et al.* The distance between each pillar has not been modified though each side has been widened. The slit on each bar permits sliding of the double grid

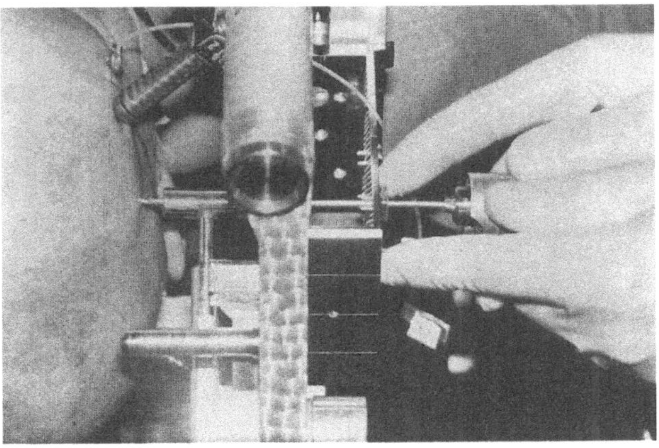

Fig. 3. Transcutaneous burr hole through a double grid and a special guide. This guide prevents any deviation of the drill even on curved surface. The drill is replaced by the coagulation probe. The tip of this probe is of 1.5 mm. The orifice in the dura produces a thigh joint around the electrode preventing leakage of the CSF

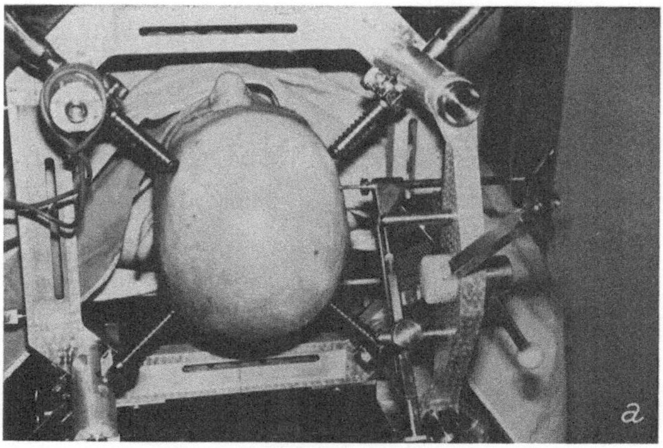

Fig. 4 a. Insertion of the bony anchor

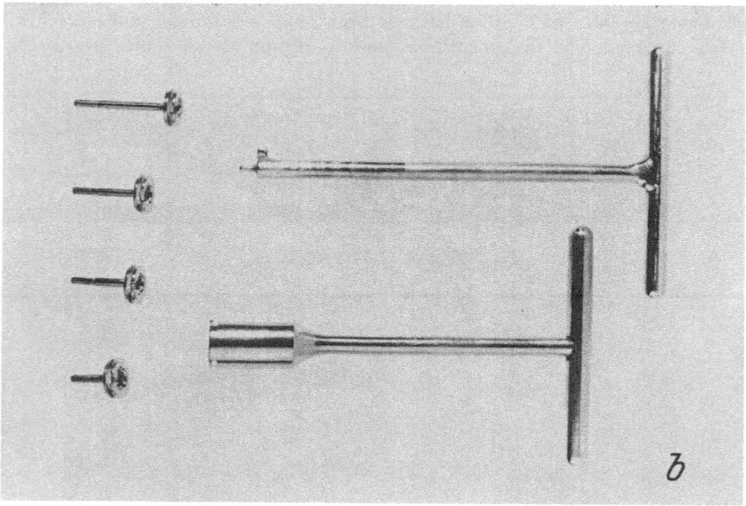

Fig. 4 b. Upper right is the bony anchor insertion device. On the left, different length of bony anchors. The tip of the anchor is slightly bigger than the diameter of the burr hole. It is pushed with force and requires the removing device on the lower right for removal

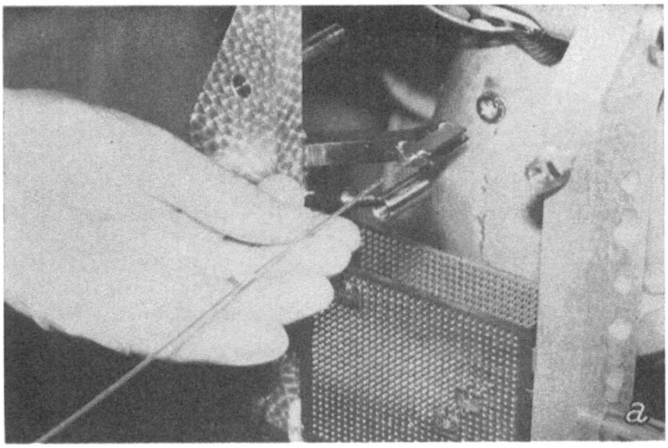

Fig. 5 a. Insertion of the electrode with its inner stylet in place through the guiding arm and anchor

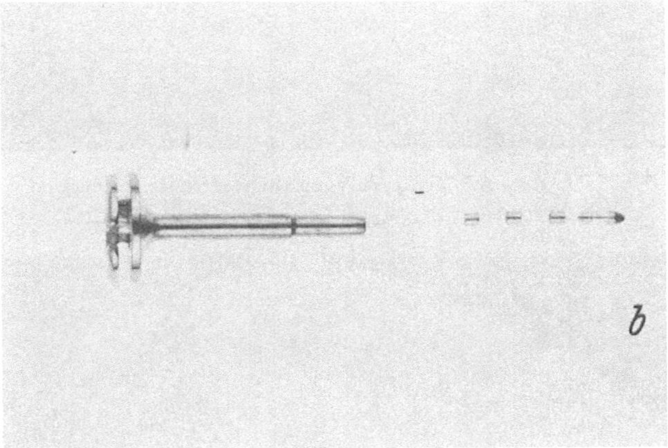

Fig. 5 b. The electrodes are made of PVC with gold rings. Each electrode carry from 4 to 15 recording plots. The external diameter is 1.5 mm. They are semirigid with the inner stylet in place for insertion and without the stylet are soft and flexible. They are water tight. Their electric impedance is less than 10 kohms

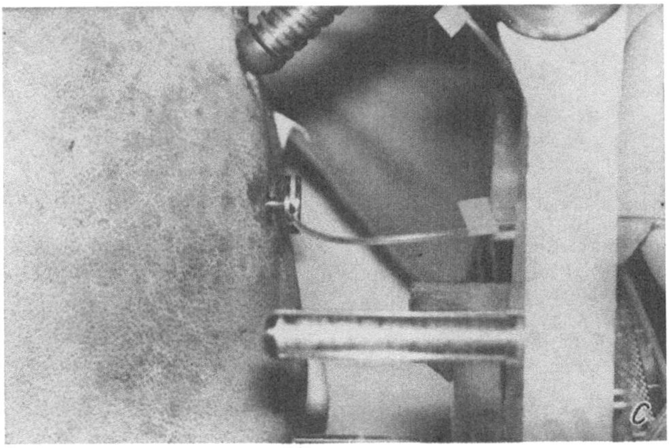

Fig. 5 c. The electrode without the stylet is flexible and can be easily, rapidly

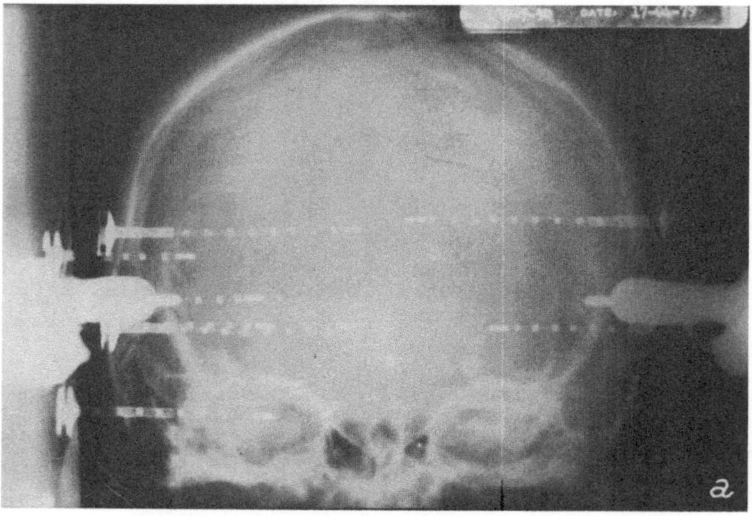

Fig. 6 a. AP X-ray showing the electrodes in place

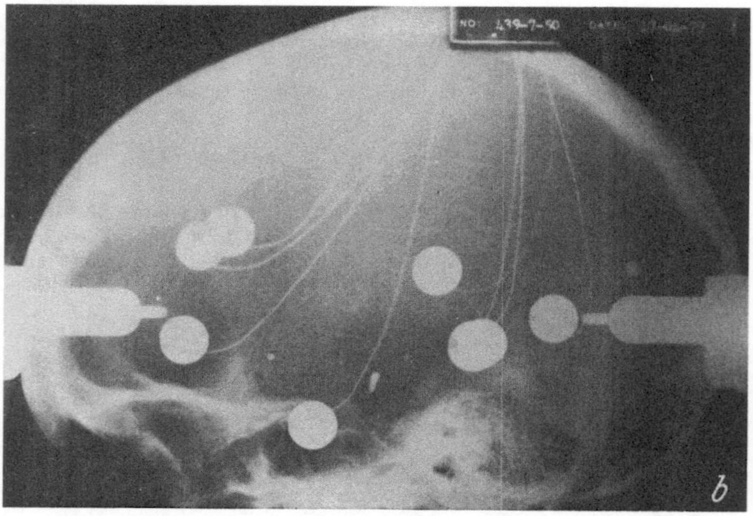

Fig. 6 b. Lateral X-ray showing bony anchors holding electrodes in place and external wire of the electrodes connected to the EEG recorder with ytrium as palliative intervention in specific cases, *e.g.*, epileptic foci in the speech or visual areas, bitemporal epilepsy, poorly defined epileptic foci, and in patients of poor somatic or psychological status.

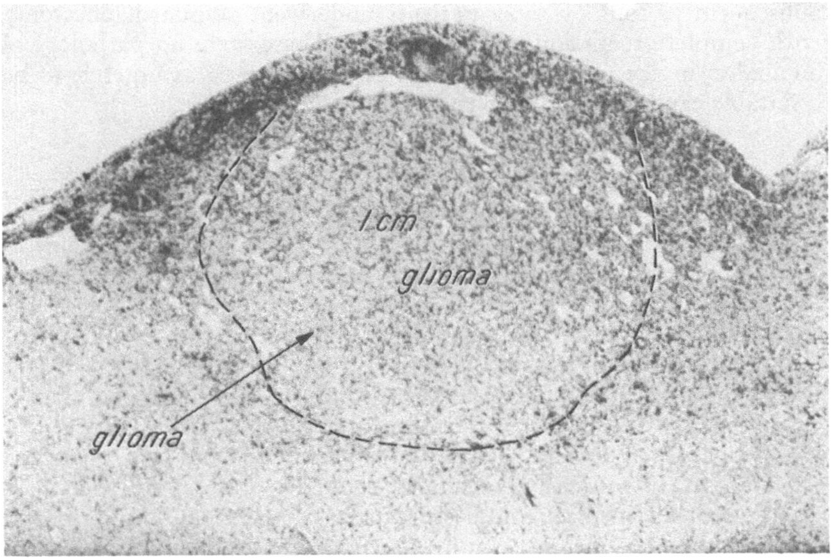

Fig. 7. 1 cm diameter glioma found in surgical specimen

Material and Methods

Our material is somewhat different. Ten of our patients were treated with open surgery, and five with stereotactic lesions. Of these five patients, three had a focus in the amygdala, one in the amygdala and hyppocampus and one in the hyppocampus.

After recording at least three spontaneous seizures on the scalp with synchronized audio-video-electroencephalography monitoring [5], a stereoencephalographic procedure was performed [1]. No significant abnormality were found and CT scan was normal. Chronic depth electrode implantation was carried out as shown on Figs. 2 to 6.

In each case, electrophysiological exploration was carried out until we had seen and recorded three spontaneous seizures with the depth electrodes. Electrical stimulation is performed before withdrawal of the electrodes. Chemical stimulation is not performed in our unit.

It was decided to create selective, small destructive lesions in the amygdala and Ammon horn in the five patients using Claude Bertrand's leucotome. Seven operations were carried out, as two patients required a second procedure in order to produce a more extensive lesion.

Results

There were no complications and patients were ambulant the following day.

There was a reduction of 50% in the frequency of the seizures. Subsequently, four of these patients underwent standard lobectomy with complete remission of the seizures. There were no pathological anomalies in the resected material. The fifth one was not felt to be a suitable candidate for open surgery.

Discussion

In spite of the small serie, we feel that some positive conclusions may be drawn from our results.

We can say that a lesion in the amygdala and hyppocampus is not sufficient to control seizures in patients with a primary focus in the amygdala and/or Ammon's horn. If it can be proved by stereo-electroencephalography that the focus lies in these regions, bigger lesions must be carried out such as those done by Talairach *et al.* [7].

In 1977, Rosene *et al.* [4] demonstrated that: "The subiculum of the primate hyppocampal formation stands at the end of a polarized sequence of intrinsic hyppocampal efferents and is the source of efferents to the medial frontal cortex, the caudal cingulate gyrus and the parahyppocampal area and amygdala in the temporal lobe. In addition, the subiculum sends subcortical efferents to the septum and diencephalon."

In view of this, larger lesions in the primary focus and perhaps in other areas should be performed. Well identified conduction pathways of the epileptic discharges could also be concomitantly destroyed provided there is evidence of ictal discharge. This is true for primary epilepsy of the limbic system and is also of great value in other type of intractable seizures.

There are some pitfalls. We have already mentioned ten other patients with primary foci in the limbic structures of the temporal lobe. They were not selected for stereotactic procedures but had a lobectomy. In the pathological specimens, we found very small benign gliomas, less than 1 cm in diameter in two patients (Fig. 7).

When first seen, these two patients had a five year history of symptoms. Without a lobectomy, the tumour would have probably grown and in a few years, we would have discovered a bigger lesion, possibly with malignant transformation.

We feel that stereotactic lesions larger than produced by leucotome should be performed provided we have proof that the epileptogenic focus is in a well defined area. Stereotactic lesions may also have a role in interrupting pathways clearly proven as participating in the epileptic discharge. Only under these conditions, will it be possible to say that stereotactic lesions are effective in a specific type of epilepsy.

References

1. Bancaud, J., Talairach, J., *et al.*, La stéréo-électro-encéphalographie dans l'épilepsie. Paris: Masson et Cie. 1965.
2. Bouvier, G., Saint-Hilaire, J. M., Vézina, J. L., Béique, R., Picard, R., La chirurgie fonctionnelle de l'épilepsie. Union Médicale du Canada *105* (1976), 1483—1485.
3. Ojemann, G. A., Ward, A. A., Jr., Stereotactic and other procedures for epilepsy. In: Advances in Neurology, Vol. 8, pp. 241—265. New York: Raven Press. 1975.
4. Rosene, D. L., Van Hoesen, G. W., Hyppocampal efferences reach widespread area of cerebral cortex and the amygdala in the rhesus monkey. Sciences *198* (1977), 315—317.
5. Saint-Hilaire, J. M., Bouvier, G., Lymburner, J., Picard, R., Mercier, M., La stéréo-électro-encéphalographie synchronisée avec l'enregistrement visuel et sonore dans l'exploration chronique de l'épilepsie. Union Médicale du Canada *105* (1976), 1538—1541.
6. Szikla, G., Bouvier, G., Hori, T., Petrov, V., Angiography of the human brain cortex, p. 273. Berlin-Heidelberg-New York: Springer. 1977.
7. Talairach, J., Bancaud, J., Szikla, G., Bonis, A., Vedrenne, C., *et al.*, Approche nouvelle de la neurochirurgie de l'épilepsie. Méthodologie stéréotaxique et résultats thérapeutiques. Société de Neurochirurgie de langue française, 24e congrès annuel, Marseilles, 25–28 juin 1974, Tome 20, Supplément 1, juin 1974, pp. 205—206.
8. Talairach, J., Szikla, G., Tournoux, P., Prossalentis, A., Borda-Ferrer, M., Covello, L., Iacob, M., Mempel, E., avec la collaboration de Buser, P., et Bancaud, J., Atlas d'anatomie stéréotaxique du télencéphale. Paris: Masson et Cie. 1967.

Acta Neurochirurgica, Suppl. 30, 161—167 (1980)

The Effect of Medial Amygdalotomy and Anterior Hippocampotomy on Behavior and Seizures in Epileptic Patients

E. Mempel*, B. Witkiewicz, R. Stadnicki, E. Łuczywek, L. Kuciński, G. Pawłowski, and **J. Nowak**

With 5 Figures

Summary

In 70 patients with epilepsy and severe behavioural disturbances with EEG changes in the temporal regions, we performed EEG investigations of deep temporal structures, temporal cortex and scalp, using Talairach's stereotactic apparatus. Taking into account the recorded changes we performed 115 stereotactic lesions on the medial amygdala (both unilaterally and bilaterally) and on the anterior hippocampus (cornu Ammonis). The results in epileptic processes were: total recovery in 11.4%, evident clinical improvement in 74.3% and no improvement in 14.3%. Similar results were obtained in behavioural disturbances. Bilateral amygdalotomy and unilateral hippocampotomy in selected cases may produce recovery or amelioration and make possible return to normal social life for epileptic patients with severe behavioural changes.

Keywords: Amygdalotomy; hippocampotomy; epilepsy-behaviour.

Introduction

From the time when amygdalotomy was introduced by Narabayashi as a treatment for epileptic cases with severe behavioural [9] disturbances in feeble-minded children, this type of treatment has become used more generally in various medical centers throughout the world [1, 2, 6, 8, 10]. In 1967 we started to use a modified procedure in the Department of Neurosurgery of the Polish Academy of Sciences. In place of total destruction of the amygdala, our procedure was limited to the destruction of its medial part, based on recent anatomical and neurophysiological data. In many cases this type of intervention was supplemented by the stereotactic exclusion of the anterior

* Department of Neurosurgery, Polish Academy of Sciences, 16 Barska str., 02–325 Warsaw, Poland.

0065-1419/80/Suppl. 30/0161/$ 01.40

part of the hippocampus (cornu Ammonis) when indicated by stereo-electroencephalographic recording (SEEG). This paper constitutes a clinical analysis of the results obtained in surgical intervention in epileptic patients with behavioural disturbances.

Material and Method

During the years 1967–1978, seventy epileptic patients with behavioural disturbances of different intensity were operated (115 stereotactic procedures). EEG abnormalities were observed only (or mainly) within the temporal regions of the brain. There were 39 men and 31 women in this group and the most numerous were patients in the 11–20 age group (Fig. 1). Drug therapy carried out in these patients in neurological and psychiatric departments and continued in ambulatory conditions did not stop the progress of the illness. The patients in our department underwent a series of EEG investigations, whilst conscious and during physiological and pharmacological sleep. All possible precautions were taken to record seizures during EEG investigations. During SEEG investigations performed under halothane anaesthesia, multilead (5 and 10) cerebral electrodes were implanted in both poles of the temporal lobes, the amygdala, the anterior and medial hippocampal complexes needle electrodes were used for scalp recording. Besides this, electrical stimulation was applied to the amygdalic and hippocampal structures to observe clinical symptoms and provoked discharges in the EEG records. In 70% of these cases investigation was undertaken under light anaesthesia, and in 30% of the cases conscious patients. If both spontaneous activity was recorded and electrical stimulation produced appropriate discharges in the amygdaloid nucleus, its medial part was destroyed, as a rule in two stages (Fig. 2). In 3 cases a bilateral amygdalotomy was carried out as a single surgical procedure. In 29 cases additional lesions were created in the anterior hippocampus (unilaterally), as suggested by SEEG investigations. In 11 cases only a unilateral amygdalotomy was carried out and this was because the condition of the patients had sufficiently improved to render a bilateral surgical procedure unnecessary. In a group of 10 patients who had previously underwent temporal lobectomy, 9 contralateral amygdalotomies and 1 amygdalotomy with anterior hippocampotomy was performed. In 3 patients, the SEEG revealed epileptic activity mainly in the hippocampus, and so the lesion was carried out only unilaterally in the cornu Ammonis.

As stated previously, the 70 patients under consideration demonstrated various degrees of behavioural disturbances. Different and changing reactions to everyday situations as well as psychotic disturbances were observed (Fig. 3). The most frequently described disturbances were: attacks of anger (37 cases), often without reasonable provocation. The same applies to symptoms of aggressiveness (42 cases), appearing in the form of verbal or physical aggression directed against the immediate environment, most often against the mother. Frequent symptoms in this group of patients were fear and anguor animi (20 cases), lasting for several hours or even several days. Fear preceded the epileptic seizures or appeared independently of them, sometimes without any motivation. A characteristic symptom in those patients was the lability of their mood, ranging from low mood (11 cases) and signs of depression (10 cases) to hypomania combined with hyper-mobility. Obnubilative states were present in 14 patients. A frequent set of symptoms in this group were pseudo-schizophrenic disturbances with visual and auditory pseudo-hallucinations. In 13 cases unprovoked flights from places of residence to hiding places happened, most often just prior to an incipient epileptic seizure. Nine patients displayed suicidal tendencies, and 5 attempted to realize these, but were prevented from

Sex	Age					
	0–10	11–20	21–30	31–40	> 40	Total
Men	2	27	8	1	1	39
Women	3	14	10	3	1	31
Total	5	41	18	4	2	70

Fig. 1. Age of patients

Bilateral amygdalotomy			Unilateral amygdalotomy			Unilateral hipocampotomy	Temporal lobectomy and		Total
one stage operation	two stages operation	with hipocampotomy	amygdalotomy only	with bilateral hipocampotomy	with unilateral hipocampotomy		amygdalotomy	amygdalotomy and hipocampotomy	
3	18	12	11	1	12	3	9	1	70

Fig. 2. Kind of surgery

Symptoms	Number of patients before surgery	Number of patients after surgery	% of improvement
Anger attacks	37	9	75.7
Verbal and motional aggresion	42	7	83.4
Fear. states of fear	20	1	95
Sedness. mood decrease	11	4	63.6
States of depression	10	3	70
Motional excitement, anxiety	30	0	100
Psycho-motional decrease	14	7	50
Obnubilation state	14	8	42.9
Pseudo-hallucinations and illusions	10	3	70
Mental and motional obsession	7	4	42.9
Suicidal ideas and attemps	9	3	66.7
Flight tendency	13	0	100
Excessive sexual excitement	8	0	100

Fig. 3. Emotional-psychotic changes

doing so. Hyper-sexuality was demonstrated in 8 cases with 3 showing a tendency to exhibitionism.

When considering the epileptic seizures it should be stated that 75% of the patients experienced different types of seizures (from 2 to 5 types). 41 patients were confirmed to have generalized seizures with maximal symptoms as well as other kinds of attacks (Fig. 4). Note should be taken of obnubilative states occuring independently from other epileptic seizures. It should be also stated that in a group of 14 cases with seizures involving affect, in the form of dysphorial be-

			Before surgery	After surgery		
				disappearing of symptoms	decrease of symptoms	reduced character of symptoms
Partial epilepsy	with simple symptoms	motor fits	28	5	13	10
		sensorial fits	1	—	1	—
		vegetative fits	5	2	2	1
	with complex symptoms	psycho-motor fits	19	7	7	5
		psycho-sensor fits	5	1	2	2
		intellectual fits	2	—	1	1
		affective fits	14	12	1	1
		obnubillation states	14	12	1	1
General epilepsy	with submaximal symptoms		27	5	15	7
	with maximal symptoms		41	10	26	5
Unilateral children fits			1	1	—	—

Fig. 4. Kinds of epileptic fits

haviour of differing intensity, in 4 patients these constituted the only symptom of illness in the presence of EEG changes in the temporal region. Moreover, the most numerous group of seizures were the motor seizures with a simple symptomatology (28 cases) and psycho-motor seizures (19 cases) with oral and motor-automatism symptoms.

Results of Surgical Treatment

Surgical treatment had a beneficial effect on the frequency and severity of epileptic fits (Fig. 4) and produced a considerable improvement in patients' behaviour (Fig. 3). In 8 patients symptoms completely disappeared and the patients did not require further anti-epileptic pharmacological treatment. Anxiety and motor excitability, hypersexuality, fear and states of fear and flight disappeared completely. Significant improvement was obtained in states of psychomotor excitation, anger and aggressiveness, which were reduced to the point where the patients were better able to control their behaviour.

A characteristic result of amygdalotomy is undoubtly the disappearance in some cases and in other a substantial reduction of pseudo-schizophrenic symptoms such as pseudo-hallucinations and illusions (70%). In 66.7% of the cases the stereotactic surgical treatment resulted in reduction of suicidal tendencies.

Beneficial effect on epileptic seizures are expressed by reduction of both their frequency and severity so that, for example, a prolonged

	Behavioural disturbances		Epileptic seizures	
	number of patients	%	number of patients	%
Recovery	8	11.4	8	11.4
Improvement	45	64.3	52	74.3
No improvement	17	24.3	10	14.3
Total	70	100	70	100

Fig. 5. Last results of the surgical treatment

tonico-clonic seizure would be reduced to the clonic phase lasting several seconds, sometimes without a total loss of consciousness, or even to just the aura without the seizure proper. Epileptic states observed before the operations also disappeared. 60% of the patients operated on were able to return to their schools (2 persons passed their matriculation exams) mostly in specialized technical schools, or to take up simple jobs or sheltered employments.

Discussion

The amygdaloid nuclei (CA) of the brain demonstrate a distinct influence on the emotions and behaviour. Neurophysiological investigations have proven that although the CA are not the source where emotions are created, they have a regulatory effect on states of fear, anger, and aggression as well as endocrinological and autonomical facets of such behaviour [4, 5]. Two efferent paths leave the medial CA region. Their fibers head towards different regions of the limbic system, and their terminations are in the hypothalamus.

Electrical stimulation of these regions provokes fear, flight and aggression, whereas stimulation of the lateral region has a restraining influence on these symptoms [3]. It is therefore logical to attack the medial CA regions to obtain positive therapeutic results in cases of emotional and behavioural disturbances. The lateral part of the CA influences endocrine regulation, sexual symptoms and normal motherhood. Its damage disrupts these functions, thus demonstrating a disinhibitory process. Furthermore, the medial CA region is characterized in the EEG by release of discharges of the highest amplitude, which also applies to the anterior hippocampus—cornu Ammonis. Both these cerebral structures are characterized by the lowest epileptogenic threshold to electrical stimulation. Therefore they can act as pace-makers for channeling epileptic fits. The lesion of the mentioned structures constitutes a filter blocking the discharges from the epileptic focus on their way to different subcortical structures. The functional change obtained in this way produces a positive control on the epileptic process and also has a beneficial effect on disturbances of normal emotional reactions.

Conclusion

1. Medial bilateral amygdalotomy and anterior unilateral hippocampotomy give beneficial medical results in selected epileptic cases with severe behavioural disturbances and epileptiform abnormalities of the electrical activity of the temporal cerebral regions.

2. The procedure brings about a reduction of excessive motor and emotional excitability as well as reduction of the course of the epileptic process, diminishing quantitatively and qualitatively different types of epileptic fits. Despite the palliative character of the above-mentioned surgical procedures it is possible in some cases to obtain a complete recovery from the symptoms (in our cases up to 11.4%).

3. Surgical procedures reducing excessive motor and emotional excitability do not simultaneously evoke adynamic symptoms and do not simultaneously deprive the patients of emotional reaction.

4. Medial amygdalotomy and anterior hippocampotomy which have a beneficial therapeutic influence on epilepsy and behavioural disturbances, do not give side effects, and in particular they do not reduce mental capacity.

5. Our observations prove that the above mentioned stereotactic procedures do not result in endocrine disturbances and contrary to the described disturbances in experimental neurophysiological investigations both pregnancy and motherhood proceed normally.

References

1. Balasubramanian, V., Ramamurthi, B., Stereotactic amygdalectomy. Proc. Austr. Ass. Neurol. *5* (1968), 277—287.
2. Chitanond, H., Stereotactic amygdalotomy in the treatment of olfactory seizures and psychiatric disorders with olfactory hallucinations. Conf. Neurol. *27* (1966), 181.
3. Fonberg, E., The inhibitory role of amygdala. Acta Biol. Exp. (Warsaw) *23* (1963), 171—179 a.
4. Gloor, P., Feindel, W., Affective behaviour and temporal lobe. In: Physiologie und Pathophysiologie des vegetativen Nervensystems (Monnier, M., ed.). Stuttgart: Hippokrates-Verlag. 1963.
5. Goddard, G., Functions of the amygdala. Psychol. Bull. *62* (1964), 2, 89.
6. Heimburger, R., Whitlock, C., Kalsbeck, J., Stereotactic amygdalotomy for epilepsy with expressive behaviour. J. Amer. Med. Ass. *198* (1966), 741.
7. Łuczywek, E., Mempel, E., Stereotactic amygdalotomy in the light of neuropsychological investigations. Acta Neurochir. Suppl. *23* (1976), 221—223.
8. Mempel, E., The influence of partial (dorso-medial) amygdalectomy on emotional disturbances and epileptic fits in humans. Present limits of neurosurgery, pp. 492—499. Prague: Avicenum. 1972.
9. Narabayashi, H., Stereotactic amygdalotomy for behaviour disorders of epileptic nature. Excerpta Med. Amst. ICS *2* (1965), 236—242.
10. Vaernet, K., Stereotactic amygdalotomy in temporal lobe epilepsy. Confin. Neurol. *34* (1972), 176—183.

Acta Neurochirurgica, Suppl. 30, 169—175

Memory and Learning in Epileptic Patients Treated by Amygdalotomy and Anterior Hippocampotomy

E. Łuczywek* and **E. Mempel**

With 2 Figures

Summary

The memory and learning capacity in patients treated for temporal epilepsy was studied. The study was performed in 55 patients, observed before and after stereotaxic amygdalotomy and hippocampotomy. Very often disturbances in memory and learning capability were present before surgery. After surgery their learning efficiency increased. Disturbances in memory tracing, as provoked by distraction, remained at the same level after neurosurgery. No decrease in general intelligence was noted.

Keywords: Amygdalotomy; anterior hippocampotomy; memory and learning.

Introduction

Many years of neurophysiological and neuropsychological studies of memory, a basic function of the brain, have confirmed the complexity of this process and its connection with almost all of the brain structures, each of which plays a specific role in the memory process [4, 11]. The extent of memory disturbance is not determined by the total amount of diseased brain tissue, but by the structure affected by the disease [2—4], The limbic system of the brain, including the hippocampus, plays a special role in the memory process. Dysfunction of the hippocampus causes general, non-specific memory disturbances such as difficulties in assimilating new material, and in memorizing current events and past events close to the time of injury of the hippocampus. It has been stressed that these disturbances concern short-term memory and learning, while long-term memory, speech and work proficiency remain unaffected [6, 9—11].

As in the Korsakow amnesis syndrome, the range of short-term memory in patients with lesions of limbic structures is not reduced.

* Department of Neurosurgery, Polish Academy of Sciences, 16 Barska str., 02-325 Warsaw, Poland.

0065-1419/80/Suppl. 30/0169/$ 01.40

However, these disturbances result in delayed reproduction, caused by the patient's susceptibility to interference [2, 4].

Among the most interesting results of studies of the memory process are those obtained in patients whose surgical treatment consists in exclusion of certain structures of the limbic system. They are patients with severe forms of epilepsy which cannot be reduced or eliminated by long-term pharmacological treatment [5, 8].

Method

The patients presented in this work were subjected to serial EEG and SEEG examinations, positive contrast ventriculography, and neurological and psychiatric examinations. The examinations were made before, immediately after and a long time after the operation, the aim being to evaluate the effect of interrupting certain deep structures of the temporal lobe on cognitive processes. The examinations were usually supplemented with a thorough history based on interviews with the patient and his family, with particular emphasis on memory and learning ability.

The psychological examination consisted of the following tests:

1. Intelligence quotient test (Wechsler scale for adults or for children);
2. Neuropsychological tests for evaluating speech, praxis and gnosis;
3. A set of tests (which could be modified and extended depending on the state of the patients) for evaluating: a) short-term memory; b) ability to act on the basis of short-term memory traces in the presence of external interference (empty distraction—30 seconds, heterogenic distraction—30 seconds); c) ability to learn word material; d) long-term memory.

In this study the authors concentrated their attention on word memory. From the dictionary of word frequency in the Polish language the authors selected a number of the most frequently occuring common nouns, paying particular attention to their length (max. 2–3 syllables) and ease of articulation. In the memory examination the patient was presented with unrelated elements—series of words, mediated verbally, and series of drawings of objects, mediated visually, and a sentence. The patient's memory was evaluated from his ability to reproduce verbally the series of words and sentences and to reproduce verbally the names of objects portrayed by the drawings (also selected acc. to the word frequency dictionary).

Material

The material in this study consists of patients hospitalized in the Department of Neurosurgery, Polish Academy of Sciences, because of severe epilepsy, mainly with temporal lobe EEG symptoms. These patients were subjected to stereotactic procedures, which consisted of exclusion by cryosurgery of the medial part of the amygdala and/or the anterior part of the hippocampus (cornu Ammonis), SEEG recording and electrical stimulation. The latter examinations indicated that the most pronounced disturbances of the bioelectrical function of the brain originated in these deep-seated structures of the temporal lobe. During the period 1967—1978 a total of 70 epileptic patients were subjected to stereotactic intervention by cryosurgery to the following structures: 1. medial part of the left amygdaloid nucleus; 2. medial parts of both amygdaloid nuclei; 3. medial parts of both amygdaloid nuclei and the anterior part of the hippocampus unilaterally; 4. anterior part of the hippocampus.

In this study the authors analyse the results obtained in 55 patients, 29 male and 26 female. All patients were of young age. The most numerous group consisted of schoolchildren and scool-leavers. The period of clinical observation ranged from 1 to 9 years.

Results

A preliminary analysis of the 55 patients examined in this study has made it possible to draw a general picture of their cognitive processes, particularly as regards mental efficiency and mnemonic capability. The results of the Wechsler test for mental efficiency performed before the operation show that 24 patients were below normal for their respective age groups, 15 of them having scores indicating mental deficiency. Comparison of the average IQ's before and after surgery indicates a slight improvement of this parameter: mean II before surgery = 77.6, after surgery 78.3 (statistically not significant). This increase in IQ score was found both in thos with normal IQ and in those whose IQ score before surgery was below normal. This is particularly marked in patients whose age at the time of surgery was more than 16 years.

The range of short-term memory in patients after surgery is slightly higher than that before the operation, as can be seen by comparing the mean values for the whole group of 55 patients. Analysis of the individual sub-groups shown that the biggest improvement was obtained in the group of patients with normal IQ scores while the group of mentally dull or deficient patients showed no significant improvement.

The data on the learning of word material are as follows: the cumulative curves of results obtained in patients after surgery are higher than those obtained in the same patients before surgical intervention (Fig. 1). This general improvement shows that the patients ability to learn word material was not impaired by the stereotactic procedure but, on the contrary, was slightly improved. It should be emphasized that 45 out of the 55 patients were subjected to left-sided amygdalotomy.

It is seen from the learning curves that both the preoperative and the post-operative learning curves are lower than normal. The patients are unable to achieve the maximum result not only at the sixth, but even at the tenth trial. However, the cumulative curve composed of post-operative results bears a closer resemblance to normal. This is best seen in the curves obtained in patients with decreased mental efficiency whose age is above sixteen years (Fig. 2). In comparison with the pre-operative curve, characterized by low values and a plateau, the post-operative curve of these patients bears a much closer resemblance to the normal curve (rise in consecutive values showing an increase in the number of memorized words). It should be stressed that only 7 out of the 55 patients examined had a normal learning curve before the operation, which means that only some of the patients without an evident decrease in general mental efficiency had normal learning ability.

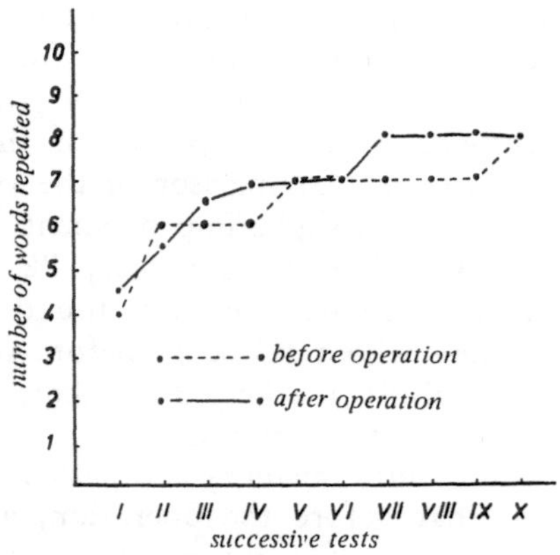

Fig. 1. Curve of verbal material learning for the whole group

The effect of interference on the short-term memory trace was investigated in 15 patients. Delayed reproduction (a 30-second-interval filled with organized activities and a 30-second-period during which the patients were asked to solve simple arithmetical problems) was investigated in a group of patients before and after surgery. The age of the patients in this group ranged from 13 to 29 years (mean age 17.9). The mental efficiency level of these patients ranged from IQ = 45 to IQ = 124 (mean IQ = 92.6).

During the first interview 10 patients complained of memory disturbances impairing their ability to assimilate new material. In seven patients complaints about memory disturbances were confirmed by low marks at school and the necessity to repeat classes. Neuropsychological examinations of these patients did not reveal any significant disturbance of gnosis or praxis. Neither did they reveal any speech disturbances typical of aphasia. In all these patients the learning curve for new material was abnormal (plateau, irregularities or falling off). There were no marked disturbances in long-term memory.

Even during the pre-operative examination the majority of the patients exhibited a narrowing of the short-term memory range, so that their reproduction of word series and of names of object presented on drawings was limited to 3 or 4 elements. Susceptibility of the memory trace to distraction was examined using sets of elements, the number of which corresponded to a patient's memory

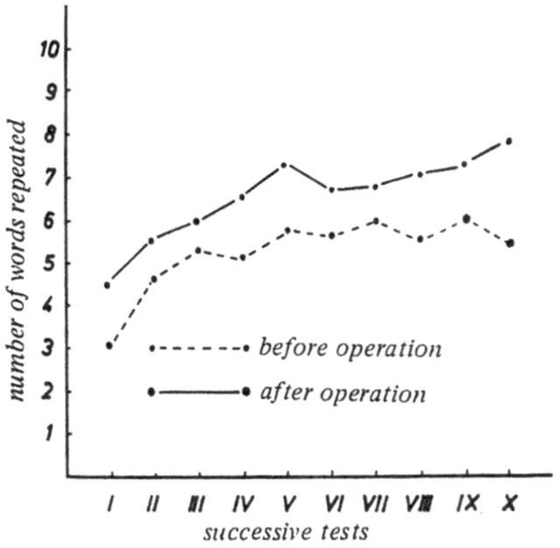

Fig. 2. Curves of verbal material learning for the whole group (results in patients aged over 16 years with low IQ)

range for a given type of material. After an interval of 30 seconds the patients were able to reproduce structuralized material (sentences) better than sets of elements. The most easily forgotten elements were words, particularly after heterogenic distraction (counting). The worst retention was observed in the three patients with the lowest IQ. It was very difficult to hold their attention to whatever they were doing. If one relates the results obtained to the method of mediating the test material one can conclude that interfering factors seem to have a smaller effect on the reproduction of material mediated visually than that mediated verbally.

After surgery the range of short-term memory increased to 4–5 elements. In patients subjected to lesions in the right hemisphere the short-term memory range corresponded to the lower limit of normal people (5 elements). A half of the patients complained of memory disturbances manifesting themselves in the form of learning difficulties. Patients subjected to lesions within the hemisphere dominant for speech showed an improvement in their ability to remember word material after heterogenic distraction. On the other hand, patients subjected to stereotactic lesions in right hemisphere (amygdalotomy and anterior hippocampotomy) showed a tendency toward intensification of memory disturbances. Memorization of structuralized material in conditions of heterogenic distraction was better, particularly in patients after left-sided hippocampotomy and amygdalotomy who, however, found it very difficult to reproduce visually mediated material.

Discussion

The memory and learning disturbances observed in these patients before stereotaxy, together with a general impairment of mental efficiency, were the result of a general dysfunction of the brain. In most of these patients epileptic seizures appeared in the first years of their lives and at the time of hospitalization the disease had lasted from several to a dozen or so years. Analysis of the results of partial hippocampotomy and amygdalotomy shows that the stereotaxic lesions had a number of favourable effects on these patients, such as elimination or a reduction in the number of epileptic seizures, reduction of emotional tension and hyperexcitability. This, in turn, had a beneficial effect on their ability to concentrate and cognitive processes [5–8]. The stereotactic procedures did not impair their function [1, 5, 7]. The increase in susceptibility of the memory trace to external interference that was observed in patients after stereotactic injury of the medial part of the amygdaloid nuclei and the anterior part of the hippocampus indicates that the limbic structures of the brain play a role in short-term memory and learning processes. It should be mentioned, however, that selective interruption of the medial part of the amygdaloid nuclei and of the anterior part of the hippocampus did not produce such extensive disturbances of short-term memory as those observed after bilateral resection of thetemporal lobes [12], or after unilateral resection with removal of the anterior hippocampus (cornu Ammonis) and the amygdaloid nucleus [9, 10].

The authors of this paper did not observe any unfavourable effects of the stereotactic procedure on the patients general mental efficiency. In some cases, an increase in IQ was observed. The patients are able to continue their education, although their learning time is longer than normal. In this connection it is worth mentioning that despite the prolonged learning time the assimilation of new material by these patients is permanent.

Conclusion

1. The stereotactic procedure had no unfavourable effect on the general mental efficiency of the patients, and in some cases it even caused a rise in IQ.

2. Memory disturbances in the form of narrowed short-term memory range and increased susceptibility of the memory trace to external interference were observed in these patients before the operation. Stereotactic lesions of the medial part of the amygdaloid nucleus in the left hemisphere resulted in improved memory performance in conditions of distraction.

3. The learning of new material by epileptic patients, which was impaired before the operation, shows a tendency to improve after surgery.

References

1. Anderson, R., Cognitive changes after amygdalotomy. Neuropsychologia *16*, 4 (1978), 439—451.
2. Kijaszczenko, N. K., Mozg i pamjat. Naruszenije proizwolnogo i nieproizwolnogo zapominanija pri lokalnych porażenijach mozga (Brain and memory. Disorders of voluntary and involuntary remembering after local brain lesions). Moskwa: MGU. 1975.
3. Klimkowski, M., Pamięć człowieka i jej mechanizmy. Analiza neuropsychologiczna (Human memory and its mechanisms, Neuropsychological analysis). Lublin: Uniwersytet M. Curie-Skłodowskiej. 1976.
4. Łuria, A. R., Nejropsichologija pamjati, Naruszenija pamjati pri głubinnych naruszenijach mozga (Neuropsychology of memory. Memory disorders after deep brain lesions). Moskwa: Pedagogika. 1976.
5. Łuczywek, E., Mempel, E., Stereotactic amygdalotomy in the light of neuropsychological investigations. Acta Neurochir. Suppl. 23 (1976), 221—223.
6. Łuczywek, E., Mempel, E., Wpływ prawostronnej hipokampotomii na pamięć i uczenie się (Effect of right-sided hippocampotomy on memory and learning ability). Neur. Neurochir. Pol. *12*, 5 (1978), 671—674.
7. Olsnes, K., Łuczywek, E., Mempel, E., Wpływ amygdalotomii na pamięć i uczenie się u chorych operowanych z powodu padaczki (Effect of amygdalotomy on memory and learning in patients treated surgically for epilepsy). Neur. Neurochir. Pol. *10*, 6 (1976), 775—780.
8. Mempel, E., The influence of partial (dorso-medial) amygdalectomy on emotional disturbances and epileptic fits in humans. Present limits of neurosurgery, pp. 492—497. Prague: Avicenum. 1972.
9. Milner, B., Disorders of memory after brain lesions in man. Neuropsychologia *6* (1968), 175—179.
10. Moroz, B. T., Limbiko-kortikalnyje miechanizmy regulacji pamjati (Limbic-cortical mechanisms of memory disorders). Żurnał Wysszej nierwnoj diejatielnosti *4* (1976), 802—809.
11. Traugutt, N. N., O miechanizmach naruszenija pamjati (About the mechanisms of memory disorders). Leningrad: Nauka. 1973.
12. Scoville, W. B., Milner, B., Loss of recent memory after bilateral hippocampal lesions. J. Neurol. Neurosurg. Psychiat. *20* (1957), 11—21.

Acta Neurochirurgica, Suppl. 30, 177—181 (1980)

Slowing of Scalp EEG After Electrical Stimulation of Amygdala in Man

L. Laitinen* and **E. Toivakka**

With 2 Figures

Summary

Electrical stimulation (60 Hz) of the amygdala in anaesthetized patients caused a predominantly ipsilateral slowing of the scalp EEG. The slowing appeared a few seconds after cessation of stimulation and lasted for 2–3 min. The frequency of the slow waves was 1–1.5 Hz and the amplitude 200–400 μV.

Introduction

In 1972 Sano *et al.* reported on a slowing of the scalp EEG activity during and after electrical stimulation of the posteromedial hypothalamus. We have observed a similar phenomenon to occur after stimulation of the amygdala. In this paper we report on our series of 27 patients in whom we studied the effects of high-frequency stimulation of the amygdala on the scalp EEG activity.

Patients and Methods

Thirteen of the 27 patients were erethistic oligophrenics (EO), 13 suffered from intractable temporal lobe epilepsy (TLE), and one from schizophrenia with aggressive episodes. Fifteen were male and 12 female. The patients' ages in the EO group ranged from 11 to 24 years (mean 15), and from 7 to 51 years (mean 23) in the TLE group. The schizophrenic patient was 31 years old.

Severe aggressive and restless behavior was the reason for surgery in the EO patients, three of whom also had had epileptic fits. The TLE patients had had frequent seizures despite heavy antiepileptic medication. The schizophrenic patient had suffered from aggressive episodes with epilepsy for 10 years. Frontal leucotomy performed elsewhere 8 years previously had been without effect.

Laitinen's stereoguide was used. Seventeen of the 27 patients were operated on under general anaesthesia. Premedication consisted of atropine. After induction

* Department of Neurosurgery, University Central Hospital, Helsinki, Finland.
Present address: Department of Neurosurgery, University Hospital, S-90185 Umea, Sweden.

0065-1419/80/Suppl. 30/0177/$ 01.00

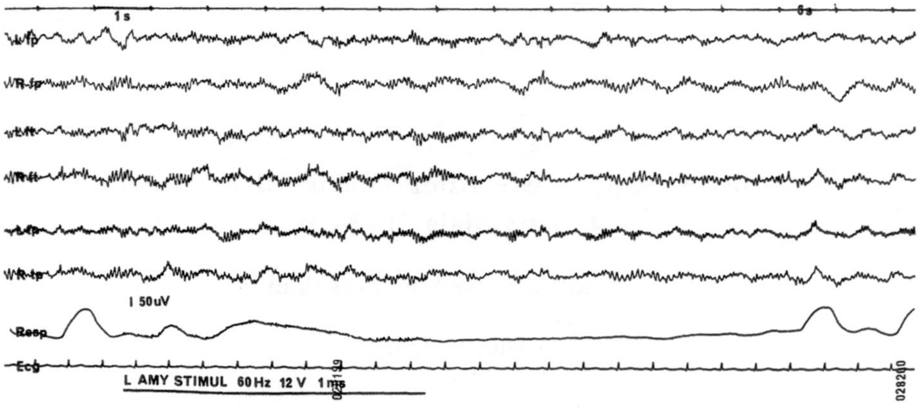

Fig. 1 a. Predominantly ipsilateral slowing produced by 60 Hz stimulation of the left amygdala. Respiratory arrest lasts for 6 sec. No slowing is visible yet

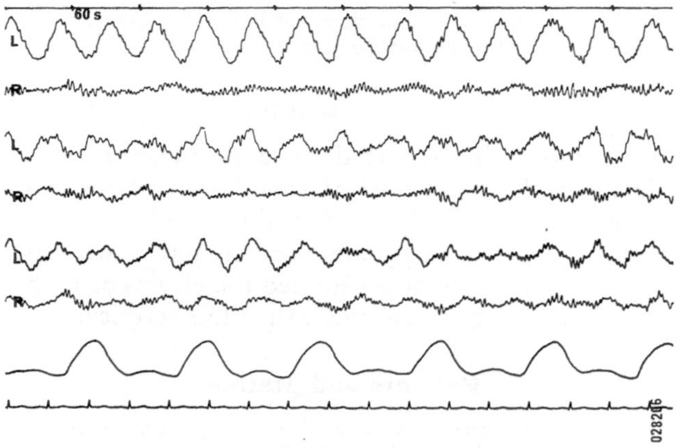

Fig. 1 b. 60 seconds later the left-sided slowing has reached its maximum intensity

Table 1. *Effect of Stimulation of Amygdala on Scalp EEG* (60 Hz, 6–15 V, 1 msec)

Diagnosis (anaesthesia)	No. of patients	Ipsilateral slowing	Bilateral slowing	No change
TLE (general)	4	2	1	1
TLE (local)	9	—	—	9
EO (general)	13	9	3	1
Schizophrenia (local)	1	1	—	—
Total	27	12	4	11

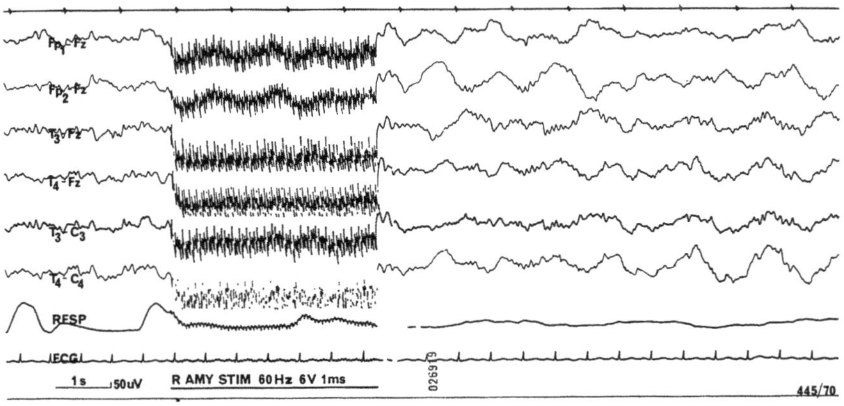

Fig. 2 a. Bilateral slowing visible already at the end of stimulation of the right amygdala

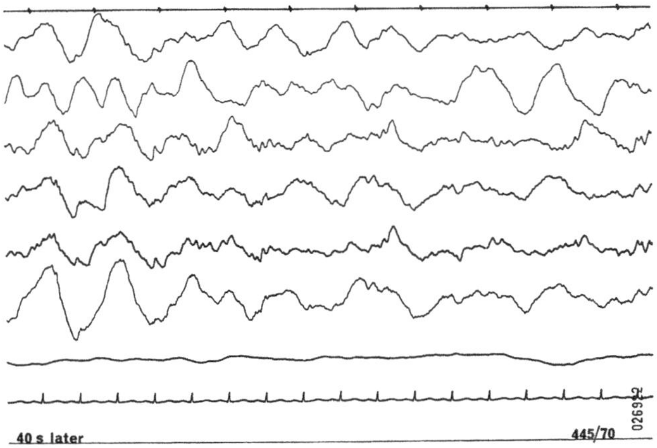

Fig. 2 b. 40 seconds later the slowing has reached its maximum. Respiration has not returned yet, but the pCO_2 has been kept within normal limits by manual ventilation

of anaesthesia with thiopentone the patients were given suxamethonium and intubated. Anaesthesia was maintained with halothane (less than 1%) and nitrous oxide-oxygen. Before the stimulation halothane was withdrawn and anaesthesia was allowed to lighten. The patients breathed spontaneously. In addition, local anaesthesia consisting of prilocaine phelypressin was injected into the scalp.

Ten patients were operated on under local anaesthesia using prilocaine phelypressin. As premedication they had received 50 mg of cyclizine lactate and some of them in addition received 5–6 mg of morphine atropine.

The patients were placed on the operating table in a supine position. The temporal horns were visualized with air insufflated through frontal burr holes into the lateral ventricles and manipulated into the temporal horns. The target in the amygdala lay 21–24 mm lateral to the midline, 5 mm behind the tip of the temporal horn and just on its dorsal margin.

A straight concentric bipolar electrode 1 mm thick with an interpolar distance of 5 mm was used. The stimulus parameters were 60 Hz, unidirectional 1 msec square wave pulses, 2–15 V and train duration of 2–11 sec.

For recording of the scalp EEG an 8-channel Beckman-Offner electroencephalograph was used.

Results

Conspicuous slowing of the ipsilateral scalp EEG with a simultaneous gradual increase of the amplitude was seen in 12 of the 13 erethistic patients operated on under general anaesthesia and stimulated with a frequency of 60 Hz (Fig. 1 a and b, Table 1). Slowing also occurred in three of those four TLE patients who underwent general anaesthesia, and in the schizophrenic patient who received local anaesthesia. In 12 cases the slowing was unilateral, ipsilateral to stimulation. In four it was bilateral, but also arose from the ipsilateral hemisphere and gradually spread over to the opposite side (Fig. 2 a and b).

The slowing usually began about 10 seconds after the cessation of stimulation. Within one minute it gradually changed to an extremely slow high-voltage activity (1–1.5 Hz, 200–400 μV) predominantly over the stimulated hemisphere, but occasionally involving both hemispheres. After two minutes the slow activity began to disappear. There were no clinical or EEG signs of epileptic discharge in connection to the slowing. The patients were kept normocapnic throughout the stimulation procedure.

In 11 patients operated on under local anaesthesia no slowing was observed. The difference may have been due to a shorter train duration and lower intensity of stimulation than in the general anaesthesia group.

Discussion

As far as we know there is no report in the literature on the slowing of cortical EEG activity after electrical stimulation of the amygdala. Narabayashi (1979), despite his vast experience with amygdalotomy, has never observed it. Sano *et al.* (1972) obtained a slowing of the scalp EEG, similar to ours, when they stimulated anaesthetized erethistic patients in the posteromedial hypothalamus. They demonstrated that the slowing spread bilaterally over the two hemispheres and also to the ipsilateral amygdala and hippocampus.

Typical features of the cortical slowing after stimulation of the amygdala are 1. its late and gradual appearance, *i.e.*, approximately 10 seconds after cessation of stimulation; 2. its propagation which is predominantly ipsilateral but may also be bilateral; 3. its frequency of 1–1.5 Hz and amplitude of 200–400 μV; 4. an asynchrony between the two hemispheres.

Anaesthesia seems to play a role in the generation of the slowing; we only observed it once in a patient operated on under local anaesthesia.

We have no explanation for the cortical slowing reported here. It may be caused by depletion of some neurotransmitters (noradrenaline?) from the stimulated area.

References

Narabayashi, H., Personal communication, 1979.

Sano, K., Sekino, H., Mayanagi, Y., Results of stimulation and destruction of the posterior hypothalamus in cases with violent, aggressive, or restless behaviors. In: Psychosurgery, pp. 57—75 (Hitchcock, E., Laitinen, L., Vaernet, K., eds.). Springfield, Ill.: Ch. C Thomas. 1972.

Acta Neurochirurgica, Suppl. 30, 183—187 (1980)

Central Stimulation Treatment of Epilepsy

M. Šramka*, G. Fritz, D. Gajdošová, and **P. Nádvorník**

With 2 Figures

Summary

Therapeutic electrical stimulation of nucleus caudatus was performed in 26 patients suffering from epilepsy. Sixteen of them had previously undergone destructive stereotactic surgery in different deep brain structures and the stimulation was indicated as an additional procedure. The results reported are related to 10 patients stimulated without any other surgical treatment. In 3 subjects stimulation of temporal lobe structures was performed as well.

Good therapeutic effects were obtained in 2 cases following caudate stimulation. Mild improvement or no effect were obtained in the other cases, including the two submitted to hippocapal stimulation.

Interesting speculation on the relationships between caudate and hippocampal electrical activity have been generated.

Introduction

The knowledge that some brain structures have a depressing influence on the motor brain activity is used for epilepsy treatment by means of central stimulation. Cooper [1, 2] started with cerebellar stimulation locating the electrodes on the surface of cerebellum by classic neurosurgical approach. We followed Cooper's experience with eight patients, but we introduced the electrodes stereotactically into the deep cerebellar structures [3]. Five years ago, in the 1974, we started with the stimulation of the head of the caudate, which is also considered to exert a depressing effect in the brain. Furthermore, we tried also direct stimulation of the same deep temporal structures involved in the epileptic process. We report here the results obtained by the stimulation of the caudate and of hippocampal structures on the epileptic seizures and on the brain epileptic electrical activity.

---

* Research Laboratory of Clinical Stereotaxy VÚHB, Bratislava, ČSSR.

0065-1419/80/Suppl. 30/0183/$ 01.00

Material and Method

Up to now, caudate stimulation has been performed in 26 patients. Sixteen of them previously underwent destructive stereotactic surgery in different deep brain structures and stimulation was indicated as an additional procedure. Only 10 patients underwent stimulation without any other surgical treatment. Two of them underwent also hippocampal stimulation. This is the group of patients considered in this report. The patients concerned are listed in Table 1. The disease had been present for a long period before the beginning of central stimulation. The clinical picture was usually very complicated and behavioral abnormalities were present in most of the cases, all of whom were refractory to drug therapy. The electrodes were introduced in the head of the caudate. Other electrodes were introduced in thalamic structures, including anterior reticular nuclei and lamina medialis, in the amygdala, and in the hippocampal gyrus, for stereoelectroencephalographic (SEEG) examination. The electrodes were left in all these structures ("chronic" examination) to monitor their activity and the effect of stimulation. In seven patients the end of the electrodes was left outside the skin to enable their connection to a stimulator or to a recorder. In three patients percutaneous stimulation was used, by means of an implanted receiver. The coordinates of the target in the caudate were 26.5 mm anterior to the midpoint of the AC-PC (intercommissural line), 3 mm below it, and 13 mm lateral to sagittal line.

A special interest was taken in the relationship between the caudate and hippocampal gyrus, which showed epileptic activity in all our patients. The electrodes were introduced symmetrically into both hemispheres to have the possibility to stimulate (simultaneously or successively) symmetrical and homologous brain structures.

Results

The effects of caudate stimulation on the epileptic syndrome were good in two cases (see Table 1): stimulation resulted in complete disappearance of seizures, normalization of the EEG and improvement of mental activity. In the other cases, the effect was limited to improvement or was alltogether lacking. Stimulation of deep structures of the temporal lack (two patients) was followed by reduction in seizure frequency in one case and by abolition of discharges in the other. We were not able to find consistent relations between the type of epilepsy or stimulation program and the results obtained.

The simultaneous stimulation of both caudate nuclei increased the pathological activity of the hippocampal structures. The effect, however, lasted only a few seconds. In some patients, the hippocampal pathological activity decreased first, than increased and finally disappeared. In some cases we performed independent stimulation of the right and left caudates. When the stimulation was made on the caudate on the same side of the hippocampus showing an abnormal electrical activity suggesting an anatomical lesion (slow waves), a bilateral decrease of the epileptic potentials was observed.

Table 1. *Review of Stimulated Epileptic Patients*

No.	Patient	Age at surgery	Implantation of electrodes	Program of stimulation	Disease before stimulation	Follow-up	Results
1	D. A. 24 years, f	7 years	17. 9. 1974 A, G.hp, Cd bilat.	Cd bilat.: 10–100 Hz, 10 V, lms, 10′, 1/d, 1 w	GM 1/m, psychomotor 10/w	4 years, 10 months	reduction of seizures
2	M. Š. 33 years, f	14 years	23. 10. 1974 A, G.hp, Cd bilat.	Cd r., Cd l.: 10 Hz, 10 V, lms, 5′, 1/d, 1 w	GM 1/m, psychomotor 1–5 d	4 years, 9 months	suppression of seizures
3	Č. V. 23 years, m	6 years	24. 1. 1975 Cd bilat.	Cd l.: 10–100 Hz, 10 V, lms, 10′, 4/d, 12 d	GM 3–5 m, aura	4 years, 6 months	without changes
4	T. A. 24 years, f	13 years	17. 4. 1977 A, G.hp, Cd bilat.	Cd bilat.: 10 Hz, 5 V, lms, 10′, 1/d, 8 d	GM 2–4/w, psychomotor 1/d, neurosis hysterica	2 years, 2 months	suppression of seizures
5	S. M. 23 years, f	17 years	13. 10. 1977 A, G.hp, Rt, H_2, Cd bilat.	Cd bilat.: 100 Hz, 10 V, lms, 10′, 1/d, 1 m	GM 6–8/m, psychomotor 8–10/d, mental changes, aura	1 year, 9 months	reduction of seizures
6	Z. R. 19 years, f	5 years	14. 10. 1977 A, G.hp, Rt, H_2, Cd bilat.	Cd bilat.: 100 Hz, 10 V, lms, 10′, 1/d, 24 d	GM 2–4/m, aura 8–10/d, akinetic seizures 5/d	1 year, 9 months	without changes
7	M. M. 18 years, m	2 years	19. 11. 1977 A, G.hp, Lm bilat.	A l., A r., Lm l.: 10–100 Hz, 3–5 V, lms, 10′, 1/d, 10 w	posttraumatic EpEEG, mental changes	1 year, 7 months	without changes
8	K. K. 27 years, m	22 years	2. 3. 1978 A, G.hp, Rt, H_2, Cd bilat.	Cd bilat.: 10 Hz, 10 V, 1 ms, 10′, 1/d, 32 d	GM 3–4/w, psychomotor 15/w, Jackson 3–4/w	1 year, 3 months	reduction of seizures
9	H. Y. 22 years, m	8 years	3. 3. 1978 A, G.hp, Cd bilat.	Cd bilat.: 10–100 Hz, 10 V, lms, 10′, 1/d, 99 d	GM 1–2/m, psychomotor 3–4/d, mental changes	1 year, 3 months	reduction of seizures
10	L. D. 22 years, m	4 years	20. 1. 1977 A, G.hp, Cd bilat.	A l., A r.: pacemaker 1 Hz, 4′, 5 V, 0.4 ms permanently, 6 m	GM 1/y, psychomotor 10–20/m, mental improved	6 months	reduction of seizures

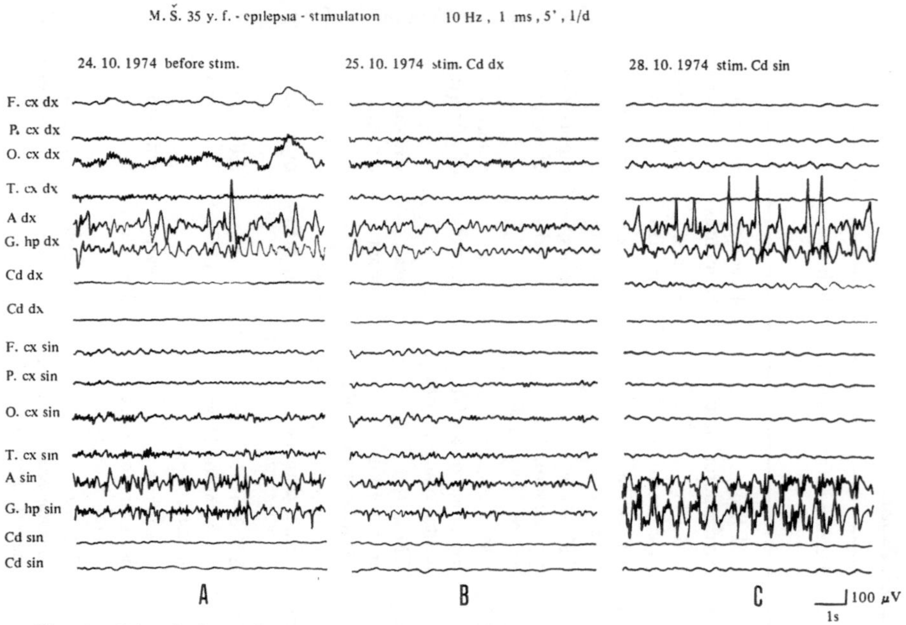

Fig. 1. Stimulation of caput nc. caudati bilat. A) Before stimulation. B) After stimulation Cd dx 1st day. C) After stimulation Cd sin 4th day. (*A* n. amygdalae; *G. hp* gyrus hippocampi; *Cd* caput nc. caudati, *F, P, O, T cx* cortex; *dx* right; *sin* left)

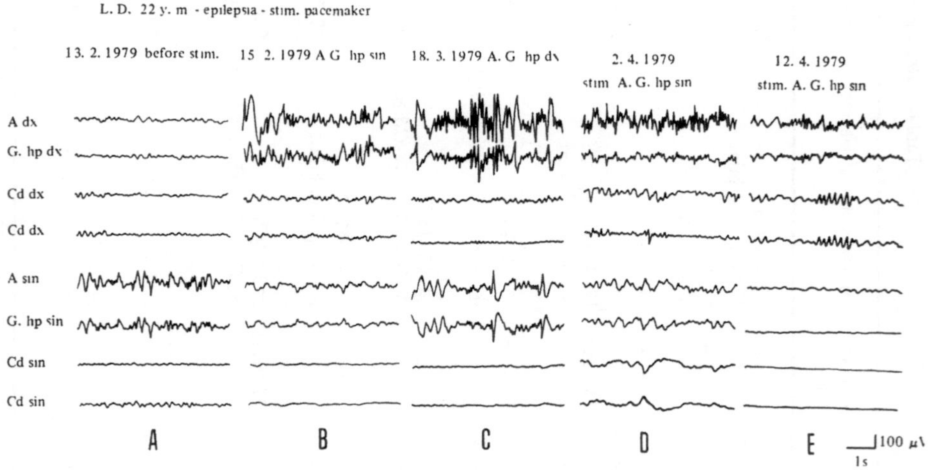

Fig. 2. Stimulation of gyrus hippocampi bilat. A) Before stimulation. B) After stimulation A, G. hp sin 2nd day. C) After stimulation A, G. hp dx 5th day. D) After stimulation A, G. hp sin 20th day. E) After stimulation A, G. hp sin 30th day. (*A* nc. amygdalae, *G. hp* gyrus hippocampi, *Cd* caput nc. caudati; *dx* right; *sin* left)

However, when the stimulation was applied to the caudate of the side of the hippocampus showing irritative electrical abnormalities, regarded as "mirror" in origin, the epileptic activity increased bilaterally (Fig. 1).

Analogous observations were made in the two patients in whom the stimulation was directly applied to the epileptic focus (*i.e.*, the hippocampal gyrus; Fig. 2) while recording from the caudate. To be noticed that in the patient showing a clinical improvement, the latter followed the stimulation of the deep temporal structures where the primary focus appeared to be located. In this case, synchronized waves were recorded from the caudate following hippocampal stimulation.

Discussion

The above observations suggest some ideas on the strategy of stimulation therapy. When the epileptic activity is present in both hippocampal gyri, it seems necessary to distinguish the side on which the electrical activity concomitant with the anatomical lesion is localized. This side may be recognized by identification of spike and wave discharges mixed with irregular slow background activity. Ipsilateral caudate or hippocampal stimulation seems to be effective in the condition. The activity of the brain structures participating in epilepsy tends to return to normal. On the other hand, with stimulation on the opposite side (the "mirror" irritative focus) the epileptic activity becomes more severe. The simultaneous stimulation of both caudates is followed initially by slow improvement. At that point synchronized depressive waves appear in the caudate. One pathophysiological explanation may be that caudate stimulation has a depressive influence on the zone of the lesion rather than on the contralateral side.

References

1. Cooper, I. S., Amin, I., Gilan, S., Waltz, J. M., The effect of chronic stimulation of cerebellar cortex on epilepsy in man. In: The cerebellum, epilepsy and behavior, pp. 113—171 (Cooper, I. S., Riklan, M., Shnider, R. S., eds.). 1974.
2. Cooper, I. S., Gilman, S., The effect of chronic cerebellar stimulation upon epilepsy in man. 98th Annual Meeting Amer. Neurol. Assoc., July 11–13, 1973, Montreal.
3. Šramka, M., Fritz, G., Galanda, M., Nádvorník, P., Some observations in treatment stimulation of epilepsy. Acta Neurochir. Suppl. 23 (1976), 257—262.

Acta Neurochirurgica, Suppl. 30, 189—192 (1980)

D. Closure

Closing Remarks

G. F. Rossi*

My task is to close this session with some remarks on the theme under discussion: "surgery of epilepsy". Time prevents me from commenting in detail on the many aspects of the subject which have been dealt with by the preceeding speakers. I will therefore limit my-self to a few, general comments.

1. First of all, let us consider the results which can be obtained today in this field of functional neurosurgery. As I said in the introduction, the main purpose of this meeting is that of examining both the progress so far achieved and the problems still to be solved. The analysis of the results of surgery appears apt to give us a good indication of both progresses and limits.

In which way can we evaluate the results of surgical treatment of an epileptic patient? The most obvious, and easy, way is to consider the effect of surgery on the occurrence and frequency of seizures. As we have heard from the papers presented, there is no doubt that surgery can bring about a remarkable reduction of seizure frequency in the great majority of patients and lead to a definitive suppression of seizures in many of them. A comparison of the surgical results presented to-day with those reported in the past shows that there has been a continuous, progressive improvement.

None the less, in all series there is still a certain percentage of cases showing only minimal benefit or no benefit at all from the surgical treatment. As I have previously, stated [1, 2], the causes of surgical failures can be many. However, the most relevant of them seems to be the difficulty we still have in precisely defining the spatial organization of the lesional-functional epileptogenic complex and the intracerebral pathways of propagation of the seizure discharge. At present, the surgical operation is based on the integration

* Institute of Neurosurgery, Catholic University, Rome, Italy.

0065-1419/80/Suppl. 30/0189/$ 01.00

of the results of electrophysiological analysis with those of the accurate study of the clinical seizure patterns and detailed neuroradiological study. These diagnostic methods can be further improved. However, it appears likely that substantial improvement is more likely to come from the development of new methods contributing to the knowledge of the cerebral events underlying epilepsy from a different angle, for instance from methods aiming at detecting local cerebral metabolic changes, as has been suggested this morning by Dr. Rasmussen and Prof. Gillingham.

A second remark on the evaluation of the results of surgery seems relevant. In my opinion, there is a considerable difference between the definitive suppression of seizures and the reduction of seizure frequency. Certainly, both results have to be regarded as positive, both of them bringing to clinical improvement. However, definitive suppression of seizures means that the patient is no longer an epileptic; reduction of seizure frequency, even when remarkable, means that the epileptic syndrome is less severe, but the patient is still epileptic. You are most certainly aware of the psychological and social implications of this difference. As a result of this, I think it advisable that when describing or reporting the results of surgical treatment, an unequivocal distinction be made between these two types of results. Likewise, when discussing the surgical approaches to epilepsy and even more when offering surgical treatment to the patient and his or her relatives, we should distinguish between the approaches permitting a complete cure of the patient and those aiming at improving his or her epileptic syndrome. As I said previously in my introduction, in my opinion the best chance of obtaining suppression of seizures is provided by the surgical approaches reported in the first part of morning session, with the object of completely removing the lesional-functional epileptogenic complex (summarized in the introduction in Fig. 1, A). This opinion appears to be supported by the results reported by the preceeding speakers. If one accepts this view, it might be suggested that the second and third types of surgical approach, namely that attempting to interrupt the pathways of propagations of the epileptic discharges and that based on cerebral or cerebellar electrical stimulation (shown in the introduction in Fig. 1, B and C), be regarded as second choice procedures, to be taken into consideration when the first one is not feasible.

2. My second general comment is to a certain extent related to the one I have just made. The problems of the epileptic patient who comes to the neurosurgeon are many. Most, if not all, of the epileptic candidates for surgery have been epileptic for years. Therefore, they have to face not only their seizures, but also the consequences of their

state on their psychological attitude and social relationships. These patients regard surgery as at the ultimate solution to their problems. This should not be forgotten by the neurosurgeon, as has been stressed this morning by Dr. Bonis. He has to prepare his patient first of all for the possibility that the presurgical examinations may not confirm the preliminary general indication for surgical treatment and, second, for the possibility that surgery will not necessarily be followed by the complete suppression of seizures. Furthermore, the work of the neurosurgeon is not over after surgery, even when seizures suppression has been obtained. The cured patient, now without seizures, may need help to resume or normalize his relationship with the community; in other words, to regard himself as a "normal" man (or woman or child). This is not an easy task. To fulfil it, the neurosurgeon needs the help of others, particularly psychologists and social workers.

3. This brings me to the next comment. Surgery of epilepsy, to be performed—as it should be—in the correct fashion, requires a complex organization, gathering people of wide experience in the many and different aspects of epileptology. The surgical act, per se, is only one, even if of relevant importance, in the many steps leading to therapeutic success. To build such an organization is obviously difficult; it requires time, motivated personnel and money. Perhaps, one of the explanation of the discrepancy between the large number of potential candidates for surgical treatment and the relatively small number of patients actually referred to the neurosurgeon (which I pointed out in my introductory remarks) can be found in the small number of neurosurgical organizations satisfying all the requirements I have just mentioned. We need more of these organizations. However, we have to be careful in building them. We must remember that there is still a diffuse skeptical attitude of the non-neurosurgical medical world towards the possibilities of surgical treatment for the epileptic patient. To defeat this, we must provide these sceptical people with the best results. And that requires the type of organization reminded above.

4. I finally come to my last comment. The neurosurgeon is well aware of the fact that the ideal means to treat epilepsy is not that of ablating the cerebral neuronal aggregates whose abnormal activity produces epilepsy, nor that of cutting the cerebral pathways conducting the discharges originating in these neurons. The ideal means would be that of correcting the functional abnormality of these cerebral neurones leaving them alive. We all look at the time when this will be possible. The neurosurgeon can contribute to it, continuing what he did in the past and does in the present times to the

development of our knowledge of epileptology. Such a time, however, is yet to come. Therefore, at present, traditional surgical treatment maintains its role, and such a role, as it clearly results from what has been reported by our speakers, seems to be still relevant.

References

1. Rossi, G. F., Considerations on the principles of surgical treatment of partial epilepsies. Brain Res. *95* (1975), 395—402.
2. Rossi, G. F., Colicchio, G., Gentilomo, A., Scerrati, M., Discussion on the causes of failure of surgical treatment of partial epilepsies. Appl. Neurophysiol. *41* (1978), 29—37.

Section II

Stereotactic Cerebral Irradiation

Acta Neurochirurgica, Suppl. 30, 195—197 (1980)

Some Comments on the INSERM Symposium on Stereotactic Cerebral Irradiations Held Friday, July 13, 1979*

G. Szikla**

The idea of organizing a Symposium on Stereotactic Cerebral Irradiations arose from several converging trends in the recent evolution of stereotactic neurosurgery. The latter might indeed offer solutions to problems arising from significant progress achieved in other fields.

Actually, the new diagnostic possibilities and essentially the generalized use of computerized tomography modifies to a great extent the problems of management of brain tumours. With increasing frequency, the CT scan discovers small lesions located in critical or vital areas of the brain.

This explains the renewed interest in precise and less traumatic techniques affording adequate and early treatment of this type of lesions. High dose focal irradiations limited to the lesion might destroy small tumours without inflicting significant damage to the adjacent brain—even in important and vulnerable areas, such as primary motor centres, speech areas etc.—provided that the heavily irradiated volume corresponds closely to that of the tumour. The indispensable precision of both localizations, namely of the tumour on one hand and of the irradiation on the other, can be obtained by stereotactic techniques only.

Both the diagnostic and the therapeutic procedures have to rely upon a close collaboration of several disciplines, all collected data being cross-correlated and mutually checked within the same stereotactic coordinate system.

* The proceedings of the Symposium are published as a separate volume in the INSERM Symposium series (Elsevier-North-Holland Biomedical Press Publ.).

** Service de Neurochirurgie Fonctionnelle, Centre Hospitalier Sainte-Anne, 1, rue Cabanis, F-75014 Paris, Cedex 14, France.

0065-1419/80/Suppl. 30/0195/$ 01.00

This opens fascinating new fields for theoretical and clinical research, *e.g.*, on the histologic or electrophysiologic correlates of CT images, or on dose-dependent changes induced by ionizing radiation in the brain etc.

Out of the four main topics three, namely

1. In vivo localization of the tumoural *target-volume*,
2. *radiosurgical techniques and dosimetry*,
3. *early and late radiation-effects*,

were devoted to such basic aspects of the stereotactic irradiations.

The general survey of the broad *indication fields* and of the achieved *results*, fourth and final panel of the Symposium, supplied a wealth of data allowing to assess present possibilities and limits of these methods.

Let us mention only some of the more important points. Unquestionably, the use of CT data in the localization and the volume assessment is a major progress in the stereotactic management of brain tumours. Several technical solutions were presented aiming to establish a common coordinate system for CT and stereotactic data. At the same time the absolute necessity of cross-correlations with other data and in particular with control biopsies was emphasized, as CT images *alone* cannot give reliable information about the nature of the tumour and can be misleading even regarding its precise 3 D delineation. Peripheral hypodensity can just as well signify perifocal oedema as it can correspond to infiltrated tissue, containing tumour cells, for example.

The second panel allowed to compare the different radiosurgical techniques and the physical dosimetry of the delivered focal stereotactic irradiations: Gamma-Unit of Leksell, the Gammamed single dose and the protracted permanent ^{192}Iridium and ^{125}Iodine implantation of Mundinger, the Bragg-peak proton radiosurgical method of Kjellberg, the association of temporary interstitial ^{192}Iridium implantation and external radiotherapy developed by Szikla and Schlienger and applied by several French stereotactic teams using the Talairach system.

The early and late effects of focal high dose irradiation, volume-dose-time correlations of radiation oedema, brain swelling and necrotic changes were discussed in the third part of the Symposium.

In the final panel, papers presenting the long term results in different indications covered a multitude of pathologic conditions: pituitary adenomas, and diabetic retinopathy (excluding however Y 90 hypophysectomy), acoustic neurinomas, inoperable AVM, solid craniopharyngiomas, pineal region tumours, secreting cystic cavities and malignant as well as lower grade gliomas.

A significant point was stated by B. Larsson: "In the era of stereotactic techniques, CT and new radiations, there seems to be no need for a demarcation line between radiosurgical treatment of small tumours and fractionated radiotherapy for infiltrating malignancies. On one hand, stereotactic surgery may benefit from the kinetical models which characterize present developments in general radiotherapy, on the other hand, radiotherapy for malignant tumours in the brain calls for the precise measures of stereotactic surgery."

For the first time, a confrontation of the different techniques, and the multidisciplinary discussion of the basic problems by stereotactic neurosurgeons, radiotherapists, radiobiologists, physicists, neurologists, physiologists and pathologists, allowed a comprehensive survey of this rapidly expanding field, which at present is clearly one of the important orientations of stereotactic surgery, both because of the great number of cases and because of the challenging problems they present.

Section III

Neurostimulation for Pain and Spasticity

Acta Neurochirurgica, Suppl. 30, 201—217 (1980)

A. Pain

Analgesia Induced by Electrical Stimulation of the Brain Stem in Animals: Involvement of Serotoninergic Mechanisms

J.-M. Besson* and **J.-L. Oliveras****

With 5 Figures

Over the last few years, many studies have centered on the analgesic effects induced by electrical stimulation of certain areas of the brain stem. Initial observations by Reynolds [63], demonstrating powerful analgesic effects induced by stimulation of the periaqueductal grey matter (PAG) in the rat, have led to subsequent studies (see ref. in [12, 23, 42, 49]). The same analgesic effects following stimulation of the PAG have now been reported in cat [43, 53], monkey [27], and man [1, 36, 64].

A point of great interest is the similarity between this type of analgesia and morphine analgesia, suggesting at least in part, that electrical analgesia might result from liberation of the endogenous morphine-like substances.

In this report we will successively consider:

The characteristics and the mechanisms mediating stimulation producing analgesia.

The relationship between electrical analgesia and morphine analgesia.

I. Characteristics and Mechanisms of Electrical Analgesia

In the rat, most of the studies have been restricted on the mesencephalic PAG. The effective sites include the whole of the

* Unité de Recherches de Neurophysiologie Pharmacologique de l'INSERM (U 161), 2 rue d'Alésia, F-75014 Paris, France.

** Chercheur I.N.S.E.R.M.

0065-1419/80/Suppl. 30/0201/$ 03.40

PAG and the neighbouring periventricular areas. In this presentation we will essentially consider the systematic mapping study which has been carried out in our laboratory on the cat [43, 53, 55, 59] with 300 stimulation sites extending from the mesencephalon to the medulla.

Methods

The animals were chronically prepared under general anaesthesia to permit the implantation of central bipolar concentric stimulating electrodes, wires for tooth pulp stimulation and electrodes for the jaw opening reflex (JOR) recording. Deep brain electrodes were made of stainless steel; the inner core was sharpened to a tip diameter of 30 μ. They were lowered between frontal planes A 2.5 to P 12 (according to the atlas of Berman [11]), within and adjacent to the periaqueductal grey matter and into different raphé nuclei rich in serotonin containing cell bodies Dorsal Raphé Nucleus (DRN); Raphé Centralis Superior (CS); Raphé Centralis Inferior (CI). This nucleus includes the nuclei raphé pontis, raphé magnus and raphé obscurus.

Brain stimulation consisted of 100–200 msec trains of either 50 Hz sine waves (15–100 μA) or monophasic rectangular pulses (0.2 msec, 100/sec, 2–10 V); in both cases stimulus trains were generally delivered at a frequency of 3/sec for several seconds to one minute.

The analgesic effects were evaluated by the responses of the animals to pinch and to the electrical stimulation of the tooth pulp:

Pinches were applied to the tail, the 4 limbs and the ears with a small hemostatic or toothed forceps. During the early stages of testing, pinch intensity was barely adequate to elicit an orienting reaction, vocalization and withdrawal. Later, if brain stimulation appeared to block such responses, pinch intensity was progressively increased to a level which in the normal cat would elicit vigorous escape attempts, attack and hissing. Brain stimulation was considered to have an analgesic effect only if all such behavioral signs were clearly and reliably absent. The magnitude of the analgesic effect was rated as powerful, moderate or weak, in relation to the intensity of the pinches at which these behaviors were abolished.

Tooth pulp, uniquely innervated by small diameter fibers (Aδ and C) is particularly effective for the study of pain processes since in humans pain is thought to be the only sensation induced by its stimulation.

Electrical stimulation of the tooth pulp was delivered via two platinum electrodes inserted through two small holes in the dentine of the upper canine, directly into the pulp. Using this kind of stimulation, we have considered two types of nociceptive behavioral responses: the J.O.R. induced by the application of a single brief electrical shock (0.2 to 2 ms) and more integrated nociceptive manifestations induced by train shocks of long duration (50 Hz, 10 sec.). The JOR reflex which corresponds to a nociceptive flexor reflex in the spinal cord [39, 73] was recorded by means of two silver wires separated for about 1 cm, wrapped around the digastric muscle ipsilateral to the tooth stimulated [60].

1. Distribution of Effective Sites and Characteristics of Analgesia

The anatomical locations of effective sites of stimulation are shown in Figs. 1 and 2.

At the level of the PAG, the points from which analgesia was obtained were essentially located in the ventral area in or close the

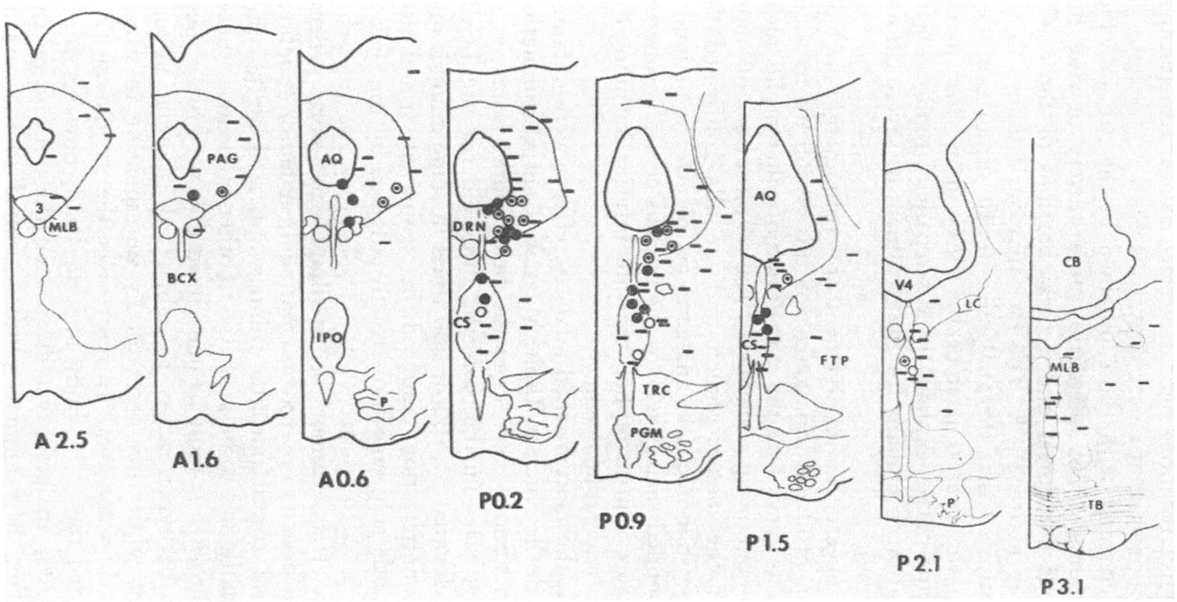

Fig. 1. Sites for electrical analgesia at the mesencephalic level in the cat. Analgesic effects: ● powerful, ⊙ moderate; ○ weak; — no analgesia. The most efficacious sites are located in the nuclei raphé dorsalis (DRN) and central superior (CS). Abbreviations according to the stereotaxic atlas of the brain stem [11]: *AQ* Aqueduct; *BCX* decussation of the brachium conjonctivum; *CB* cerebellum; *CS* nucleus central superior; *DRN* dorsal raphé nucleus; *FTP* paralemniscal tegmental field; *IPO* posterior interpeduncular nucleus; *MLB* medial longitudinal bundle; *PAG* periaqueductal grey matter; *TRC* tegmental reticular nucleus. (Modified from Oliveras *et al.*, ref. 55)

nucleus raphé dorsalis, rich in serotoninergic cell bodies. Frequently, stimulation of sites adjacent to this region or stimulation in dorsal PAG elicited aversive reactions such as directed attack, fear (escape), apparent pain, and prominent motor disturbances.

These results contrast with those obtained in the rat, in which analgesia was obtained from stimulation at a variety of sites distributed throughout the dorsal and ventral portions of the caudal periaqueductal grey matter [48, 50]. The fact that our findings in the cat clearly demonstrated that the analgesic sites of stimulation were strictly located in the ventral part of the PAG in or close to the DRN could perhaps partly explain the discrepancies reported with deep brain stimulation in humans for the treatment of severe chronic pain (see this volume).

This location suggests the involvement of serotoninergic mechanisms in stimulation producing analgesia, for this reason we have investigated the effects elicited by the stimulation of other raphé nuclei rich in serotonin-containing neurones. The exploration of more posterior areas of the mesencephalon and medulla confirmed the importance of the raphé nuclei in analgesia as the effective stimulation zones corresponded successively to the nucleus centralis superior followed by the more ventral raphé: centralis inferior including the nuclei raphé pontis and raphé magnus.

Without doubt, the most marked analgesic effects were obtained from sites located in the Nucleus Raphé Magnus. Central stimulation totally blocked, in almost every case, the behavioural responses to intense peripheral pinch. Furthermore the threshold for the J.O.R. was considerably elevated by 100 or 200 times in some animals and the nociceptive manifestations induced by trains of stimulation delivered in the tooth pulp was also strongly affected by the central stimulation.

The analgesic effect cannot be attributed to more general stimulation-evoked deficits in sensory, emotional, or motor functions since during central stimulation the animals appeared alert, calm, able to walk normally and to be attentive to other innocuous stimuli (touch, visual, auditory). It must be underlined that very often these animals seemed to be hyperreactive to light tactile stimulation such as touch or air jet, while they were totally unresponsive to strong pinches applied in the same area. In most cases, the peripheral field of analgesia included the entire body and the head; however for a few sites in the PAG, analgesia was clearest on the tail and on the posterior limbs. For these animals pinches applied to the ears of forelimbs evoked entirely normal defensive and aggressive reactions. Generally the analgesic effect of brain stimulation could be seen

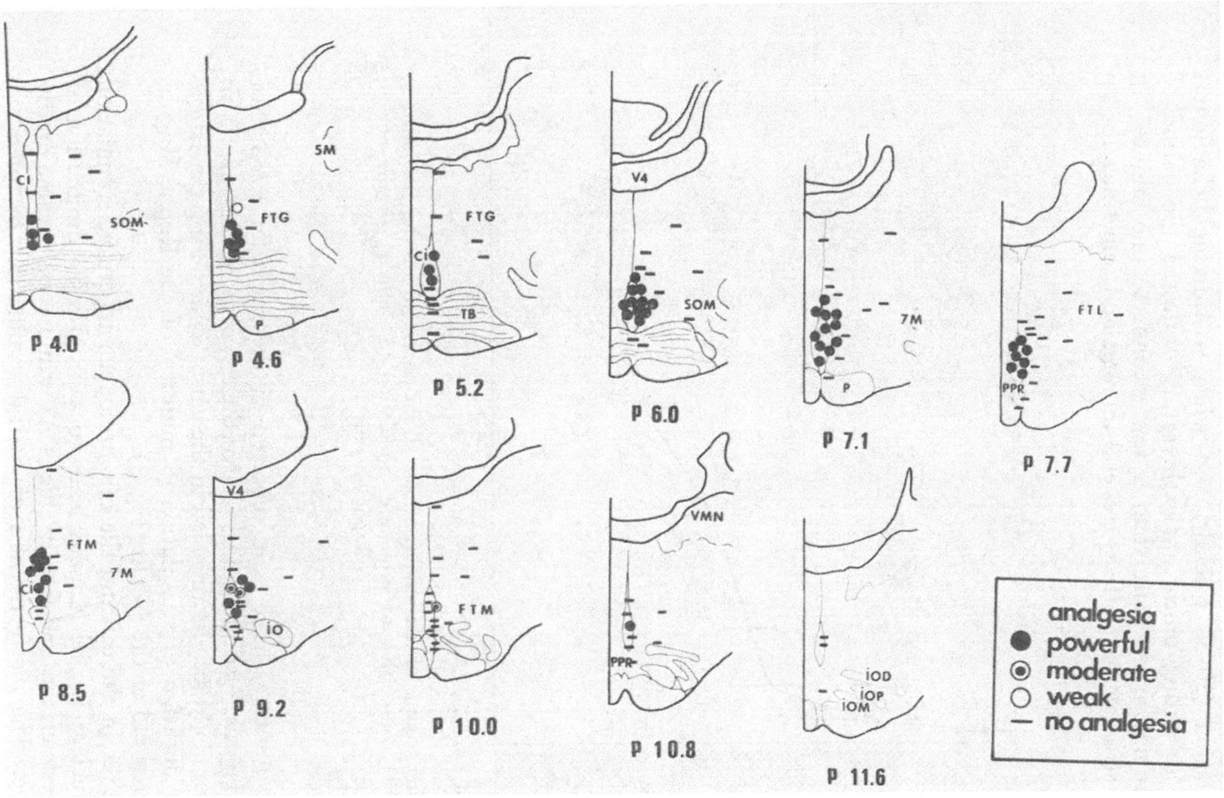

Fig. 2. Sites for electrical analgesia at the level of the medulla in the cat. Strong analgesic effects were essentially obtained by stimulation of the nucleus centralis inferior (principally the nucleus Raphé Magnus). Abbreviations according to the stereotaxic atlas of the brain stem [11]: *CI* Nucleus centralis inferior; *FTG* giganto-cellular tegmental field; *FTL* lateral tegmental field; *FTM* magnocellular tegmental field; *IO* inferior olive; *P* pyramidal tract; *PPR* post pyramidal raphé nucleus; *SOM* medial nucleus of the superior olive; *TB* trapezoid body; *5 M* motor trigeminal nucleus; *7 M* facial nucleus medial division. (Modified from Oliveras *et al.*, ref. 55)

approximatively 10 seconds after stimulation onset. For brief periods of stimulation (20–30 seconds) and when considering behavioural reactions to strong pinch, analgesia rarely outlasted the period of brain stimulation by more than a few seconds to one minute. In contrast, stronger post effects (several minutes and sometimes for up

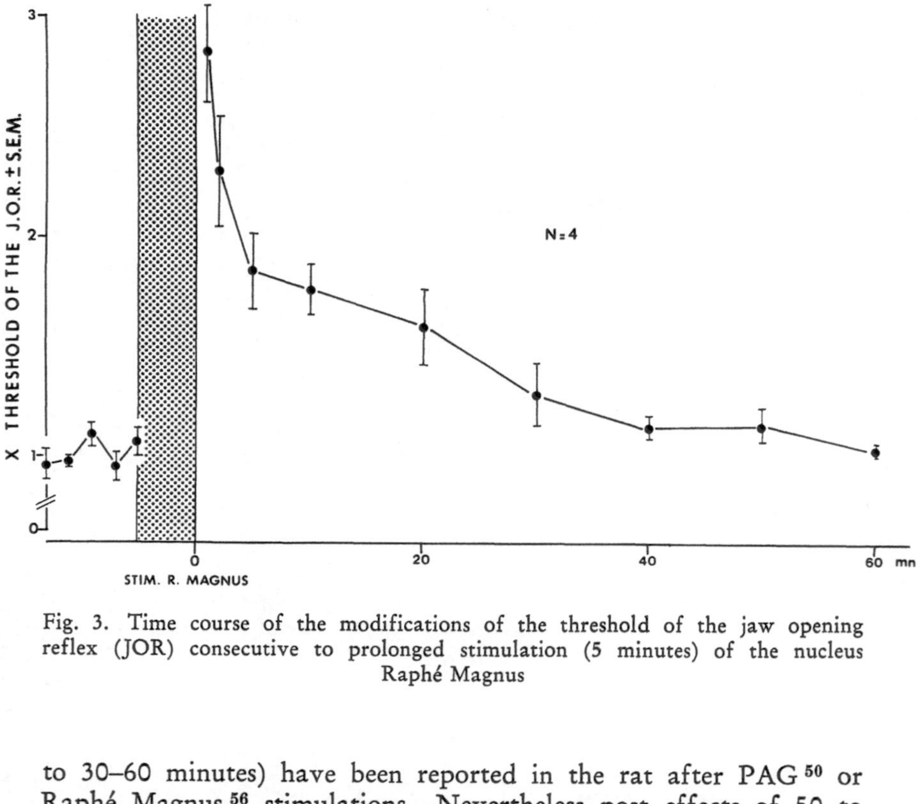

Fig. 3. Time course of the modifications of the threshold of the jaw opening reflex (JOR) consecutive to prolonged stimulation (5 minutes) of the nucleus Raphé Magnus

to 30–60 minutes) have been reported in the rat after PAG [50] or Raphé Magnus [56] stimulations. Nevertheless post effects of 50 to 60 minutes could also be revealed in the cat by considering the effects of longer duration of stimulation (5 minutes) of the Raphé Magnus on the threshold of the J.O.R. (Fig. 3).

However in the cat and the rat, prolonged repetitive stimulation of the Nucleus Raphé Magnus leads to a progressive diminution of the analgesic effects and finally (Fig. 4 A), stimulation became totally ineffective. The ineffectiveness of central stimulation, or tolerance, persisted as long as the testing continued and also for several hours after the initiation of the prolonged stimulation periods. In several

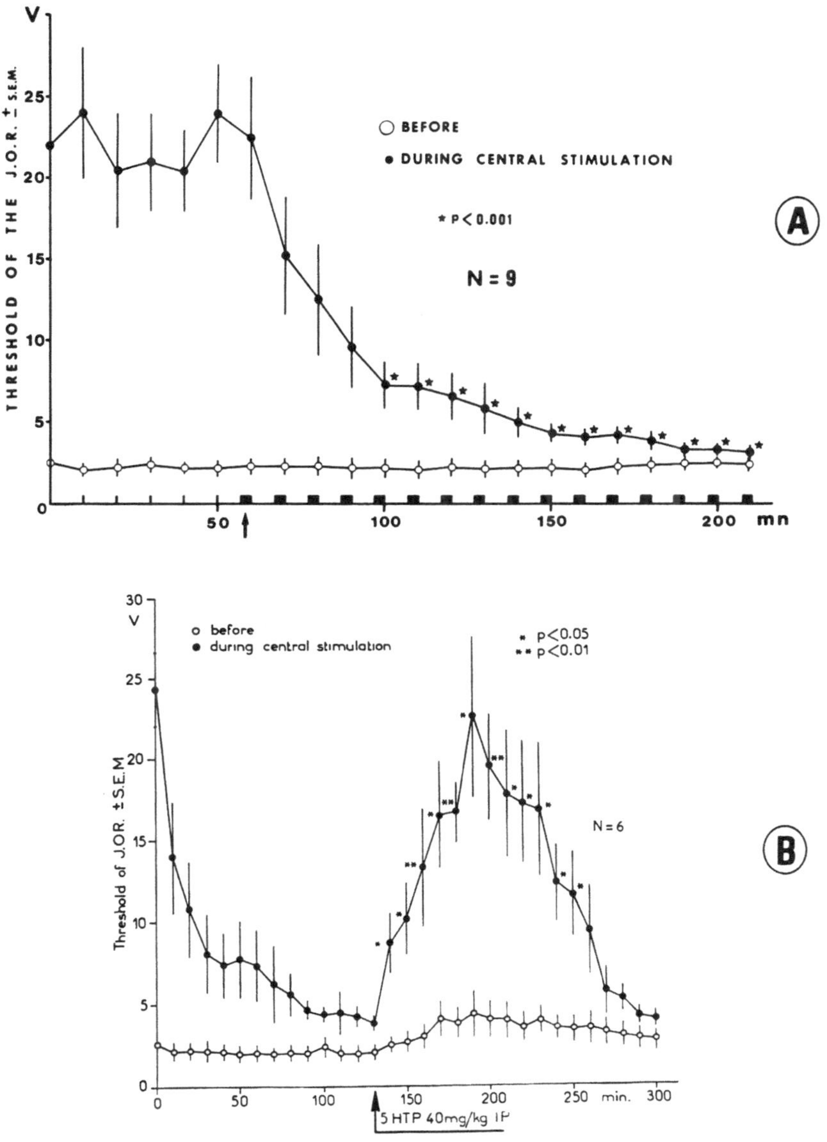

Fig. 4. Tolerance to central stimulation of the nucleus Raphé Magnus. A) Threshold of the JOR during Raphé stimulation was constantly obtained. Then (at the left the duration of the central stimulation was 10 seconds and the large increase of the JOR during Raphé stimulation was constantly obtained. Then (at the arrow) central stimulation was delivered during 3 minutes each 10 minutes. In this case note that the central stimulation became less and less effective. B) Threshold of the JOR before and during central stimulation. In these experiments (6 cats), the central stimulation was applied for 3 minutes during 10 minutes. Note the progressive disappearance of the efficacy of central stimulation and its restoration after administration of 5-HTP. (Modified from Oliveras *et al.*, ref. 57)

animals we noticed that a recovery period of several days was required before unequivocal analgesia and could again be induced [57].

Tolerance to PAG stimulation was also reported in the rat [47] but in addition, our experiments in the cat demonstrate that the administration of 5-Hydroxytryptophan (5-HTP; 40 mg/kg/IP), a serotonin precursor, totally restores the analgesic effect induced by Raphé Magnus stimulation (Fig. 4 B). It is of considerable interest to emphasize the fact that tolerance to PAG stimulation in humans [36] is reduced by dietary supplementation with L-Tryptophan [35].

II. Mechanisms Mediating Analgesia

It is generally admitted that analgesia is an active phenomenon that results, at least partly, from the activation of descending inhibitory systems, which in turn block the transmission of nociceptive messages at the spinal level. This idea is supported by the suppression of certain nociceptive reflexes in the rat and in the cat by central stimulation [50, 60]. A more direct argument has been put forward by our groups [43, 53]. Stimulation of the PAG and of the nucleus raphé dorsalis induces a powerful inhibition on some dorsal horn neurones involved in nociception. These results have been confirmed by other teams at the level of the trigeminal system [44, 70, 71, 82].

Similarly stimulation of the Nucleus Raphé Magnus powerfully inhibits dorsal horn neurones responses to noxious natural stimulation [10, 24, 30, 40]; this inhibitory action has also been demonstrated on neurones at the origin of ascending pathways such as the spinothalamic [51, 78] and spinoreticular [52] tracts. These results are in good agreement with anatomical studies demonstrating massive spinal projections from the Nucleus Raphé Magnus [7, 8, 13, 14, 16, 46, 54]. Interestingly lesion of this nucleus [54] strongly decreased the 5-HT amount in the superficial layers of the spinal cord where thin afferent fibers are known to project. There is, as yet, no evidence for direct descending spinal pathways from the PAG or the Raphé dorsalis. Further negative evidence is that lesions of the DRN do not alter spinal serotonin levels [54]. In contrast, projections from the PAG to the NRM have been described [22, 45, 67] and it is quite possible that the analgesic effects of PAG stimulation are mediated via the Raphé Magnus.

The involvement of descending control systems in analgesia is also strongly suggested by behavioural experiments in the rat [8, 9] which have described a reduction in the analgesic efficacy of PAG stimulation following bilateral destruction of the dorsolateral funiculus of the cord which contains some descending fibers from the

Raphé Magnus. They went on to show that a unilateral lesion of the funiculus blocked the analgesic effects of the stimulation on the side of the body ipsilateral to the lesion whilst sparing the contralateral analgesic efficacy. In agreement with these results are the recent electrophysiological demonstrations that a similar funicular lesion will block Raphé Magnus inhibitions on dorsal horn neurones [24, 78]. The indisputable conclusion from these results is that the analgesic effects of central stimulation are mediated, at least partly, by the activation of these descending inhibitory systems.

These results clearly demonstrate that the Raphé Nuclei, rich in serotonergic cell bodies, seem to play a basic role in the mechanism of electrical analgesia. The involvement of serotonin has been more directly tested by the following electrophysiological and behavioural studies:

Iontophoretic application of serotonin depressed the activity of dorsal horn neurones, including those at the origin of the spinothalamic tract [10, 32, 38, 62].

The analgesia induced by PAG stimulation [31] and the inhibitory effects on dorsal horn neurones following DRN stimulation [29] can be strongly attenuated by LSD which blocks the activity of serotonergic neurones.

In the rat, the administration of the serotonin synthesis inhibitor, p-CPA, blocks the analgesic effects of stimulation only from electrodes near the DRN; the analgesia reappears after administration of 5-Hydroxytryptophan [2]. In addition, recent electrophysiological experiments have shown that the inhibitory effects induced by stimulation of the Nucleus Raphé Magnus on the responses of dorsal horn neurones evoked by C fibres activation, were strongly affected after depletion of 5-HT induced by p-CPA [65].

We have already mentioned that the tolerance to the stimulation of the Nucleus Raphé Magnus was reversed by administration of 5-HTP.

Thus, inhibitory effects of central stimulation, whether measured behaviourally in the awake animal or electrophysiologically in the spinal cord of the anaesthesized preparation, seem to depend upon the integrity of serotoninergic transmission systems.

III. Analogies Between Stimulation Producing Analgesia and Morphine Analgesia

These relationship have been extensively reviewed by several groups [12, 23, 42, 49, 81]. Consequently, we just want to mention the essential findings.

a) As stimulation producing analgesia, morphine analgesia is strongly reduced in animals treated with p-CPA [17, 21, 41, 76, 77]. Correspondingly the analgesia is facilitated after intraventricular or systemic injection of 5-HTP [72, 75]. The analgesia induced by microinjection of morphine into the PAG [79] and the Nucleus Raphé Magnus [18] is notably reduced after administration of cinanserin, a blocker of serotonin receptors.

The analgesic effects of morphine are reduced or abolished by lesions of the PAG but including the mesencephalic raphé nuclei [25, 68, 69, 80] and also by Raphé Magnus lesions [61, 80]. The most marked effects are produced by these Raphé Magnus lesions.

On the basis of the previously discussed descending projections of the NRM, it seems that the analgesic action of morphine is to some extent dependent on the integrity of bulbospinal serotonergic systems. This hypothesis is strongly supported by a marked reduction in morphine analgesia following dorsolateral funicular lesions which destroy the pathways descending from the Raphé Magnus [8, 9]. These experiments agree well with those using injections of 5,6-dihydroxytryptamine into the lateral ventricles to pharmacologically lesion serotonin terminals at the spinal level without altering brain stem monoamines. This reduction of spinal serotonin is accompanied by a strong diminution in the analgesic effects of morphine [26, 77].

b) Powerful analgesia can be produced by microinjection of morphine at the level of the periaqueductal and periventricular grey matter (ref. in [81]) and into the Raphé Magnus [81]. In these experiments, the effective doses of morphine (few microgrammes) are between 1,000 and 2,000 times less than those necessary by intramuscular or subcutaneous routes. Furthermore, local microinjection of naloxone into the PAG and the NRM can reduce the analgesic effect of systemic morphine.

c) Tolerance can be demonstrated for both types of analgesia and finally, there are phenomena of cross-tolerance between electrical analgesia and morphine analgesia: analgesia produced by stimulation of the PAG is considerably less pronounced when the animal has previously been made tolerant to morphine [47]. In the same way, the analgesic effects produced by administration of morphine are strongly reduced by previous prolonged electrical stimulation of the Nucleus Raphé Magnus [56].

d) The periventricular grey matter, PAG and Raphé Nuclei dorsalis and medianus are relatively rich in morphine receptors [6, 34, 74] and recent work using the immunofluorescence technique has shown that the periaqueductal and periventricular areas, the ventrolateral PAG and the NRM contain some cell bodies rich in enkephalin [33].

e) The analgesia produced by stimulation of the PAG in the rat [3], the regions around the third ventricle in man [1, 36] and the Raphé Magnus in the cat [57] (Fig. 5) is reduced or abolished by the administration of opiate antagonist Naloxone. In animals, the effect of Naloxone is more pronounced when acting on analgesia produced by Raphé Magnus. These behavioural studies correlate well with

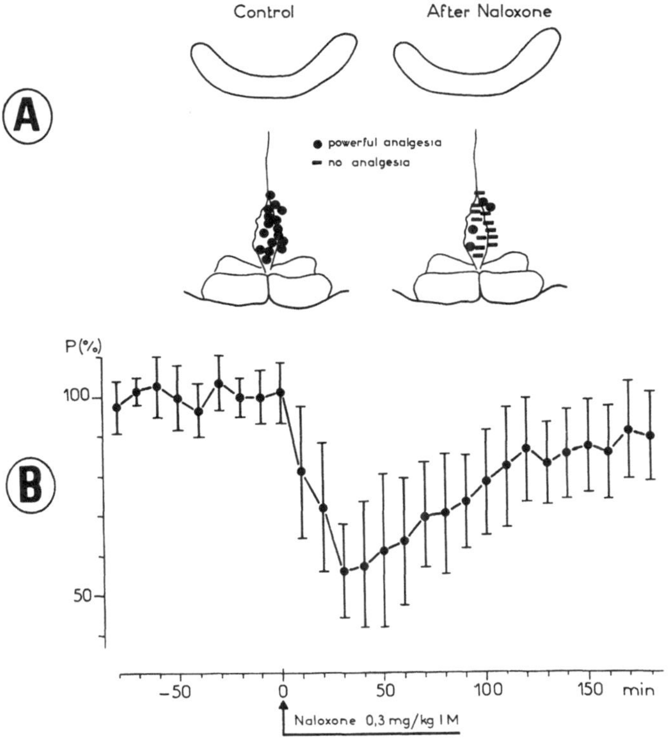

Fig. 5. Effects of Naloxone on the analgesic effects induced by stimulation of the nucleus Raphé Magnus in the cat. A) Analgesia tested by the pinch test: the stimulation of 12/16 sites became totally ineffective after Naloxone (0.3 mg/kg I.M.). B) Analgesia tested by the jaw opening reflex: general findings obtained in 14 cats. For each animal the successive values of the increase of the threshold of the JOR, tested every 10 minutes, were expressed by the ratio T'/T (T' = threshold during central stimulation; T = threshold before central stimulation). The average value of the 9 ratios obtained before naloxone administration was used as a reference (100%) to normalize each individual ratio before and after naloxone injection. Then, these normalized values obtained in 14 different cats were averaged. Each dot of the graph represents this mean value ± safety interval 5% (P). (Modified from Oliveras *et al.*, ref. 58)

electrophysiological studies which have given a demonstration of both the descending inhibitory systems emanating from the Raphé Magnus and the involvement of opiate mechanisms in this effect by the attenuation by Naloxone of the effects of Raphé Magnus stimulation on the C fiber response of dorsal horn neurones in the intact rat [66]. However two groups [15, 19, 20] found no effect of naloxone.

The suppression of electrical analgesia by Naloxone can be explained on the basis of the presence of morphine-like endogenous substances in the ventral nervous system. In addition, it seems likely that an electrical stimulation releases these substances and that Naloxone acts as an antagonist by an action of the opiate receptors. The β-endorphin [4, 37] or enkephalin like material [5] concentrations in human cerebrospinal fluid have been reported to be increased by PAG stimulation; however, there is no clear experimental evidence in animals.

In conclusion, these results suggest the existence of an endogenous neuronal system capable of modulating the transmission of painful messages. This powerful system, located in the periaqueductal, periventricular and raphé nuclei areas can be activated by morphine and electrical stimulation. The posterior areas of the brain stem, notably the Raphé Magnus, seem play a major role in these mechanisms.

It has been shown that analgesia can partly result from the activation of a raphé spinal system. These descending serotonergic systems, mostly originating in the Nucleus Raphé Magnus have dense projections in the dorsal horn of the spinal cord, particularly at the level of the substantia gelatinosa of Rolando. The mechanisms by which they influence the transmission of pain is as yet, not clear.

Acknowledgement

This work was supported by l'Institut National de la Santé et de la Recherche Médicale (I.N.S.E.R.M.) A.T.P. 39-76-71.

References

1. Adams, J. E., Naloxone reversal of analgesia produced by brain stimulation in the human. Pain *2* (1976), 161—166.
2. Akil, H., Mayer, D. J., Antagonism of stimulation-produced analgesia by p-CPA, a serotonin synthesis inhibitor. Brain Res. *44* (1972), 692—697.
3. Akil, H., Mayer, D. J., Liebeskind, J. C., Antagonism of stimulation-produced analgesia by naloxone, a narcotic antagonist. Science *191* (1976), 961—962.
4. Akil, H., Richardson, D. E., Barchas, J. D., Li, C. H., Appearance of β-endorphinlike immunoreactivity in human ventricular cerebrospinal fluid upon analgesic electrical stimulation. Proc. Natl. Acad. Sci. (Wash.) *75* (1978), 5170—5172.

5. Akil, H., Richardson, D. E., Hughues, J., Barchas, J. P., Enkephalin-like material elevated in ventricular cerebrospinal fluid of pain patients after analgesic focal stimulation. Science *201* (1978), 463—465.
6. Atweh, S. F., Kuhar, M. J., Autoradiographic localization of opiate receptors in rat brain. II. The brain stem. Brain Res. *129* (1977), 1—12.
7. Basbaum, A. I., Clanton, C. H., Fields, H. L., Three bulbospinal pathways from rostral medulla of the cat: an autoradiographic study of pain modulating systems. J. comp. Neurol. *178* (1978), 209—224.
8. Basbaum, A. I., Clanton, C. H., Fields, H. L., Opiate and stimulus produced analgesia: functional anatomy of a medullospinal pathway. Proc. Nat. Acad. Sci. (Wash.) *73* (1976), 4685—4688.
9. Basbaum, A. I., Marley, N. J. E., O'Keefe, J., Clanton, C. H., Reversal of morphine and stimulus-produced analgesia by subtotal spinal cord lesions. Pain *3* (1977), 43—56.
10. Belcher, G., Ryall, R. W., Schaffner, R., The differential effects of 5-hydroxytryptamine, noradrenaline and Raphé stimulation on nociceptive and non-nociceptive horn interneurones in the cat. Brain Res. *151* (1978), 307—321.
11. Berman, A. L., The Brain Stem of the Cat. A Cytoarchitectonic Atlas with Stereotaxic Coordinates. Madison, Wisc.: Univ. of Wisconsin Press. 1968.
12. Besson, J. M., Le Bars, D., Oliveras, J. L., L'analgésie morphinique: données neurobiologiques. Ann. Anesth. Franç. XIX, *5* (1978), 343—369.
13. Bobillier, P., Seguin, S., Petitjean, F., Salvert, D., Touret, M., Jouvet, M., The raphé nuclei of the cat brain stem: a topographical atlas of their efferent projections as revealed by autoradiography. Brain Res. *113* (1976), 449—486.
14. Brodal, A., Taber, E., Walberg, F., The raphé nuclei of the brain stem in the cat: II. Efferent connections. J. comp. Neurol. *114* (1960), 239—359.
15. Carstens, E., Klumpp, D., Zimmermann, M., The opiate antagonist, Naloxone, does not affect descending inhibition from midbrain of nociceptive spinal neuronal discharges in the cat. Neurosci. Letters *11* (1979), 323—327.
16. Dahlström, A., Fuxe, K., Evidence for the existence of monoamine neurons in the central nervous system. II. Experimentally induced changes in the intraneuronal amine levels of bulbospinal neuron systems. Acta physiol. scand. *64*, Suppl. 247 (1965), 5—36.
17. Dewey, W. L., Harris, L. S., Howes, J. F., Nuite, J. A., The effect of various neurohumoral modulators on the activity of morphine and the narcotic antagonists in the tail-flick and phenylquinone tests. J. Pharmacol. Exp. Ther. *175* (1970), 435—442.
18. Dickenson, A. H., Oliveras, J. L., Besson, J. M., Role of the nucleus raphé magnus in opiate analgesia as studied by the microinjection technique in the rat. Brain Res. *170* (1979), 95—111.
19. Duggan, A. W., Griersmith, B. I., Inhibition of the spinal transmission of nociceptive information by supraspinal stimulation in the cat. Pain *6* (1979), 149—161.
20. Duggan, A. W., Hall, J. H., Headley, P. M., Griersmith, B. T., The effect of Naloxone on the excitation of dorsal horn neurons of the cat by noxious and non-noxious cutaneous stimuli. Brain Res. *138* (1977), 185—189.
21. Fennessy, M. R., Lee, J. R., Modification of morphine analgesia by drugs affecting adrenergic and tryptaminergic mechanisms. J. Pharm. Pharmacol. *22* (1970), 930—935.
22. Fields, H. L., Anderson, S. D., Evidence that raphé-spinal mediate opiate and midbrain stimulation-produced analgesia. Pain *5* (1978), 333—349.

23. Fields, H. L., Basbaum, A. I., Brain stem control of spinal pain transmission neurons. Ann. Rev. Physiol. *40* (1978), 193—221.

24. Fields, H. L., Basbaum, A. I., Clanton, C. H., Anderson, S. D., Nucleus raphé magnus inhibition of spinal cord dorsal horn neurons. Brain Res. *126* (1977), 441—453.

25. Garau, L., Mulas, M. L., Pepeu, G., The influence of raphé lesions on the effect of morphine on nociception and cortical Ach output. Neuropharmacology *14* (1975), 259—263.

26. Genovese, E., Zonta, N., Mantegazza, P., Decreased antinociceptive activity of morphine in rats pretreated intraventricularly with 5.6-dihydroxytryptamine a long-lasting selective depletor of brain serotonin. Psychopharmacology *32* (1973), 359—364.

27. Goodman, S. J., Holcombe, V., Selective and Prolonged Analgesia in Monkey Resulting from Brain Stimulation. In: Advances in Pain Research and Therapy, Vol. 1, pp. 495—502 (Bonica, J. J., Albe-Fessard, D., eds.). 1976.

28. Görlitz, B., Frey, H., Central monoamines and antinociceptive drug action. Europ. J. Pharmacol. *20* (1972), 171—180.

29. Guilbaud, G., Besson, J. M., Oliveras, J. L., Liebeskind, J. C., Suppression by LSD of the inhibitory effect exerted by dorsal raphé stimulation on certain spinal cord interneurons in the cat. Brain Res. *61* (1973), 417—422.

30. Guilbaud, G., Oliveras, J. L., Giesler, G., Jr., Besson, J. M., Effects induced by stimulation of the centralis inferior nucleus of the raphé on dorsal horn interneurons in cat's spinal cord. Brain Res. *126* (1977), 355—360.

31. Hayes, R. L., Newlon, P. G., Rosecrans, J. A., Mayer, D. J., Reduction of stimulation-produced analgesia by lysergic acid diethylamide depressor of serotonergic neural activity. Brain Res. *122* (1977), 367—372.

32. Headley, P. M., Duggan, A. W., Griersmith, B. T., Selective reduction by noradrenaline and 5-hydroxytryptamine of nociceptive responses of cat dorsal horn neurones. Brain Res. *145* (1978), 185—189.

33. Hökfelt, T., Ljungdahl, A., Terenius, L., Elde, R., Nilsson, G., Immunohistochemical analysis of peptide pathways possibly related to pain and analgesia: enkephalin and substance P. Proc. Natl. Acad. Sci. (Wash.) *74* (1977), 3081—3085.

34. Hong, J. S., Yang, H. Y. T., Fratta, W., Costa, E., Determination of methionin enkephalin in discrete regions of rat brain. Brain Res. *134* (1977), 383—386.

35. Hosobuchi, Y., Tryptophan reversal of tolerance to analgesia induced by central gray stimulation. Lancet 2 (1978), 47.

36. Hosobuchi, Y, Adams, J. E., Linchitz, R., Pain relief by electrical stimulation of central gray matter in humans. Science *197* (1977), 183—186.

37. Hosobuchi, Y., Rossier, J., Bloom, J. E., Guillemin, R., Stimulation of human periaqueductal gray for pain relief increase immunoreactive beta-endorphin in ventricular fluid. Science *203* (1979), 279—281.

38. Jordan, L. M., Kenshalo, D. R., Martin, R. F., Haber, L. H., Willis, W. D., Depression of primate spinothalamic tract neurons by iontophoretic application of 5-hydroxytryptamine. Pain *5* (1978), 135—142.

39. Keller, O., Vycklicky, L., Sykova, E., Reflexes from Aδ and Aα trigeminal afferents. Brain Res. *37* (1972), 330—332.

40. Le Bars, D., Menétrey, D., Besson, J. M., Effects of morphine upon the lamina V type cell activities in the dorsal horn of decerebrate cat. Brain Res. *113* (1976), 293—310.

41. Lee, J. R., Fennessy, M. R., The relationship between morphine analgesia and the levels of biogenic amines in the mouse brain. Europ. J. Pharmacol. *12* (1970), 65—70.
42. Liebeskind, J. C., Giesler, G., Jr., Urca, G., Evidence Pertaining to an Endogenous Mechanism of Pain Inhibition in the Central Nervous System. In: Sensory Functions of the Skin in Primates, pp. 561—573 (Zotterman, I., ed.). Pergamon Press. 1976.
43. Liebeskind, J. C., Guilbaud, G., Besson, J. M., Oliveras, J. L., Analgesia from electrical stimulation of the periaqueductal gray matter in the cat: behavioral observations and inhibitory effects on spinal cord interneurons. Brain Res. *50* (1973), 441—446.
44. Lovick, T. A., West, D. C., Wolstencroft, J. H., Interactions Between Brain Stem Nuclei and the Trigeminal System. In: Pain in the Trigeminal Region, pp. 307—317 (Anderson and Matthews, eds.). Elsevier: North-Holland Biomedical Press. 1977.
45. Lovick, T. A., West, D. C., Wolstencroft, J. H., Responses of raphé spinal and other bulbar raphé neurones to stimulation of the periaqueductal gray in the cat. Neurosci. Letters *8* (1978), 45—49.
46. Martin, R. F., Jordan, L. M., Willis, W. D., Differential projections of cat medullary raphé neurons demonstrated by retrograde labelling following spinal cord lesions. J. comp. Neurol. *182* (1978), 77—88.
47. Mayer, D. J., Hayes, R., Stimulation-produced analgesia: development of tolerance and cross-tolerance to morphine. Science *188* (1975), 941—943.
48. Mayer, D. J., Liebeskind, J. C., Pain reduction by focal electrical stimulation of the brain: an anatomical and behavioral analysis. Brain Res. *68* (1974), 73—93.
49. Mayer, D. J., Price, D. D., Central nervous system mechanisms of analgesia. Pain *2* (1976), 379—404.
50. Mayer, D. J., Wolfe, T. L., Akil, H., Carder, B., Liebeskind, J. C., Analgesia from electrical stimulation in the brainstem of the rat. Science *174* (1971), 1351—1354.
51. McCreery, D. B., Bloedel, J. R., Reduction of the response of cat spinothalamic neurons to graded mechanical stimuli by electrical stimulation of the lower brain stem. Brain Res. *97* (1975), 151—156.
52. Menétrey, D., Chaouch, A., Besson, J. M., Location and properties of lumbar spinoreticular tract neurons in the rat. Neurosci. Letters J. Neurophysiol. (in press).
53. Oliveras, J. L., Besson, J. M., Guilbaud, G., Liebeskind, J. C., Behavioral and electrophysiological evidence of pain inhibition from midbrain stimulation in the cat. Exp. Brain Res. *20* (1974), 32—44.
54. Oliveras, J. L., Bourgoin, S., Hery, F., Besson, J. M., Hamon, M., The topographical distribution of serotoninergic terminals in the spinal cord of the cat: Biochemical mapping by the combined use of microdissection and microassay procedures. Brain Res. *138* (1977), 393—406.
55. Oliveras, J. L., Guilbaud, G., Besson, J. M., A map of serotoninergic structures involved in stimulation producing analgesia in unrestrained freely moving cats. Brain Res. *164* (1979), 317—322.
56. Oliveras, J. L., Hosobuchi, Y., Bruxelles, J., Passot, C., Besson, J. M., Analgesic effects induced by electrical stimulation of the nucleus raphé magnus in the rat: interaction with morphine analgesia. Abstracts 7th international Congress of Pharmacology (Paris), Vol. 1, No. 280, 1978.

57. Oliveras, J. L., Hosobuchi, Y., Guilbaud, G., Besson, J. M., Analgesia electrical stimulation of the feline nucleus raphé magnus: development of tolerance and its reversal by 5-HTP. Brain Res. *146* (1978), 404—409.
58. Oliveras, J. L., Hosobuchi, Y., Redjemi, F., Guilbaud, G., Besson, J. M., Opiate antagonist, naloxone, strongly reduces analgesia induced by stimulation of a raphé nucleus (centralis inferior). Brain Res. *120* (1977), 221—229.
59. Oliveras, J. L., Redjemi, F., Guilbaud, G., Besson, J. M., Analgesia induced by electrical stimulation of the inferior centralis nucleus of the raphé in the cat. Pain *1* (1975), 139—245.
60. Oliveras, J. L., Woda, A., Guilbaud, G., Besson, J. M., Inhibition of the jaw opening reflex by electrical stimulation of the periaqueductal gray matter in the awake, unrestrained cat. Brain Res. *72* (1974), 328—331.
61. Proudfit, H. K., Anderson, E. G., Morphine analgesia: blockade by raphé magnus lesions. Brain Res. *98* (1975), 612—618.
62. Randić, M., Yu, H. H., Effects of 5-Hydroxytryptamine and bradykinin in cat dorsal horn neurones activated by noxious stimuli. Brain Res. *111* (1976), 197—203.
63. Reynolds, D. V., Surgery in the rat during electrical analgesia induced by focal brain stimulation. Science *164* (1969), 444—445.
64. Richardson, D. E., Akil, H., Pain reduction by electrical brain stimulation in man: chronic self-stimulation in the periaqueductal gray matter. J. Neurosurg. *47* (1977), 184—194.
65. Rivot, J. P., Chaouch, A., Besson, J. M., Caractéristiques électrophysiologiques et pharmacologiques du contrôle exercé par le noyau raphé magnus sur la transmission spinale des messages nociceptifs. J. Physiol. (Paris) (in press).
66. Rivot, J. P., Chaouch, A., Besson, J. M., The influence of Naloxone on the C fiber response of dorsal horn neurons and their inhibitory control by raphé magnus stimulation. Brain Res. *176* (1979), 355—364.
67. Ruda, M. A., Autoradiographic examination of the efferent projections of the midbrain central gray in the cat. Ph.D. Dissertation, University of Pennsylvania (1976).
68. Samanin, R., Gumulka, M., Valzelli, L., Reduced effect of morphine in midbrain raphé lesioned rats. Europ. J. Pharmacol. *10* (1970), 339—343.
69. Sasa, M., Munekiyo, K., Osumi, Y., Takaori, S., Attenuation of morphine analgesia in rats with lesions of the locus coeruleus and dorsal Raphé Nucleus. Europ. J. Pharmacol. *42* (1977), 53—62.
70. Sasa, M., Munekiyo, K., Takaori, S., Dorsal raphé stimulation produced inhibitory effect on trigeminal nucleus neurons. Brain Res. *101* (1975), 199—207.
71. Sessle, B. J., Dubner, R., Greenwood, L. F., Lucier, G. E., Descending influences of periaqueductal gray matter and somatosensory cerebral cortex on neurones in trigeminal brain stem nuclei. Canad. J. Physiol. Pharmacol. *54* (1976), 66—69.
72. Sewell, R. D. E., Spencer, P. S. J., Modification of the antinociceptive activity of narcotic agonists and antagonists by intraventricular injection of biogenic amines in mice. Brit. J. Pharmacol. *51* (1974), 140P—141P.
73. Sherrington, C. S., Reflexes elicitable in the cat from pinna, vibrissae and jaws. J. Physiol. (Lond.) *51* (1917), 404—431.
74. Snyder, S. H., Simantov, R., The opiate receptor and opioid peptides. J. Neurochem. *28* (1977), 13—20.
75. Sparkes, C. G., Spencer, P. S. G., Antinociceptive activity of morphine after injection of biogenic amines in the cerebral ventricles of the conscious rat. Brit. J. Pharmacol. *42* (1971), 230—241.

76. Tenen, S. S., Antagonism of the analgesic effect of morphine and other drugs by p-chlorophenylalanine, a serotonin depletor. Psychopharmacologia (Berl.) *12* (1968), 278—285.
77. Vogt, M., The effect of lowering the 5-hydroxytryptamine content of the rat spinal cord on analgesia produced by morphine. J. Physiol. (Lond.) *236* (1974), 483—498.
78. Willis, W. D., Haber, L. H., Martin, R. F., Inhibition of spinothalamic tract cells and interneurons by brainstem stimulation in the monkey. J. Neurophysiol. *40* (1977), 968—981.
79. Yaksh, T. L., Du Chateau, J. C., Rudy, T. A., Antagonism by methysergide and cinanserin of the antinociceptive action of morphine administered into the periaqueductal gray. Brain Res. *104* (1976), 367—372.
80. Yaksh, T. L., Plant, R. L., Rudy, T. A., Studies of the antagonism by raphé lesions of the antinociceptive action of systemic morphine. Eur. J. Pharmacol. *41* (1977), 399—408.
81. Yaksh, T. L., Rudy, T. A., Narcotic analgetics: CNS sites and mechanisms of action as revealed by intracerebral injection techniques. Pain *4* (1978), 299—359.
82. Yokota, T., Hashimoto, S., Periaqueductal gray and tooth pulp afferent interaction on units in caudal medulla oblongata. Brain Res. *117* (1976), 508—512.

Acta Neurochirurgica, Suppl. 30, 219—227 (1980)

The Current Status of Analgesic Brain Stimulation

Y. Hosobuchi*

Summary

This paper reviews the author's nine years of experience in analgesic brain stimulation. During this time, of 22 patients with pain of peripheral origin who were treated with periaqueductal gray (PAG), stimulation 16 achieved successful control of pain. Of 40 patients who presented with deafferentation pain, 16 were able to control their dysesthesia by brain stimulation of the subcortical somatosensory region alone; follow-up was over a long period. The mechanism of deafferentation pain is poorly understood and the effectiveness of subcortical somatosensory electrical stimulation to relieve such pain is based on empirical observation. The analgesia produced by PAG stimulation appears to be mediated by the release of beta-endorphin from the anterior hypothalamus. The released beta-endorphin binds to the opiate receptors in the PAG and activates the descending pain-inhibitory pathway. However, the repetitive stimulation of this serotonergic system produces tolerance to its analgesic effect, due to a decreased rate of serotonin turnover. Loading of the serotonin precursor by dietary supplementation of the essential amino acid L-tryptophan reverses this tolerance.

Keywords: Brain stimulation; endorphin; serotonin; analgesia.

Introduction

Since my initial report on the stimulation of N. Posterior ventralis medialis (PVM) of the thalamus for the control of facial anaesthesia dolorosa in 1973 [11], two subcortical areas have been used as the loci of electrical stimulation for analgesia in humans. First, the somatosensory areas (medial lemniscus, sensory nuclei of thalamus—both PVM and Posterior ventralis lateralis (PVL)—and the posterior limb of the internal capsule) were stimulated for the control of deafferentation pain [1, 11, 14, 16]. Second, the periaqueductal and periventricular areas (PAG) were selected as the stimulation sites for pain originating from peripheral noxious stimuli [10, 18]. This report reviews the results obtained, since 1970, from the stimulation of both these areas in 62 patients.

---

* Department of Neurological Surgery, University of California, San Francisco, CA 94143, U.S.A.

0065-1419/80/Suppl. 30/0219/$ 01.80

Materials and Methods

The subjects selected for this review are 62 patients in whom the author implanted brain electrodes for control of their pain between January 1970 and December 1978. They have been followed for 6 months to 9½ years.

The patients selected for this procedure were experiencing severe and chronic intractable pain. Medication, including opiates in large doses, was ineffective in controlling their pain. The analgesic brain stimulation technique was chosen over ablative surgical procedures because of the nature of their pain, since the latter procedure was not likely to reduce their pain, and carries the increased risk of neurological deficit that can be more disturbing than the original pain.

Table 1. *DBS Results: Deafferentation Pain*

	Total number	I.C.	S.Th.	Med. Lemn.	Initial results		Internalized results	
					Success	Failure	Success	Failure
Thalamic pain	11	11			6	5	4	2
Anaesthesia dolorosa	9		9	1 °	4 * °	5	3	1
Post-herpetic neuralgia	3		3		1	2	1 *	
Brachial plexus lesion	4	2	1	1	3	1	2 *	1
Paraplegia	6	5		1	2	4	1	1
Phantom limb pain	2	2			1	1	1 *	
Post-cordotomy dysaesthesia	5	4		1	4	1	4 *	
Total	40	24	13	4	21	19	16	5

Abbreviations: *DBS* deep brain stimulation; *I.C.* internal capsule; *S.Th.* sensory thalamus; *Med. Lemn.* medial lemniscus.

* Patients having total or almost complete pain relief with less than 6 months of stimulation (a total of 7 patients, 3 with post-cordotomy dysaesthesia).

° One patient had a good result with S.Th. (VPM) stimulation for 11 months, then developed a nodal current leak. A new electrode was inserted into the Med. Lemn. but stimulation controlled her pain for only 3 months.

Forty patients were suffering from deafferentation pain (Table 1), and the other 22 patients had pain of peripheral origin (Table 2). A detailed description of the multicontact electrodes implanted in the brain, the stereotactic coordinates of the stimulation site, and surgical technique has been published elsewhere [1, 10, 11]. A wire connected to the implanted electrodes was brought to the external surface of the body temporarily to test the analgesic effectiveness of brain stimulation. It was internalized when its effectiveness was apparent to both the patient and our medical staff.

Results

Brain stimulation was considered to be therapeutically successful only if the patient was able to control the pain by stimulation alone, or with additional disulfiram, L-tryptophan, or mild sedatives. If any analgesic agents except salicylates or acetaminophen were needed in addition, brain stimulation was considered to be a failure.

Table 2. *DBS Results: PAGS for Pain of Peripheral Origin*

Etiology of pain	Number of patients	Results *		Comments on failures
		Success	Failure	
Cancer	5	3	2	one case, not internalized: L-tryptophan-reversible. Another case, total tolerance after 2 months
Chronic low back pain	14	12	2	one case, subgaleal infection. Another case, total tolerance after 20 months
Non-malignant abdominal pain	1		1	one case, total tolerance after 14 months
Atypical facial pain	1	1		
Osteoporosis of spine	1		1	one case, total tolerance after 4 months
Total	22	16	6	

* All but one [21] were internalized.

As summarized in Table 1, only 50% of the patients with deafferentation pain had their electrodes internalized. Of those, only 15 were considered to be successful on a long-term basis; however, 7 of these 15 patients reported total or nearly total disappearance of their original dysaesthesia within 6 months of continuous stimulation (the earliest disappearance occurred in 2 weeks). Pain has never recurred in these patients and they no longer need brain stimulation. This observation is in accord with the results reported by Mazar [14]. Overall, postcordotomy dysaesthesia responded well to brain stimulation, despite our original report that the results in facial anaesthesia dolorosa were rather disappointing [11].

None of the patients with deafferentation pain responded to PAG stimulation (Table 3). Stimulation of the posterior limb of the internal capsule produced a better response than stimulation of the sensory nuclei of the thalamus. Despite limited experience with stimulation of the medial lemniscus, as suggested by Mundinger [16], this site may be worth exploring in the future for this difficult pain syndrome.

In contrast to deafferentation pain, pain of peripheral origin responded well to PAG stimulation. This technique's long-term results continue to improve since the introduction, in recent years, of the adjunctive use of disulfiram and L-tryptophan to reverse tolerance to the analgesic effect of PAG stimulation. These drugs also potentiate analgesia produced by stimulation and thus reduce the frequency of stimulation required. The results of PAG stimulation are summarized in Table 2.

The causes of failure in analgesic brain stimulation are listed in Table 4. A delayed death occurred (4 months postoperatively) in one patient with ventricular haemorrhage due to myocardial infarction.

Discussion

The analgesic effect of stimulation of the subcortical somatosensory area on deafferentation pain was discovered empirically. The neurophysiological basis of deafferentation pain is still unknown, although one common characteristic is poor response to opiates. Further discussion of analgesic brain stimulation for the control of deafferentation pain can be found in previous publications [1, 11, 14].

Significant relief from severe, intractable pain of peripheral origin is obtained by electrical stimulation of the PAG [10, 18], which induces an increase in the endorphin concentration in cerebrospinal fluid [2, 12, 15]. The effectiveness of PAG stimulation is, however, compromised by the development of tolerance [10]; it has been reported that this entails a cross-tolerance to opiates [10]. Analgesia induced by PAG stimulation is totally reversed by the specific opiate antagonist Naloxone [2, 10].

Analgesia induced by PAG stimulation is potentiated by disulfiram, which inhibits noradrenalin synthesis and thus prevents the development of tolerance. Once tolerance develops, however, it can be reversed only by abstinence from PAG stimulation, and not by disulfiram [13]. Stimulation-induced analgesia is known to be: 1. mediated by the descending pain-inhibitory system originating from the raphé nuclei of the brain stem, and 2. serotonergic [3]. On this basis, the author administered L-tryptophan, a precursor of serotonin (5-HT), to stimulation-tolerant patients. Dietary supplementation with 4.5 gm L-tryptophan daily reversed the tolerant state [9].

The endorphin concentration in human cerebrospinal fluid (CSF) has been reported to be increased by PAG stimulation [2, 12, 15]. In the rat brain, fibres immunoreactive for beta-endorphin project from cell bodies in the basal tuberal hypothalamus into the PAG [4]. Along this pathway, the fibres are denser around the wall of the third ventricle, especially near its anterior aspect. Since the

Table 3. *DBS Results: Target-Point Analysis for Deafferentation Pain*

	Long-term success vs. total implantations	Rate of success
I.C.	9/24	37.5%
S.Th.	3/13	23%
Med.Lemn.	3/4	75%
PAG	0/17	0%

Table 4. *The Causes of Failure in Somatosensory Target*

A. Initial phase	
No pain relief	9
Unable to locate target	3
Electrode shift	2
Increased pain by stimulation	2
Ventricular haemorrhage	2
Huge cortical veins	1
B. Late phase	
No pain relief	3
Pain increased by stimulation	1
Infection (subgaleal abscess and meningitis)	1

anterior part of the rat hypothalamus exhibits the highest concentration of assayable beta-endorphin [21], it seems quite possible that the beta-endorphin found in human CSF could come from beta-endorphin-containing cells densely pocked in the anterior hypothalamus. Electrical stimulation of the PAG may cause the release of beta-endorphin from the anterior hypothalamus by antidromic stimulation. The analgesic action may then be initiated by the binding of the released beta-endorphin to opiate receptors in the PAG.

The delay of a few minutes between the onset of PAG stimulation and the initiation of analgesia in humans [10] suggests that a humoral component or neuromodulator, such as beta-endorphin, is involved. Following PAG stimulation, beta-endorphin is released into human ventricular CSF, where there is a simultaneous elevation in the level of 4,5 K-ACTH. We have, in fact, ample evidence to suggest that pro-opiocortin (31 K-ACTH), the common precursor of beta-endorphin and 4,5 K-ACTH, is released in humans by PAG stimulation [8]. Rose and co-workers demonstrated that PAG stimulation in dogs induced a delayed elevation of levels of ACTH in the blood [19] (and, interestingly, that stress-induced release of ACTH was inhibited by electrical stimulation of the locus ceruleus and the nucleus sublocus

Table 5. *Beta-Endorphin Level in Ventricular Fluid (pg/ml)*

Patient	Immediately after implantation				Tolerance stage				After L-Tryptophan treatment (4.5 gm/qd, 2 wks)			
	Control	15′ *	30′ **	60′ ***	Control	15′	10′	60′	Control	15′	10′	60′
A	60	220	160	110	62	129	91	80	278	641	765	580
B	NC				70	61	76	55	241	710	1,013	NC
C	NC				40	91	77	108	276	966	1,011	1,065
Blood level of trypto-phan	1.2–1.6 mg/dl				1.1–1.6 mg/dl				1.9–2.7 mg/dl			

Control—CSF sample prior to stimulation.
* CSF sample immediately after 15 min PAG stimulation.
** CSF sample 30 min after the cessation of stimulation.
*** CSF sample 60 min after the cessation of stimulation.
NC CSF sample not collected.

ceruleus, or noradrenergic centre [20]. Because of the multitude of neuronal connections from the PAG to the anterior hypothalamus, the release of 31 K-ACTH may not simply be mediated by antidromic activation of beta-endorphin-containing neurons, but may be due to orthodromic stimulation of other neuronal connections. Our preliminary study (Table 5) shows that the basal ventricular fluid level of beta-endorphin is significantly reduced in stimulation-tolerant humans, and PAG stimulation of these patients produces only a small rise in their ventricular fluid level of beta-endorphin. Normal beta-endorphin levels and response to PAG stimulation appear, however, to be restored by dietary supplementation with L-tryptophan (Table 5). This observation, if correct, suggests that the effect of PAG stimulation on the hypothalamus may well be mediated by serotonergic neurones.

It is probable that chronic PAG stimulation induces a depressed rate of serotonin turnover in these serotonergic neurones. The reported cross-tolerance to opiates can be explained by the fact that serotonin and opiates have common descending pain-inhibitory pathways from brain stem raphé nuclei to the spinal dorsal root entry zone. Despite the development of tolerance to stimulation, the pain still responds to a higher dose of opiates because of the opiate's direct action at the spinal level.

Table 6. *5-HIAA in CSF Tolerance to Opiate and During Stimulation to Produced Analgesia (SPA): The Effects of Probenecid*

	No. of cases tested	Baseline (ng/ml)	After 4 hours of probenecid (ng/ml)
Control	4	28 ± 1	120 ± 7
After L-tryptophan 4.5 gm/day/2 wks		40 ± 4	211 ± 14
Opiate-tolerant	4	25 ± 25	59 ± 6
After L-tryptophan 4.5 gm/day/2 wks		39 ± 5.1	209 ± 8
SPA tolerant	2	27	64
After L-tryptophan 4.5 gm/day/2 wks		40	212

Since it is known that the rate of serotonin synthesis in the neurones is determined by the enzyme tryptophan-hydroxylase [6], we assume that loading the system with a serotonin precursor by dietary supplementation with L-tryptophan serves to enhance the rate of metabolic turnover of serotonin [5]. It is highly probable that what induces this tolerance to chronic stimulation is decreased turnover of serotonin in both the rostral and caudal systems. A further indication of involvement of the caudal limb or the descending pain-inhibitory system is the development of cross-tolerance to opiates in stimulation-tolerant individuals; the pain *does* still respond to higher doses of opiates because of the opiate's "direct action at the spinal level" [3]. Neff, Tozer, and Brodie demonstrated that the active transport of 5-hydroxyindolacetic acid (5-HIAA) (the main degradation product of 5-HT) from the brain to the bloodstream could be blocked by probenecid, so that the rate of accumulation of 5-HIAA in CSF could be used to calculate the turnover rate of 5-HT in the central nervous system [17]. Our recent preliminary study using a probenecid technique shows the marked depression of 5-HT turnover in opiate-tolerant cancer patients and PAG stimulation-tolerant patients. The reversal of the tolerant state by the administration of the serotonin precursor L-tryptophan is accompanied by a marked increase in 5-HT turnover (Table 6) [22].

It is thus apparent that analgesia produced by PAG stimulation closely resembles that of opiates. It is the author's contention, therefore, that if the patient is to be benefitted by PAG stimulation, he or she must have total relief of pain by the analgesic action of opiate, not by its euphoric action [7]. On this basis, the patient can be screened by intravenously administering morphine before electrode implantation surgery to forecast the outcome of PAG stimulation. The patient who has developed tolerance to opiates or the patient suffering from deafferentation pain will not obtain total pain relief either by morphine [7] or by PAG stimulation.

Acknowledgement

The author wishes to thank Dr. Floyd E. Bloom of the Salk Institute for his kind assistance in performing the radioimmunoassay for beta-endorphin.

References

1. Adams, J. E., Hosobuchi, Y., Fields, H., Stimulation of internal capsule for relief of chronic pain. J. Neurosurg. *41* (1975), 740—744.
2. Akil, H., Richardson, D. E., Hughes, J., Barchas, J. P., Enkephalin-like material elevated in ventricular cerebrospinal fluid of pain patients after analgesic focal stimulation. Science *201* (1978), 463—465.
3. Basbaum, A. L., Field, H. L., Endogenous pain control mechanisms: Review and hypothesis. Anal. Neurol. *4* (1978), 451—462.
4. Bloom, F., Battenberg, E., Rossier, J., Ling, N., Guillemin, R., Neurons containing beta-endorphin in rat brain exist separately from those containing enkephalin: immunocytochemical studies. Proc. Natl. Acad. Sci. U.S.A. *75* (1978), 1591—1595.
5. Fernstrom, J. D., Nortman, R. J., Control of brain serotonin levels by the diet. Adv. Biochem. Psychopharmacol. *11* (1974), 133—142.
6. Gal, E. M., Poczik, M., Marshall, F. D. J., Hydroxylation of tryptophan to 5-hydroxytryptophan by brain tissue in vivo. Biochem. Biophys. Res. Commun. *12* (1963), 39.
7. Hosobuchi, Y., Pain Control by Activation of the Endorphin System by Periaqueductal Gray Stimulation. In: Current Concepts in the Treatment of Pain. Springfield, Ill.: Ch. C Thomas (in press).
8. Hosobuchi, Y., Elevation of Beta-Endorphin-Like Substances and Pro-Opiocortin (31 K ACTH). In: Alteration in Brain Function, pp. 57—63 (Hitchcock, E. R., ed.). Elsevier: North Holland. 1979.
9. Hosobuchi, Y., Tryptophan reversal of tolerance to analgesia induced by central gray stimulation. Lancet *2* (1978), 47.
10. Hosobuchi, Y., Adams, J. E., Linchitz, R., Pain relief by electrical stimulation of centray gray matter in humans. Science *197* (1977), 183—186.

11. Hosobuchi, Y., Adams, J. E., Rutkin, B., Chronic thalamic stimulation for the control of facial anesthesia dolorosa. Arch. Neurol. *29* (1973), 158—162.
12. Hosobuchi, Y., Rossier, J., Bloom, J. E., Guillemin, R., Stimulation of human periaqueductal gray for pain relief increases immunoreactive beta-endorphin in ventricular fluid. Science *201* (1979), 279—281.
13. Hosobuchi, Y., Wemmer, J., Disulfiram inhibition of development of tolerance to analgesia induced by central gray stimulation in humans. Eur. J. Pharmacol. *43* (1977), 385—387.
14. Mazars, G. J., Intermittent stimulation of nucleus ventralis posterolateralis for intractable pain. Surg. Neurol. *4* (1975), 93—95.
15. Meyerson, B. A., Boethius, J., Terenius, L., Wahlstrom, A., Paper presented at the third meeting of the European Society for Stereotaxic and Functional Neurosurgery, Freiburg, September 19, 1977.
16. Mundinger, F., Results of brain stimulation presented at 3rd European Workshop on Neurostimulation. Mégève, France, March 30—31, 1979.
17. Neff, N. H., Tozer, T. N., Brodie, B. B., Application of steady state kinetics to studies of the transfer of 5-hydroxyindolacetic acid from brain to plasma. J. Pharmacol. Exp. Ther. *158* (1967), 214—218.
18. Richardson, D. E., Akil, H., Pain reduction by electrical brain stimulation in man: Chronic self-stimulation in the periaqueductal gray matter. J. Neurosurg. *47* (1977), 184—194.
19. Rose, J. C., Goldsmith, P. C., Lovinger, R., Anbert, M. C., Kaplan, S. L., Ganong, W. F., Effect of electrical stimulation of canine diencephalon on the secretion of ACTH, growth hormone (GH), and prolactin (P). Neuroendocrinology *23* (1979), 223—235.
20. Rose, J. C., Goldsmith, P. C., Ganong, W. F., Inhibition of stress-induced ACTH secretion by electrical stimulation of the brain stem in dogs. Fed. Proc. *35* (1976), 1172.
21. Rossier, J., Vargo, T. M., Minick, S., Ling, N., Bloom, F. E., Guillemin, R., Regional disassociation of beta-endorphin and encephalin contents in rat brain and pituitary. Proc. Natl. Acad. Sci. U.S.A. *74* (1977), 1562—1565.
22. Van Praag, H. M., Korf, J., Monoamine Metabolism in Depression: Clinical Applications of the Probenecid Test. In: Serotonin and Behavior (Barchas, J., Usedin, E., eds.). New York: Academic Press. 1973.

Acta Neurochirurgica, Suppl. 30, 229—237 (1980)

Biochemistry of Pain Relief with Intracerebral Stimulation

Few Facts and Many Hypotheses

B. A. Meyerson*

Summary

On the basis of data obtained from subprimates subjected to acute pain stimuli, it has been hypothesized that the suppression of chronic pain in man during stimulation in the periventricular region involves endogenous opioid mechanisms. However, there is at present no direct and unequivocal proof that the pain relief in man is necessarily and entirely dependent upon such mechanisms. There exist several putative substances with opiate-like properties but they are difficult to identify. The assay methods lack specificity and cross-reactions are common. There are only a few studies published on the influence of intracerebral stimulation in man on the CSF-content of opioid substances; the changes observed are inconsistent, and data are only given on patients having satisfactory pain relief. Furthermore, measurements have been made only during the course of a few hours and nothing is reported on the relationship between the changing concentrations of the substance and the level of pain. The observation that Naloxone may reverse the effect of intracerebral stimulation has become the keystone in postulating common mechanisms for stimulation-produced pain relief and morphine analgesia. The fact, that Naloxone is sometime ineffective or has to be used in huge, and unphysiological, doses is generally disregarded. There are a number of substances which may serve as neurotransmittors in pain transmission and pain inhibition but their mode of action in the generation and suppression of chronic pain is entirely unknown. Data collected from various European clinics covering more than 200 patients subjected to intracerebral stimulation show that the outcome of this treatment is highly unpredictable. Intracerebral stimulation as a clinically useful treatment of chronic pain can not be further developed unless hard data on its biochemical background in man are provided.

Keywords: Pain; brain stimulation; endorphin.

One of the main reasons why stimulation-produced analgesia (SPA) in animals, as well periventricular stimulation for pain in patients, has come into the focus of interest in pain research is the fact

---

* Department of Neurosurgery, Karolinska sjukhuset, S-104 01 Stockholm-60, Sweden.

0065-1419/80/Suppl. 30/0229/$ 01.80

that both these phenomena have been linked to the discovery of neurotransmitters or neuromodulators with morphine-like properties. Today, a host of data has accumulated on the biochemical background to SPA in animals, and it has been proven beyond doubt that the endogenous opioids are at least partially involved. It has been taken for granted that similar mechanisms are responsible for pain relief with periventricular stimulation in man. It is not until the last two years that some data have been available to substantiate this assumption. However, we have to realize that most of the evidence presented is still indirect. In this article, these recent data will be briefly reviewed. Unfortunately, very little can at present be said about the neurohumoural basis for other types of central nervous stimulation for pain, such as stimulation of the lemniscal system at the level of the dorsal columns of the spinal cord or of the sensory nuclei of thalamus as well as of the sensory part of the internal capsule. At present, there is nothing indicating that endogenous opioids are involved [22].

The analysis of the possible physiological mechanisms for pain relief during periventricular stimulation is primarily based on data derived from experiments on animals, almost exclusively on subprimates. Caution is warranted when applying animal data to man, and therapeutic periventricular stimulation and SPA in animals are in some respects fundamentally different. It suffices here to point out two of these differences. First is the rather trivial—though often neglected—fact that SPA in animals refers to acute, induced pain whereas in patients one is dealing with chronic pain. There are conflicting reports about pain thresholds and tolerance in patients during periventricular stimulation but in any case such effects are minimal and not at all comparable to what can be achieved in animals, which are rendered analgetic in the true sense of the word [8, 11, 27]. Secondly, in virtually all animal experiments stimulation has been performed in the periaqueductal region and in the raphé nuclei complex deep in the brain stem. For obvious reasons these regions are not accessible in the patient where stimulation has been restricted to the caudal part of the diencephalon and sometimes to the border region of the rostral mesencephalon. In animals the site of stimulation is critical [23]. This is the case also in patients, particularly with regard to medio-lateral location [1, 20, 21]. There are hardly any data on the extent of the area susceptible to stimulation in subhuman primates and it is not until recently that the diencephalic region has been explored in the rat [28]. That study is of particular interest as it demonstrated that analgesia could be evoked with stimulation applied to sites homologous to those where pain relief may be obtained in patients.

Distribution of Receptors and Endogenous Opioids

In animals there are several lines of evidence that support the involvement of the endogenous opioids in SPA. One is the overlap in the anatomical distribution of opioid receptors and of loci susceptible to stimulation. In man, there are no detailed maps available on the distribution of the opioid receptors, and data are given only on relatively extensive regions of the brain [29]. Thus, receptors are abundant in the limbic system but also in the periaqueductal grey. The medio-basal part of the posterior thalamus, being the preferred site for stimulation in patients, has not been mapped. An indirect method of demonstrating the presence of opioid receptors is to study the effects of microinjection of morphine. This has actually been done in the monkey and it was found that morphine-susceptible loci were present also in the medio-basal thalamus [26].

There are hardly any data published on the distribution of the endogenous opioids in man, and only approximate estimations of the relative content of endorphins and enkefalins in large compartments of the brain have been made. There is a need for detailed mapping data, such as those published by Hökfelt *et al.* [15], which show the exact location of neurons or groups of neurons containing a particular substance. That would make possible a meaningful correlation to the effective stimulatory sites in patients and allow conclusions as to possible mechanisms behind the pain relief.

Tolerance to Stimulation

There is much evidence that morphine-analgesia and SPA have common mechanisms and this suggests that endogenous opioids are involved in SPA. Cross-tolerance between morphine-analgesia and SPA has been demonstrated in animals [19] and has occasionally been observed in patients with periventricular stimulation [14, 20]. Cross-dependency may also occur as illustrated by one of our patients who was highly dependent upon narcotics but could exchange entirely the intake of opiates for continuous stimulation [21].

Tolerance both to stimulation and to repeated administration of endorphin in the cerebral ventricles has been described in animals, and in patients tolerance to stimulation is common [14]. As a matter of fact this constitutes a serious problem and imposes restriction for the use of the stimulator. It has been shown that one link in the descending pain controlling pathways, activated by periaqueductal stimulation and relayed via the nucleus raphé magnus, is serotonergic (ref. see [6]). Hence, stimulation of this system would be expected to increase the content of serotonin in the CSF. No such observations have been published and occasional measurements that we have done on lumbar CSF have not disclosed any consistent changes *. Tolerance to stimulation in animals can readily be reversed by the administration of the serotonin precursor, 5-hydroxytryptophan [24]. Hosobuchi has later reported that a daily intake of L-tryptophan may counteract the development of tolerance to stimulation in patients [9].

Considering the animal data it is not unexpected that tolerance is common in patients. What is maybe of even more interest with regard to the discussion of the possible mechanisms for pain relief with periventricular stimulation is the observation that tolerance does not always develop, and there are some rare patients who retain the effect of stimulation over years. The absence of tolerance may be compatible with the notion that pain relief is not necessarily dependant upon the involvement of morphinomimetic mechanisms.

Naloxone

The observation that the morphine-antagonist, Naloxone, may reverse the effect of intracerebral stimulation, both in animal and man, has become the keystone in postulating common mechanisms for stimulation-produced pain relief and morphine-analgesia [25]. However, the effects of Naloxone are very complex indeed. Results of studies on the effect of Naloxone on experimental, acute pain in man are inconsistent. Thus, for instance, in pain-insensitive individuals Naloxone may result in hyperalgesia whereas the contrary is the case in the pain-sensitive individual [5]. It has also been recently reported that Naloxone at low doses produces analgesia but hyperalgesia at high doses [17]. Interestingly, it was also found that Naloxone can block the placebo effect, which of course has to be taken into account when the pain relieving effect of stimulation is assessed also on the basis of Naloxone-reversal.

The population of opioid receptors are far from homogenous and there exist many different types of receptors specialized for various opioid peptides and differing in affinity to exogenous opioids [18, 30]. Consequently, they differ in affinity also to opioid competitors such as Naloxone. There are a number of experimental studies reporting that SPA is only partially reversed, or even totally unaffected by systemic administration of Naloxone [7]. In the clinical literature there is only one report, that of Adams [7], which gives detailed data on the dose-response relationship when Naloxone is given to a patient with periventricular stimulation. Otherwise, it is just stated briefly that

* Positive evidence for augmentation of CSF-serotonin is presented in this volume by Hosobuchi.

the pain relieving effect is reversible with Naloxone [11], although huge doses sometimes have to be used. It is obvious that with very high doses there is a considerable risk that non-specific blocking effects are produced. In eight of our patients Naloxone has been administered double-blind in doses of 0.4–4.0 mg subsequent to periventricular stimulation. In most a definite reversal was observed. However, it may be of particular significance that one patient who experienced a complete pain relief did not respond although a dose of 3.6 mg was given (to be published). Again, this observation may be indicative of mechanisms other than those linked with endogenous opioids in pain relief. This problem has been delt with in more detail in a recent and clarifying review by Basbaum and Fields [4]. Of interest in this connection are descending pathways which bypass interposed inhibitory enkefalin containing neurons in the dorsal horn of the spinal cord. Furthermore, there are pathways originating in the locus coerulius being rich in catecholamine containing neurons which presumably also are part of the pain modulating system. These, and other, findings have led to the assumption that the descending pain inhibiting system is partially Naloxone-insensitive. The physiological and biochemical mechanisms subserving the control of pain is thus much more complex than has generally been presumed.

Endogenous Opioids and Release with Stimulation

In the discussion of the possible role of endogenous opioids in SPA, as well as in periventricular stimulation in patients, reference is almost exclusively made to beta-endorphin and the enkefalins; sometimes these substances are delt with as being an entity. The fact that there exist a number of other substances which are putative ligands to opiate-receptors, although structurally not yet defined, is often neglected. The physiological significance of these substances with regard to pain and pain modulation is entirely unknown. The structural relationship between the endorfins and the enkefalins is now common knowledge. The 91 amino acid beta-lipotropin contains the sequences constituting the endorphins and met-enkefalin. However, the identity of the precursor to met-enkefalin is not known with certainty although its amino acid sequence is also present in beta-endorphin. Of particular interest is the fact that beta-endorphin is found in the same cells in the pituitary that contain ACTH and that they originate from the same precursor, proopiocortin (31 K). The precursor for leu-enkefalin has not yet been identified. The anatomical distribution of the endorphins and the enkefalins, which have been assumed to be of prime importance for pain modulation, indicates that there exist at least three different systems represented by: 1. the enkefalins which are widely distributed in the brain, 2. beta-endorphin found in hypothalamic neurons projecting caudally toward the posterior periventricular region, and 3. the pituitary beta-endorphin system. Although, some of the naturally occurring opioids have been structurally identified there are several difficulties involved in the quantitative analysis in these substances. Generally, radio-receptor or radioimmuno assays are used but specificity is a problem and cross-reactions are common. Therefore, these substances are generally referred to as being enkefalin-like and endorphin-like.

A straight-forward and rational experiment for the demonstration of the relation between endogenous opioids and SPA in animals would be to monitor, on a long-term basis, their release in CSF during repeated sessions of stimulation concomitant with assessment of the analgesia produced. Surprisingly, to the best of my knowledge there is only one such study published (see ref. in [3]). Instead, this experimental approach has been used in a few clinical studies published during the last two years. Ventricular CFS has been collected in connection with periventricular stimulation during the course of the electrode implantation operation. Hosobuchi *et al.* [13] have reported on the release of beta-endorphin-like substances. What is of particular interest is that in three of the patients the stimulating electrode was located in the internal capsule and in these the endorphin content was unchanged. In contrast, the specimens obtained from three other patients with stimulation in the periventricular region showed a significant increase in the beta-endorphin content following the stimulation. All six patients had good pain relief as assessed during the operation. Similar results have been published by Akil *et al.* [2]. It should be noted that there are some preliminary reports on the analgetic effect of human beta-endorphin given intraventricularly [12]. There is also a report on the release of enkefalin-like material (similar to met-enkefalin) in ventricular CSF following stimulation [3]. The relative increase was considerably less than that of beta-endorphin. On the other hand, Hosobuchi *et al.* [13] did not find any immuno-reactivity to leu-enkefalin. Nevertheless, we are faced with the findings that both substances, beta-endorphin and enkefalin, are released as a result of stimulation suggesting that they are linked to neuronal systems the activation of which is responsible for pain relief. This gives rise to several questions: are there two—or more—systems that operate in a synergistic fashion or is it one and the same system in which both substances serve as transmittors or modulators. This latter possibility seems less probable in view of the different anatomical distribution of endorphins and enkefalins. One may even ask which of these substances is the crucial one? It should be mentioned that the first report on measurements in man of opiate receptor active material in connection with periventricular stimulation was given 1977 at the meeting in Freiburg [22] (see also [20]), when we presented some preliminary results obtained in collaboration with Terenius and Wahlström in Uppsala. A significant increase of this material in lumbar CSF was found to be present 1–2 hours after stimulation in a couple of patients. Our results, however, appear less consistent than those later published. Common to the studies performed on intraventricular CSF is that data are reported only from patients who have had good pain relief with stimulation. Therefore, we do not know for certain whether a release of endogenous opioids may also occur just as a result of stimulation in this particular region, and thus whether it is specifically linked to the phenomenon of pain relief. Furthermore, specimens for analysis could only be taken during a relatively short period of time. Thus, it has not been possible to establish any dose-response relationship, and we do not know anything about the time course of return to baseline and its time relation to re-appearance of pain. It should also be noted that there are considerable difficulties involved in the evaluation of pain relief during the course of a stressful situation such as a brain operation. The stress factor, however, has been discussed by Hosobuchi [10] who has shown that stimulation produces not only an increase of the beta-endorphin-like content in ventricular CSF but also of the other fragments of the precursor common to beta-endorphin and ACTH. There remains the possibility that the augmentation of the beta-endorphin content following stimulation is part of a stress-induced ACTH-release.

Recently, data have been collected from various European and some non-European clinics on the outcome of deep brain stimulation for pain [16]. It appeared that the results were highly inconsistent and patients having the same pain diagnosis could respond differently to stimulation. This is difficult to explain as is the fact that the surgical approach is identical in patients with both good and bad results. In this presentation I have tried to indicate some of the gaps in our knowledge of the biochemistry of stimulation-produced control of pain in man. The filling of these gaps is surely a prerequisite for helping us to select the appropriate patients and to use the proper stimulation technique.

Acknowledgement

The author wishes to acknowledge the valuable criticism and advice provided by Doctor Agneta Wahlström.

References

1. Adams, J. E., Naloxone reversal of analgesia produced by brain stimulation in the human. Pain *2* (1976), 161—166.
2. Akil, H., Richardson, D. E., Barchas, J. D., Li, C. H., Appearance of beta-endorphin-like immunoreactivity in human ventricular cerebrospinal fluid upon analgesic electrical stimulation. Proc. Natl. Acad. Sci. (U.S.A.) *75* (1978), 5170—5172.
3. Akil, H., Richardson, D. E., Hughes, J., Barchas, J. D., Enkephalin-like material elevated in ventricular cerebrospinal fluid of pain patients after analgetic focal stimulation. Science *201* (1978), 463—465.
4. Basbaum, A. I., Fields, H., Endogenous pain control mechanisms: review and hypothesis. Ann. Neurol. *4* (1978), 451—462.
5. Buchsbaum, M. S., Davis, G. C., Bunney, W. E., Naloxone alters pain perception and somatosensory evoked potentials in normal subjects. Nature *270* (1977), 620—622.
6. Fields, H. L., Basbaum, A. I., Brainstem control of spinal paintransmission neurons. Ann. Rev. Physiol. *40* (1978), 217—248.
7. Gebhart, G. F., Toleikis, J. R., An evaluation of stimulation-produced analgesia in the cat. Exp. Neurol. *62* (1978), 570—579.
8. Gybels, I., Cosyns, P., Modulation of clinical and experimental pain in man by electrical stimulation of the thalamic periventricular gray. In: Sensory function of the skin in primates, with special reference to man, pp. 521—530 (Zottermann, Y., ed.). Oxford-New York: Pergamon Press. 1976.
9. Hosobuchi, Y., Tryptophan reversal of tolerance to analgesia induced by central gray stimulation. The Lancet 2 (8079) (1978), 47.
10. Hosobuchi, Y., Elevation of beta-endorphin-like substances and pro-opiocortin (31 K ACTH) by periaqueductal gray stimulation (pags) in humans. In: Modern concepts in psychiatric surgery, pp. 57—64 (Hitchcock, E. R., Ballantine, H. T., Meyerson, B. A., eds.). Amsterdam-New York-Oxford: Elsevier: North-Holland. 1979.
11. Hosobuchi, Y., Adams, J. E., Linchitz, R., Pain relief by electrical stimulation of the central gray matter in humans and its reversal by naloxone. Science *197* (1976), 183—186.
12. Hosobuchi, Y., Li, C. H., A demonstration of the analgesic activity of human beta-endorphin in six patients. Proc. Second World Congr. Pain (Montreal) 1978 (Abstr.).
13. Hosobuchi, Y., Rossier, J., Bloom, F. E., Guillemin, R., Stimulation of human periaqueductal gray for pain relief increases immunoreactive beta-endorphin in ventricular fluid. Science *203* (1979), 279—281.
14. Hosobuchi, Y., Wemmer, J., Disulfiram inhibition of development of tolerance to analgesia induced by central gray stimulation in humans. Eur. J. Pharmacol. *43* (1977), 385—387.
15. Hökfelt, T., Ljungdahl, Å., Terenius, L., Elde, R., Nilsson, G., Immunohistochemical analysis of peptide pathways possibly related to pain and analgesia: Enkephalin and substance P. Proc. Natl. Acad. Sci. (U.S.A.) *74* (1977), 3081—3085.
16. Lazorthes, Y., (Ed.), European study on deep brain stimulation. Résumé of 3rd European workshop on electrical neurostimulation, Mégève, March 30—31, 1979 (in mimeo).
17. Levine, J. D., Gordon, N. C., Fields, H. L., Naloxone dose dependently produces analgesia and hyperalgesia in postoperative pain. Nature *278* (1979), 740—741.

18. Lord, J. A. M., Waterfield, A. A., Hughes, J., Kosterlitz, H. W., Endogenous opioid peptides: Multipel agonists and receptors. Nature *267* (1977), 495—499.
19. Mayer, D. J., Hayes, R. L., Stimulation-produced analgesia: Development of tolerance and cross-tolerance to morphine. Science *188* (1975), 941—943.
20. Meyerson, B. A., Boëthius, J., Carlsson, A. M., Percutaneous central gray stimulation for cancer pain. Proc. 7th Symp. World Soc. Stereotact. Function. Neurosurg., São Paulo, 1977. Appl. Neurophysiol. *41* (1978), 57—65.
21. Meyerson, B. A., Boëthius, J., Carlsson, A. M., Alleviation of malignant pain by electrical stimulation in the periventricular periaqueductal region. Pain relief as related to stimulation sites. In: Advances in pain research and therapy, Vol. 3, pp. 525—533 (Bonica, J. J., Liebeskind, J. C., Albe-Fessard, D. G., eds.). New York: Raven Press. 1979.
22. Meyerson, B. A., Boëthius, J., Terenius, L., Wahlström, A., Endorphin mechanisms in pain relief with intracerebral and dorsal column stimulation. 3rd Meet. Eur. Soc. Stereotact. Function. Neurosurg., Freiburg, 1977 (Abstr.).
23. Oliveras, J. L., Besson, J. M., Guilbaud, G., Liebeskind, J. C., Behavioral and electrophysiological evidence of pain inhibition from midbrain stimulation in the cat. Exp. Brain Res. *20* (1974), 32—44.
24. Oliveras, J. L., Hosobuchi, Y., Guilbaud, G., Besson, J. M., Analgesic electrical stimulation of the feline nucleus raphe magnus: Development of tolerance and its reversal by 5-HTP. Brain Res. *146* (1978), 404—409.
25. Pert, A., Walter, M., Comparison between naloxone reversal of morphine and electrical stimulation induced analgesia in the rat mesencephalon. Life Sci. *19* (1976), 1023—1032.
26. Pert, A., Yaksh, T., Sites of morphine induced analgesia in the primate brain: Relation to pain pathways. Brain Res. *80* (1974), 135—140.
27. Richardson, D. E., Akil, H., Pain reduction by electrical brain stimulation in man. Chronic self-administration in the periventricular gray matter. J. Neurosurg. *47* (1977), 184—194.
28. Rhodes, D. L., Liebeskind, J. C., Analgesia from rostral brain stem stimulation in the rat. Brain Res. *143* (1978), 521—532.
29. Simon, E. J., Hiller, J. M., The opiate receptors. Ann. Rev. Pharmacol. Toxicol. *18* (1978), 371—394.
30. Terenius, L., Opioid peptides and opiates differ in receptor selectivity. Psychoneuroendocrin. 2 (1977), 53—58.
31. Terenius, L., Endogenous peptides and analgesia. Ann. Rev. Pharmacol. Toxicol. *18* (1978), 189—204.
32. Terenius, L., The opioid receptors and their ligands. In: Central regulation of the endocrine systeme, pp. 137—148 (Fuxe, K., Hökfelt, T., Luft, R., eds.). New York-London: Plenum Press. 1978.

Acta Neurochirurgica, Suppl. 30, 239—243 (1980)

Control of Dyskinesias Due to Sensory Deafferentation by Means of Thalamic Stimulation

G. Mazars*, L. Merienne, and C. Cioloca

Summary

Intermittent stimulation of the parvocellular portion of the nucleus ventralis posterolateralis (V.P.L.) by means of chronically implanted electrodes and stimulus generator was performed in 124 patients for the control of chronic intractable pain. Among these, 11 showed spontaneous abnormal movements within the painful area: 6 post amputation "jumping stumps"; 4 pseudothalamic syndromes and 1 Von Benedikt's syndrome following a cerebrovascular accident. Electrical stimulation of the V.P.L. was able to control both pain and abnormal movements in all cases. The technique was applied with an equally good result in a case of choreoathetotic syndrome without pain but with severe sensory disturbances following a demyelinating process. Attempts made to control action tremor, parkinsonism and other dyskinesias not associated with sensory deafferentation in 12 cases failed. The same mechanism seems to be responsible for pain and dyskinesia in cases of sensory deafferentation, and thalamic stimulation might work as a substitute for sensory information delivered to the nucleus ventralis posterolateralis.

Keywords: Pain; thalamus; dyskinesia; electrostimulation.

During the past 17 years our experience with intermittent stimulation of the nucleus ventralis posterolateralis (I.T.S.) for the control of pain drew our attention to the effect on certain types of dyskinesias often associated with pain. There is now good evidence that sensory deafferentation produces spontaneous abnormal movements and that these dyskinesias can be controlled by posterior thalamic stimulation in the same way as deafferentation pain [1—4].

Material and Methods

The nucleus ventralis posterolateralis (V.P.L.) is stimulated by means of gold or platinum bipolar electrodes placed stereotactically in the parvocellularis portion of the V.P.L. somatotopically corresponding to the site of pain: 8–9 mm from

* Neurosurgical Department "A", Centre Hospitalier Sainte-Anne, 1, rue Cabanis, F-75674 Paris, Cedex 14, France.

0065-1419/80/Suppl. 30/0239/$ 01.00

the midline for the face, 11–12 mm for the arm and 15–16 mm for the leg. The best electrode placements were parallel to the sagittal plane with a point of entry near the vertex.

The electrode placement was checked by stimulation with 10 Hz, 0.1 to 1 ms. and 2 volts which should produce paraesthesias in the area concerned with the pain or the abnormal movement. Therapeutic stimulations were carried out with 10 Hz, 1 ms, 0.2 to 0.9 volt over 2 to 3 minutes; this could be repeated 1 to 5 times over a 24 hours period [4, 5].

Implantable stimulators were used with sealed in batteries and a magnetic switch that worked only when a magnet was held in front of the stimulator which was generally implanted in the subclavian area. Experience shows that these parameters of stimulation will neither harm the thalamic tissue nor induce paresthesias and yet provide a fully effective control of pain in adequately selected cases.

Initially, I.T.S. was devised for the control of pain: 124 patients have been implanted during the past 17 years. It soon became evident that only sensory deafferentation pain could be controlled by this method [3, 5].

Results

Post-amputation pain, phantom limb pain, and hyperpathia or spontaneous pain irradiating over the stump have been fully controlled in 23 out of 24 patients. The phantom "shrinks" and vanishes within 1 to 14 weeks.

Abnormal movements of the stump were an important feature in six of our patients: 3 had random jerking and short spells of tremor of the stump at rest or induced by voluntary movements; 3 had a more severe "jumping stump" with permanent rapid (10 per second) tremor increased by pressure, movements and posturing. Control of tremor could be partially obtained by holding the stump in two patients.

Although pain was partially controlled by morphine and intravenous imipramine, jerking was still present in all cases.

In all of these six patients full control of pain was achieved from the very first stimulation; pain vanished after 1 to 3 minutes of stimulation. In addition, all the spontaneous abnormal movements ceased at the same time without any motor defect. Recurrence of pain was associated with return of tremor after 6 to 28 hours and a new stimulation could stop pain and tremor for the same length of time. Adequately spaced stimulations were used by all patients to prevent recurrence of pain and tremor [7].

Dyskinesias are also a common feature among patients with "thalamic syndrome" of hyperpathia and spontaneous diffuse pain involving the contralateral side. This often follows a cerebrovascular accident and is associated with sensory defects and spontaneous abnormal movements in the paretic limb which may be due to a lesion of the posterior thalamus. We had two such cases and as might be expected, stimulation at V.P.L. or in the internal capsule failed to produce paraesthesias or relieve the pain.

Indeed, we have reported four cases where, in spite of a "thalamic pain syndrome", the patients had an intact thalamus and electrical stimulation with 2 v. produced paraesthesias and with 1 v. for 3 minutes controlled the diffuse burning pain and hyperpathia. In all of these cases, the abnormal movements stopped following stimulation for several hours [6]. One of these patients who developed hyperpathia of the left arm and thorax following a moderate left hemiparesis was unable to stretch his hand because of continuous athetotic movements. Following I.T.S., pain was completely controlled and the hand dyskinesia no longer present; causalgia and hyperpathia which had made rehabilitation impossible was no longer a problem, and almost normal motor function was restored in a matter of 3 weeks. This excellent result was maintained for almost two years until a new cerebrovascular accident resulted in total hemiplegia.

Two more patients have a history of left hemiparesis, hemianopia and hyperpathia with spontaneous, "unbearable" burning pain and continuous choreo-athetotic movements of small amplitude in the paretic hand: Electrode placements in the hand area of the V.P.L. and routine 3 minute stimulations 2 to 4 times daily have controlled both the painful syndrome and the dyskinesia of the upper extremity; in addition, both cases have had considerable improvement of spasticity and of motor function.

The fourth patient has a somewhat different story: he developed a left middle cerebral artery thrombosis in March 1975; after three months, the motor recovery was almost complete but he developed hyperpathia and deep diffuse, spontaneous pain involving his right leg; spontaneous and permanent movements of the toes added to the discomfort of the patient and were controlled only by opiates. On clinical examination, deep sensibility and discriminative sensibility were impaired over the whole leg but no motor weakness nor visual field defect could be demonstrated making the site of the lesion questionable. One year later, the patient was implanted with a thalamic stimulator and from the very first stimulation has been painfree; spontaneous movements of the toes have stopped and the opiates were withdrawn on the same day without problems. In one case labelled as Von Benedikt's syndrome, a partially obstructed basilar artery was demonstrated in a 68 years old lady; following the acute stage, she developed some burning pain over the hip and the right leg and abnormal movements of the right leg gradually increasing in amplitude. The patient was more disturbed by the dyskinesia which affected her gait than by the pain. Deep sensibility and discriminative sensibility were impaired over the lower right half of the body without loss of motor power. At the sixth month, we decided to implant a thalamic stimulator since the patient's condition showed no improvement: 3 daily stimulations of 3 minutes each are able to control pain as well as abnormal movements and the patient is now able to walk unaided.

In view of these encouraging results, we decided to implant a 33 years old man with multiple sclerosis who subsequently developed hemiballistic movements, choreoathetotic movements of the left arm, hemianopia, diplopia and a severe loss of deep and superficial discriminative sensibility over the left arm, no pain developed in spite of the sensory deafferentation.

Stimulations carried out at 12 mm from the midline in the V.P.L. controlled the abnormal movements for 6 hours on each occasion and the patient has adopted a rate of six daily stimulations to prevent recurrence of the dyskinesia, although the sensory deficit is too severe for any normal use of the hand. This evidence of control of some dyskinesias by means of posterior thalamic stimulation might suggest a possible extension of other cases. We have taken the opportunity to try the effect of I.T.S. on patients who were candidates for a coagulation of the lateral thalamic nucleus; Parkinson's disease [4], congenital choreoathetosis [1], Wilson's disease [1] and action tremor [3]. No improvement was recorded in these cases and coagulation of the nucleus ventralis lateralis was done with the usual good result.

Discussion

The striking point is that all the cases where abnormal movements were controlled by posterior thalamic stimulation showed some evidence of sensory discrepancy in the limb affected by the dyskinesia. This sensory deafferentation is either peripheral in origin as in amputations, or central as in cerebrovascular accidents and in demyelinating diseases; dyskinesias not associated with sensory deafferentation failed to respond to thalamic stimulation. Suppression of pain is apparently not the direct reason for interruption of the abnormal movements since, in one case pain was missing and in the other cases, opiates failed to stop the abnormal movements. It seems that the cybernetic control of segmental position of the extremities is deeply affected by the lack of some sensory information and that posterior thalamic stimulation provides a temporary substitute for the missing sensory informations.

References

1. Mazars, G., Mérienne, L., Cioloca, C., Traitement de certains types de douleurs par des stimulateurs thalamiques implantables. Neurochirurgie *20* (1974), 117—124.
2. Mazars, G., Mérienne, L., Cioloca, C., Stimulations thalamiques intermittentes. Rev. Neurol. *128* (1973), 273—279.
3. Mazars, G., Intermittent stimulation of nucleus ventralis posterolateralis for intractable pain. Surg. Neurol. *4* (1975), 93—95.
4. Mazars, G., Mérienne, L., Cioloca, C., Emploi de stimulateurs thalamiques dans le traitement de certains types de douleurs. Ann. Médec. *73* (1975), 145—148.
5. Mazars, G., Chirurgie de la douleur, I vol., 164 p. Paris: Masson & Cie. 1975.
6. Mazars, G., Mérienne, L., Résultats de la stimulation thalamique intermittente dans le traitement des séquelles douloureuses des accidents vasculaires cérébraux. Rev. Neurol. *136* (1977).
7. Mazars, G., Mérienne, L., Chacon, C., Contribution à la physiopathologie et au traitement des "épilepsies des moignons". Rev. Neurol. 1979. In Press.

Acta Neurochirurgica, Suppl. 30, 245—258 (1980)

Deep Brain Stimulation in Mesencephalic Lemniscus Medialis for Chronic Pain

F. Mundinger* and **J. F. Salomão**

With 4 Figures

Summary

Stereotactic deep brain stimulation (DBS) with chronically implanted special devices intermittently activated by the patient himself has led to a new concept in the treatment of chronic central pain, such as the thalamic pain syndrome, herpes-zoster neuralgia, anaesthesia dolorosa, radicular and plexus lacerations, stump pain with and without causalgia and cancer pain.

Our results in 32 cases (March 31, 1979) with lemniscus medialis stimulation, including the specific and nonspecific somatosensory nuclei or periaqueductal gray matter show in 53% of our cases, a reduction of pain of over 50%. The follow-up period was 47 months. These results are better than those obtained from stimulating only one of the systems.

Mesencephalic lemniscus medialis DBS, introduced by one of the authors (Mundinger), leads to a functional blockade of spinothalamic, lemniscus medialis and spino-reticular systems. In cases where a positive morphine test had been done previously, endorphine secretion also plays a role. It is assumed that the effect of endorphine production lasts longer than the stimulation itself, especially in periaqueductal mesencephalic gray matter and medial pulvinar stimulation.

The treatment of severe chronic intractable pain, which is not treatable with any other method, still presents problems today. Here we are primarily dealing with stump causalgia with and without phantom limb pain, trigeminal and intercostal neuralgia (for example, anaesthesia dolorosa after herpes zoster), thalamic syndrome caused by cerebrovascular, and chronic pain of malignant growth, late radiation damage and traumata (plexus rupture, paraplegia). These patients are tormented with continuous burning and radiating pain to the point where it is no longer bearable. The pain impulses are primarily conducted from the site of the pain in the periphery in the

* Abteilung Stereotaxie und Neuronuklearmedizin (Director: Prof. Dr. F. Mundinger), Neurochirurgische Universitätsklinik, Hugstetter Straße 55, D-7800 Freiburg i. Br., Federal Republic of Germany.

0065-1419/80/Suppl. 30/0245/$ 02.80

Table 1 A. *Deep Brain Stimulation*

No. of cases	Clinical diagnosis	Localization of pain	Brain target	Follow-up (in months)	Results
1. A. J., 43 years, ♀	anaesthesia dolorosa	right side of face V 1–3	lemniscus medialis left	23. 1. 1978/14 months	+
2. A. P., 68 years, ♂	phantom pain after leg amputation right 1943	phantom pain right sole of foot	lemniscus medialis left	29. 6. 1978/10 months	++
3. A. P., 34 years, ♂	phantom pain after ex-articulation of right upper arm 1977 with plexus brachialis	phantom pain right arm/hand	centrum medianum M.f.a.p left	15. 5. 1975/4 years	++
4. B. W., 38 years, ♂	phantom pain after traumatic plexus and root evulsion 1960 and amputation of left arm	phantom pain left hand and finger	medial pulvinar V.c.p.e to dorsal nucleus right	17. 11. 1975/28 months	++
5. B., M., 78 years, ♂	chronic pain syndrome in face and right hand with spastic hemiparesis after apoplectic insult 1975	right side of face and right hand	lemniscus medialis left	30. 12. 1977/15 months	++
6. Bl. H., 48 years, ♂	stump and phantom pain after thigh amputation left	phantom pain big and little toes, stump pain	lemniscus medialis right	11. 5. 1978/10 months	++
7. Bl. K., 63 years, ♀	anaesthesia dolorosa right side of face	right side of face V 1–3	lemniscus medialis left	29. 8. 1977/18 months	++

8. Br. Fr., 69 years, ♂	trigeminal neuralgia after herpes-zoster infection 1967	V 2–3 left	V.c.pc.i right	6. 9. 1976/30 months	+
9. B. H., 49 years, ♂	chronic pain of right side of face	V_2 right	V.c.pc.i centrum medianum mfa u. p left	23. 7. 1976/32 months	+++
10. B. F., 58 years, ♂	anaesthesia dolorosa right V 1–3	V_{1-3} right	lemniscus medialis left	19. 4. 1978/11 months	+
11. E. A., 51 years, ♂	traumatic myelopathy with chronic pain syndrome of left paralytic arm	left arm	lemniscus medialis right	27. 4. 1978/—	0 removal
12. E. G., 53 years, ♂	chronic pain syndrome right V 1–2 after gunshot injury	right orbital cavity	lemniscus medialis left	21. 12. 1977/15 months	+++
13. F. H., 30 years, ♂	causalgiform pains with paraplegia of legs at L_1 following trauma	legs, right and left	central mesencephalic gray right	24. 4. 1975/4 years	+
14. G. A., 57 years, ♀	chronic pain syndrome of right side of body accompanying condition following operation of left side acusticus-neurinoma 1972	right side of body	pulvinar left	8. 8. 1977/19 months	+
15. H. Fr., 38 years, ♂	atypical face pain right side	V_{1-2} right	lemniscus medialis left	16. 11. 1976/28 months	+++
16. J. Fr., ♂	pain syndrome after plexus injury combined with root evulsion of upper cervical medulla with complete plegia of right arm	right arm, particularly hand	centrum medianum left	4. 6. 1975/4 years	++

Table 1 A (continued)

No. of cases	Clinical diagnosis	Localization of pain	Brain target	Follow-up (in months)	Results
17. Kl. S., 42 years, ♂	chronic pain syndrome of left hand following plexus evulsion 1962	left hand, left arm	lemniscus medialis right	13. 9. 1977/18 months	+
18. Kr. J., 69 years, ♂	anaesthesia dolorosa ac-comp. malignoma apoplex 5 days after implantation	V_{1-2}	lemniscus medialis left	13. 5. 1977/22 months	0
19. K. E., 57 years, ♀	chronic pain syndrome of right side of face	V_{1-3} right	lemniscus medialis left	14. 6. 1977/9 months	+
20. L. G., 47 years, ♂	phantom and stump pain after amputation below elbow right	phantom pain right (thumb, index and middle fingers) stump pain right	centrum medianum V.pc. arm left	27. 9. 1976/30 months	+
21. M. C., 51 years, ♂	chronic pain syndrome after apoplectic insult 1972	right side of body	lemniscus medialis left	10. 8. 1978/7 months	+
22. M. H., 34 years, ♂	chronic pain syndrome after car accident 1969 with plexus evulsion left	left side of neck and left arm	lemniscus medialis right	26. 5. 1977/22 months	+
23. N. A., 59 years, ♂	stump and phantom pain right after amputation at right thigh	stump pain right calf and heel right	lemniscus medialis left	10. 8. 1977/19 months	+
24. Pf. H., 41 years, ♂	chronic pain syndrome (phantom and stump pain) after root evulsion of left cervical vertebra 1964 with hemiplegia of left arm	phantom pain (finger, wrist) left, slight stump pain	lemniscus medialis right	16. 10. 1978/5 months	+++

25. P. Kl., 32 years, ♂	pain syndrome particularly on left side following traumatic transverse lesion of the cord with paraplegia at LW_2	both legs, left right	lemniscus medialis right	16. 5. 1977/22 months	+++
26. P. D., 42 years, ♀	anaesthesia dolorosa left	V_{1-3} left	lemniscus medialis right	1. 6. 1977/21 months	+++
27. Sch. E., 68 years, ♀	trigeminal neuralgia left V_{1-3} after herpes-zoster infection	V_{1-3} left	lemniscus medialis right	15. 10. 1976/27 months	++
28. Schw. O., 69 years, ♂	chronic pain syndrome accentuated in right leg after infarct of art. cerebri poster. left	right thigh	lemniscus medialis left	27. 5. 1977/20 months	+
29. Sch. S., 42 years, ♀	traumatic monoparesis of right leg with pain following gunshot injury	right leg	lemniscus medialis left	20. 6. 1977/21 months	++
30. Wn. H., 44 years, ♂	chronic pain syndrome left hand, spastic tetraparesis, accentuated in leg, operation acc. to Cloward 1972	left hand	lemniscus medialis right	19. 4. 1978/11 months	+
31. H. K., 49 years, ♂	pain syndrome of left side of body following apoplectic insult	left arm, left leg	mediolateral pulvinar right	2. 1. 1979/2 months	+++
32. E. A., 74 years, ♂	chronic therapy-resistant pain syndrome of left arm following plexus evulsion and root lesion	left arm	lemniscus medialis right	27. 2. 1979/1 month	+

The following criteria were used in evaluating the results: 0 No effect. + Improvement (up to 50%), pain improved, no more analgesics or only occasionally. ++ Improvement (up to 70%), no analgesics, but still slightly handicapped due to pain, fit to work. +++ Practically free of pain (> 70%), no analgesics, completely fit to work, good general condition.

spinothalamic tract into the brain. In the region of the posterior thalamus, the pain impulses divide into circuits for pain experience, pain discrimination and pain sensation. These circuits flow over the cerebral cortex and through the subcortex. During pain, these circuits are in a state of superexcitation [5, 22]. The thin c-fibres, which function as slow conductors towards the brain, are said to conduct the impulses for chronic pain are transformed primarily in the specific and nonspecific pain nuclei.

Table 1 B. *Results of DBS in Lemniscus medialis (22 cases)*

		0	(+)	+	++	+++
Anaesthesia dolorosa		1	2	1	2	3
Causalgia		1	—	1	1	—
Phantom and stump pain		—	1	—	2	1
Spinal cord injuries		—	—	1	1	1
Thalamic syndrome		—	1	1	1	—
Total	N	2	4	4	7	5
	%	9.3	18.1	18.1	31.8	22.8
					54.5 (++ and +++)	

In the last few years, inspired among others by Melzak and Wall's "Gate Control" theory [7], methods have been developed which no longer sever the pain conducting system definitively (sections or coagulation of the peripheral nerves [19], severance of nerve roots [15], of the antero-lateral column in the spinal cord [8, 16], of the trigeminal nerve root tract [21]). Instead, these methods attempt to interrupt with high frequency stimulation the interaction between the fast conducting medullated alpha-delta-2 fibres, which are responsible for the acute or initial pain, and the above mentioned slow-conducting c-fibres. Further conduction of the pain impulses into the brain is thereby prevented and the patient is relieved of his pain.

Transcutaneous neuronal stimulation by means of skin electrodes and dorsal column stimulation (DCS) by the epidural or intradural implantation of electrodes on the spinal column [17, 18, 20] make it possible to intermittently block chronic continuous pain in 10 to 60% of the patients (with the exception of herpes zoster neuralgia as well as the thalamic syndrome with its impaired central regulatory circuits between the cortical and subcortical pain conducting systems of pain experience and pain sensation [9]). In the meantime it has turned out

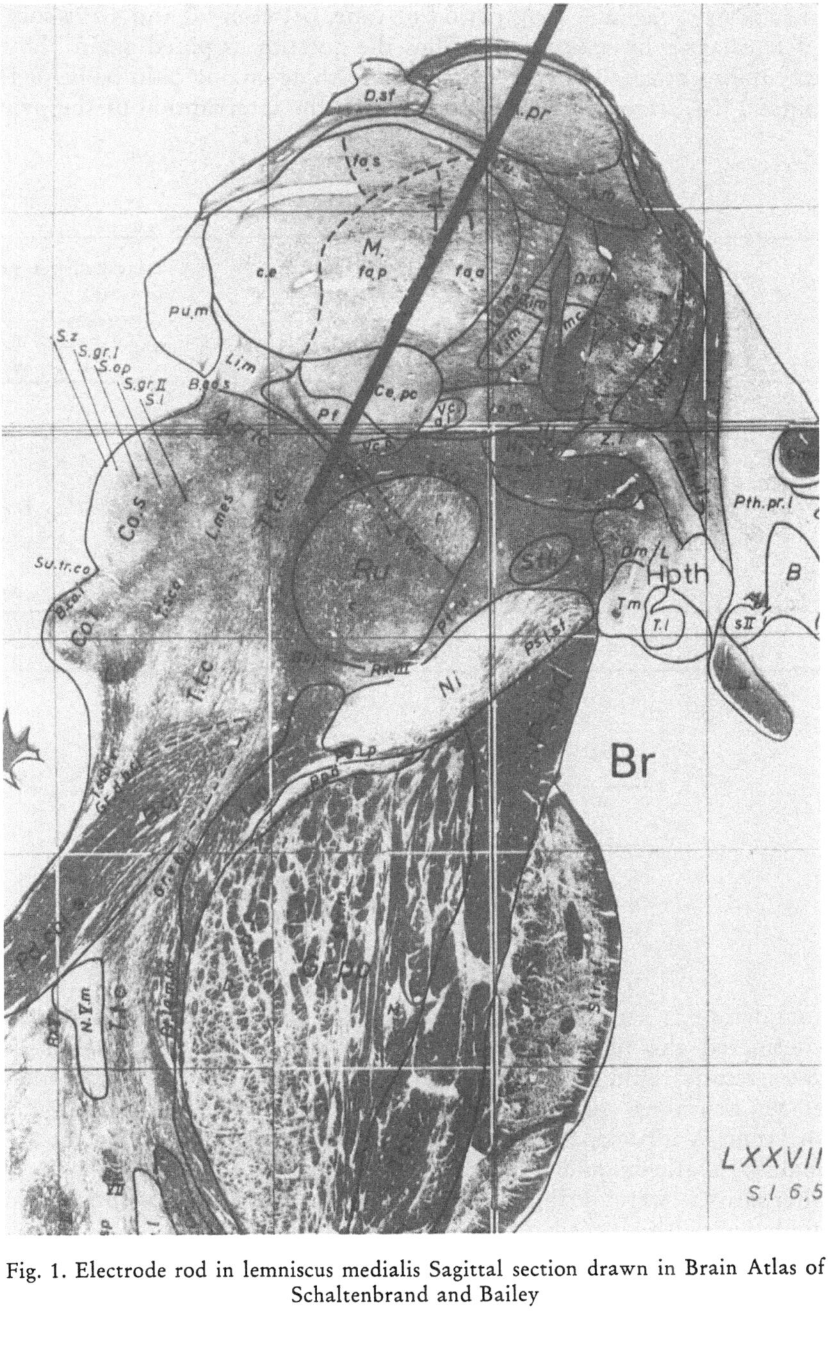

Fig. 1. Electrode rod in lemniscus medialis Sagittal section drawn in Brain Atlas of Schaltenbrand and Bailey

that after a variably long period of time, between 90 and 40% complete relapses have occurred. Thus the question is posed again: how can these patients who are tormented with agonizing pain be helped? Since 1954, stereotactic coagulation with the interruption of the pain

Table 2

	Centrum medianum (4 cases)					Med. pulvinar (3 cases)					Periaqueductal. gray (2 cases)				
	0	(+)	+	++	+++	0	(+)	+	++	+++	0	(+)	+	++	+++
Anaesthesia dolorosa	—	—	—	—	1										
Causalgia	—	—	—	1	—						—	—	1	—	—
Stump/phantom	—	1	—	1	—	—	—	—	1	—					
Spinal cord injury											—	—	1	—	—
Thalamic syndrome						—	1	—	—	1					
N	—	1	—	2	1	—	1	—	1	1	—	—	2	—	—

Table 3. *DBS Results in Chronic Pain (32 cases)*

	0	(+)	+	++	+++
N	2	7	6	10	7
%	6.3	21.9	18.8	24.3	21.7

conducting systems in the thalamus and mesencephalon [9] has been considered the ultimate course. With this method, pain relief or good results could be achieved in the long run (with 42% of herpes-zoster neuralgia cases, 32% stump and phantom limb pain, 70% thalamic syndrome, 90% malignant growth pain [12, 13]. For the remaining patients and for those who suffered a relapse, the only alternatives were sedatives, psychotropic drugs, neuroleptics and analgesics with all their consequences. Suicide was not a rarity among these patients. Deep brain stimulation (DBS), also for these cases, has opened up a further therapeutic dimension for the brain [1, 11].

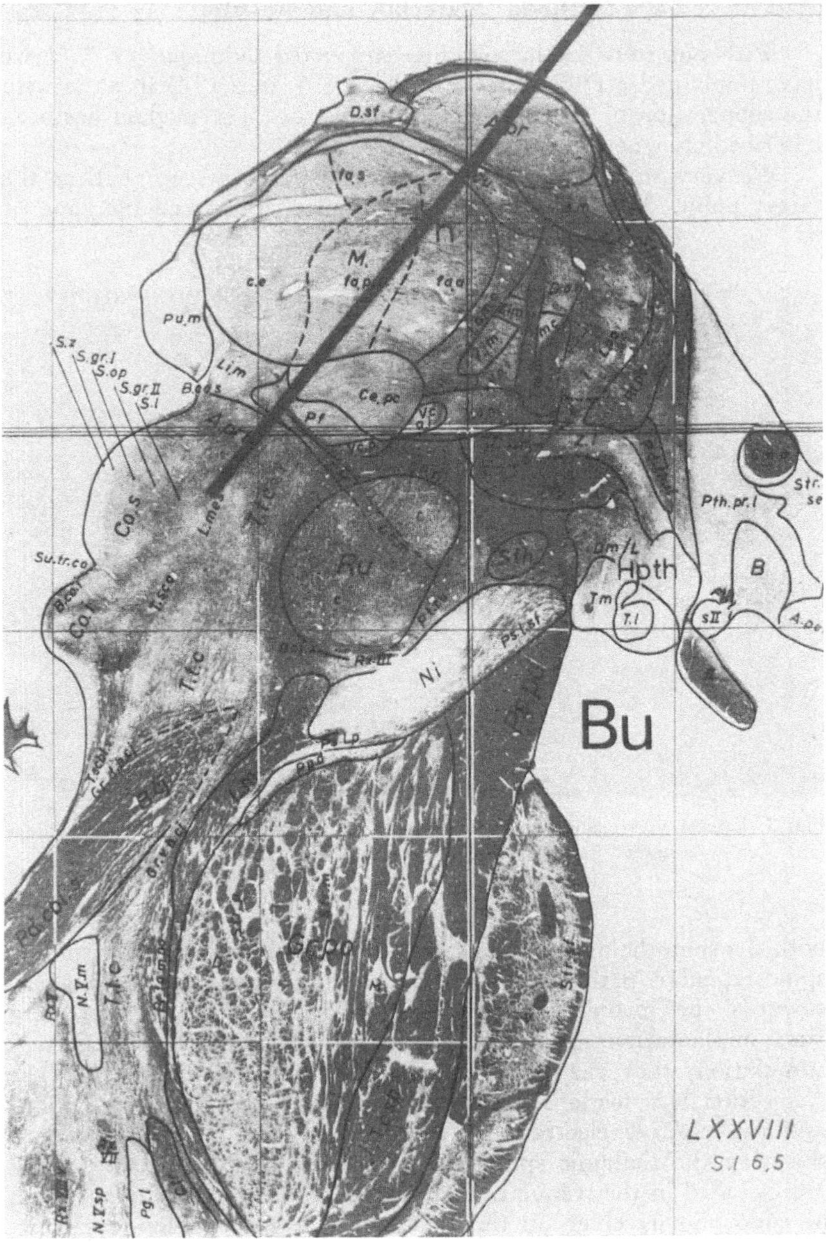

Fig. 2. The same as Fig. 1 in vertical section

Methods, Material, and Results

With our stereotactic computer-supported technique [2–4, 6, 14] we have implanted a DBS system (Medtronic®) since 1975 in parts with the cooperation of C. Ostertag and E. Milios. The method has been described elsewhere [10].

We very soon chose the lemniscus medialis mesencephali as the target point. We tried to produce stimulation induced blockade of

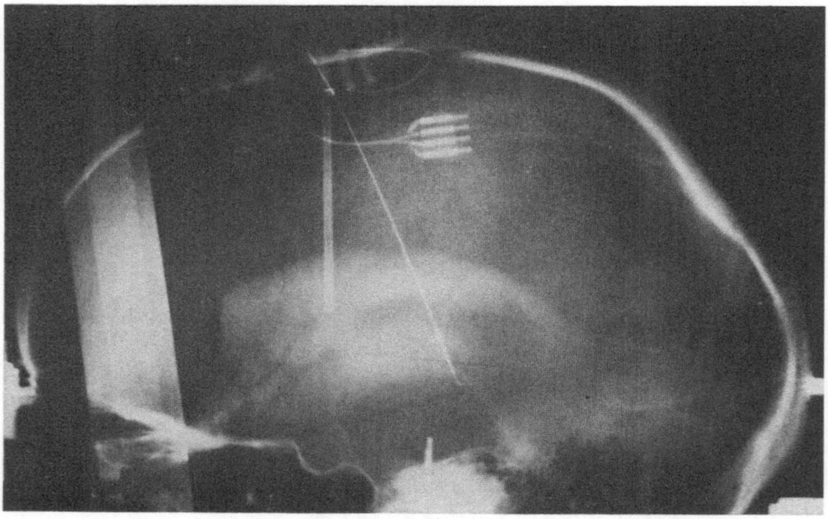

Fig. 3. Lateral view. Superimposed X-ray with lemniscus medialis as target determined in ventriculogram and implanted DBS-electrode

both the spinothalamic system and the lemniscus medialis system and spino-reticular pathways including the afferent systems that run towards the medial pulvinar (Figs. 1 and 2). After the very first implantations we noticed, on the basis of the intermittent stimulation, that the pain suppression was more effective if the connection was made between the negative 0-pole (= target point) and the positive electrode 3, which is situated 12 mm above. In this way the thalamic specific and unspecific somatosensory nuclei are included in the stimulation circuit. According to the distribution of endorphin receivers in the area of the mesencephalon, perioqueductal gray matter and the caudal thalamus, there is a secondary effect of endorphine release caused by the stimulation. This works better than with the 0 electrode in the centrum medianum and with the connection between 0 and 3 if the dorsal-medial nuclei areas are also hit; or attempts to produce endorphin by periaqueductal gray stimulation.

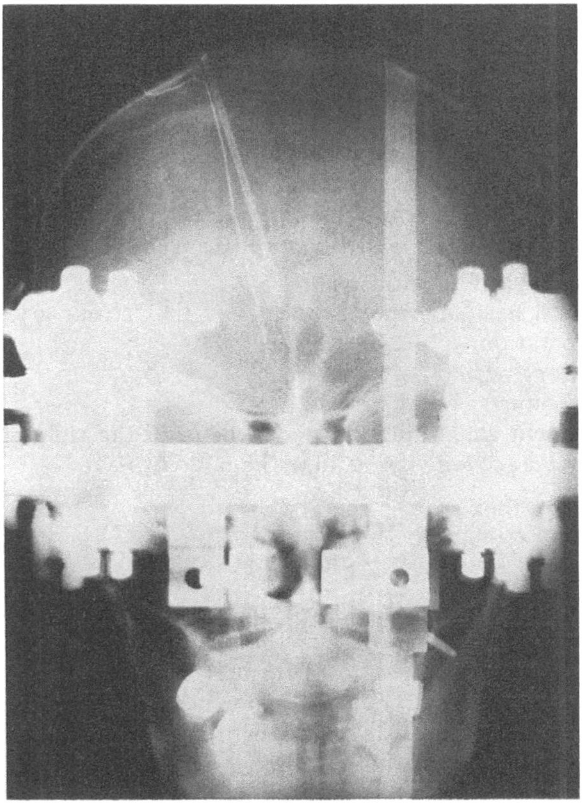

Fig. 4. Anterior-posterior view of Fig. 3

All the patients experience, depending on the intensity of stimulation tingling paraesthesia, sometimes accompanied by warm sensation. Because of the somatotopic relationship of the lemniscus medialis, one can achieve the beginning and the maximum intensity of the tingling paraesthesia is first felt in the extremities affected or the trigeminal area.

According to our experiences, the homunculus is in an area of the lemniscus medialis that reaches up to 5 mm caudally, beginning from below the posterior commissure and which lies between 2 and 5 mm below the caudally extended base line (foramen Monro posterior commissure). The medio-lateral extension is from 6.5 to 11 mm. The homunculus lies caudal to rostral (head to foot) is positioned diagonally with its face representation and extremities turned inwards medio-caudal-basal to latero-rostro-dorsal (Figs. 3 and 4).

Complications:

a) Technical; 6 patients.

2 indurative eczema in the area of the most severe stimulation paraesthesia (anaesthesia dolorosa).

1 suture dehiscence over the underlying receiver.

1 plexus brachialis irritation along the connector cable.

1 intracerebral shifting of the brain electrode.

b) Neurological: 5 patients.

1 Cerebral haemorrhage in the area of the "stroke artery" 2 days after the operation.

1 transitory occulomotor paresis.

2 focal seizures.

1 permanent slight tingling paraesthesia in the right side of face and right hand accompanying anaesthesia dolorosa.

Mortality: 0 cases.

Results

The data of the patient, clinical diagnosis, location of pain, target point (0-electrode) and the date of the operation with follow-up time and the results are compiled in the form of brief histories.

A comparison of our 22 cases, in which DBS was performed in the lemniscus medialis with inclusion of the specific and unspecific somatosensory nuclei, with the other 4 cases where DBS was done in the centrum medianum, the 3 cases in the pulvinar and the one cases in the periaqueductal stratum-griseum-mesencephali does not seem possible as there are not enough cases to warrant an accurate comparison.

The first European cooperative study on deep brain stimulation for pain, introduced in the 3rd European Workshop on Electrical Neurostimulation in Megève, March 30/31, 1979, and compiled by P. Meyerson with 203 cases, shows for deafferentiated pain, pain relief of more than 50%, in the periaqueductal gray matter 33% (57 cases), in the VPM 40%, in the internal capsula 36%. These results do not match the results that we have been able to obtain now with DBS with the inclusion of the lemniscus medialis mesencephali.

References

1. Adams, J., Hosobuchi, Y., Fields, H. L., Stimulation of internal capsule for relief of chronic pain. J. Neurosurg. *41* (1974), 740—744.
2. Birg, W., Mundinger, F., Computer calculations of target parameter for a stereotactic apparatus. Acta Neurochir. (Wien) *29* (1973), 123—129.
3. Birg, W., Mundinger, F., Computer programmes for stereotactic neurosurgery. 6th Symposium of the International Society for Research in Stereoencephalotomy. Tokyo 1973. Confin. neurol. (Basel) *36* (1974), 326—366.
4. Birg, W., Mundinger, F., Calculation of the position of a sideprotruding electrode tip in stereotactic brain operations using a stereotactic apparatus with polar coordinates. Acta Neurochir. (Wien) *32* (1975), 83—87.
5. Hassler, R., Central interactions of the system of the rapidly and slowly conducted pain. Advanc. Neurosurg. *3* (1975), 143—149.
6. Hoefer, T., Mundinger, F., Birg, W., Reinke, M., Computer calculation to localize subcortical targets in plane X-rays for stereotactic neurosurgery. 6th Symposium of the International Society for Research in Stereoencephalotomy, Tokyo, 1973. Confin. neurol. (Basel) *36* (1974), 334—340.
7. Melzak, R., Wall, P. D., Pain mechanism. A new theory. Science *150* (1965), 975—979.
8. Müke, R., Correia, A., Potentials and limits of percutaneous cervical cordotomy. Advanc. Neurosurg. *3* (1975), 195—198.
9. Mundinger, F., Stereotaktische Operationen am Gehirn. Grundlagen-Indikationen-Resultate. Stuttgart: Hippokrates. 1975.
10. Mundinger, F., Die Behandlung chronischer Schmerzen mit Hirnstimulatoren. Dtsch. med. Wschr. *102* (1977), 1724—1729.
11. Mundinger, F., Die stereotaktisch-funktionelle Behandlung des Schmerzes durch intracerebrale Ausschaltung und Stimulation. Jahrestagung des Berufsverbandes Westfälischer Nervenärzte e. V., Bad Salzuflen, 1976. In: Aktuelle Probleme der Neuropsychiatrie, pp. 88—103 (Gottschaldt, M., Grass, H., Brock, M., eds.). Berlin-Heidelberg-New York: Springer. 1978.
12. Mundinger, F., Becker, P., Long term results of central stereotactic interventions for pain. Advanc. Neurosurg. *3* (1975), 237—241.
13. Mundinger, F., Becker, P., Late results of central stereotactic interventions for pain. IInd Meeting of the European Society for Stereotactic and Functional Neurosurgery, Madrid 1975. Acta Neurochir. Suppl. *24* (1977), 229.
14. Mundinger, F., Reinke, M.-A., Hoefer, Th., Birg, W., Determination of intracerebral structures using osseous reference points for computer aided stereotactic operations. Appl. Neurophysiol. *38* (1975), 3—22.
15. Penzholz, H., Menzel, J., Hagenlocher, H. U., Results of surgical treatment of idiopathic trigeminal neuralgia using different operative techniques. Advanc. Neurosurg. *3* (1975), 320—327.
16. Piotrowski, W., Panitz, C., Results after open cordotomy. Advanc. Neurosurg. *3* (1975), 174—177.
17. Ray, Ch. D., Control of pain by electrical stimulation. A clinical value of dorsal column stimulation (DCS). Advanc. Neurosurg. *3* (1975), 216—224.
18. Shealy, C. N., Mortimer, J. R., Reswick, J. B., Electrical inhibition of pain stimulation of the dorsal columns. Preliminary clinical report. Anesth. Analg. Curr. Res. *46* (1967), 489.
19. Siegfried, J., Results of percutaneous controlled thermocoagulation of the Gasserian ganglion in 300 cases of trigeminal pain. Advanc. Neurosurg. *3* (1975), 287—295.

20. Winkelmüller, W., Dietz, H., Stolke, D., The clinical value of dorsal column stimulation (DCS). Advanc. Neurosurg. *3* (1975), 225—228.
21. Wüllenweber, R., Distelmaier, P., Results of treatment of trigeminal neuralgia by the operations of Dandy. Advanc. Neurosurg. *3* (1975), 316—319.
22. Zimmermann, M., Neurophysiological models for nociception, pain and pain therapy. Advanc. Neurosurg. *3* (1975), 199—205.

Acta Neurochirurgica, Suppl. 30, 259—268 (1980)

Electrical Stimulation of the Central Gray for Pain Relief in Human: Autopsy Data

J. Gybels*, R. Dom, and P. Cosyns*****

With 5 Figures

Summary

Anatomicpathological studies are reported of 5 brains in which electrical stimulation of the periventricular—periaqueductal gray was applied for the treatment of chronic pain. It was found that the recommended target was reached in 4 cases (only 1 case out of 5 was successful as far as pain relief is concerned). PtIr electrodes caused little tissue reaction. The chronic stimulation had not provoked lesions observable by light-microscopy.

Keywords: Chronic pain; electrical stimulation of central gray; autopsy data.

Introduction

In 1978, one of us reviewed what had been published in the clinical literature on pain relief by electrical stimulation of the central gray (Gybels 1979). It appeared from this survey that good to total pain relief was obtained in 19 patients out of 30, or 63%, while we obtained 1 good result in 8 patients. The most plausible explanation for the discrepancy between our results and those published could be that in both series of patients different structures were being stimulated. The only way to make certain of target localization is through autopsy material. We obtained an autopsy in 5 patients out of 8 (the deaths were not related to the procedure). We studied these 5 brains with the following questions in mind: 1. What target structure was stimulated, and what was the electrode trajectory? 2. What was the reaction of the brain to the presence of an electrode? 3. What was the reaction of the brain to chronic electrical stimulation?

* Department of Neurology and Neurosurgery, A. Z. Sint Rafaël, Kapucijnenvoer 35, B-3000 Leuven, Belgium.
** Unit of Neuropathology, University of Leuven, Belgium.
*** Department of Psychiatry, University of Leuven, Belgium.

0065-1419/80/Suppl. 30/0259/$ 02.00

Clinical Material

1. In Table 1 are summarized the data relevant to the influence of high medial brainstem and medial thalamic stimulation on pathological chronic and experimental acute pain in the 5 patients. More details about these patients can be found in Cosyns and Gybels (1979). As can be seen from Table 1, the majority of the cases are concerned with cancer of the head (cases 1, 2, 3, and 5); in case 4 and 5 the pain can be termed somatogenic, while in cases 1, 2, and 3 there was some involvement of the cranial nerves, either due to a previous operation to relieve the pain (cases 2 and 3), or to an infiltration of cranial nerves by the disease process (case 1 and 2).

Table 1

Case	Diagnosis	Previous oper. in NS	Follow-up	Chronic p.				Acute p.				Electrode material
				1	2	3	4	A	B	C	D	
1. D. F.	infiltration l. basis of skull by pituitary adenocarc		6 months			+		+	—	0	—	stainless steel
2. D. R. T.	infiltration l. basis of skull due to cylindroma of nasal cavity	thermo-coagul. of Gasserian ganglion	17 months	+				+	0	—	+	PtIr (90/10)
3. R. D.	r. facial pain due to Ca. of maxilla and tongue	thermo-coagul. of Gasserian ganglion	9 months	+				+	0	—	0	PtIr (90/10)
4. V. S. C.	r. hip pain due to metastasis of breast Ca.		2 weeks					0	0	0	0	Pt
5. J. N.	infiltration of basis of skull due to Ca. maxillar sinus		3 weeks	+				0	0	0	0	Pt

1 = no relief, 2 = minimal relief, 3 = good relief, 4 = total relief. A = noxious electrical stimulation, B = radiating heat, C = contact heat, D = submax. effort Tourniquet, 0 = not tested.

2. Vegetative phenomena, such as sweating, redness, changing patterns of respiration, and changes of mood, such as anxiety, could commonly be evoked in all the cases; the sensation of warmth or cold, which is regarded as a good indicator of analgesic sites (Richardson and Akil 1977), was observed in all the cases. For case 5, those phenomena were elicited only with very high current intensity (25–30 mA).

3. Stimulation parameters were as follows: a train of biphasic pulses was used, pulse duration was usually 200 µsec, both low frequency (10–30 csec) as high frequency (80–120 csec) was used, intensity of stimulating current was just below or at the threshold for vegetative or subjective phenomena (usually 0.5–2 mA); the patients were instructed to turn on the stimulator 4 times a day during 20 minutes, and to determine themselves the stimulus parameters which afforded the best pain relief.

Table 2

Autopsy data				Planned	
Case	Endpoint of trajectory	Distance to midline	Distance to ventr. wall	Distance to midline	Distance to ventr. wall
1. D. F.	C. P.	3.85 mm	2.00 mm	4 mm	2 mm
2. D. R. T.	P. G.	2.10 mm	0.75 mm	3 mm	1 mm
3. R. D.	C. P.	2.80 mm	1.70 mm	5 mm	2 mm
4. V. S. C.	P. G.	1.90 mm	0.90 mm	2 mm	1 mm
5. J. N.	C. P.	intra-ventricular	intra-ventricular	4 mm	0 mm

Autopsy Data

1. Targets

As can be seen in Table 2, in 4 cases the target was localized in the periventricular or periaqueductal gray. In cases 1, 3, and 5, the endpoint was near the posterior commissure. In case 5, the electrode was situated in the third ventricle, just at the posterior commissure. In cases 2 (Fig. 2) and 4, the end-lesion was found at the upper pontine level in the periaqueductal gray matter.

Comparison between intended target and autopsy findings shows that the stereotactic outline is quite satisfactory for 4 cases.

2. Trajectories

The electrode trajectory, along which electrical stimulation was applied to the brain is visualized for cases 1 (Fig. 1), 3 (Fig. 3), and 4 (Fig. 4) on 4 vertico-frontal sections, level 1 being most caudal, level 4 most rostral.

In case 1, the trajectory is somewhat more laterally situated than was aimed for. The target structure however was reached.

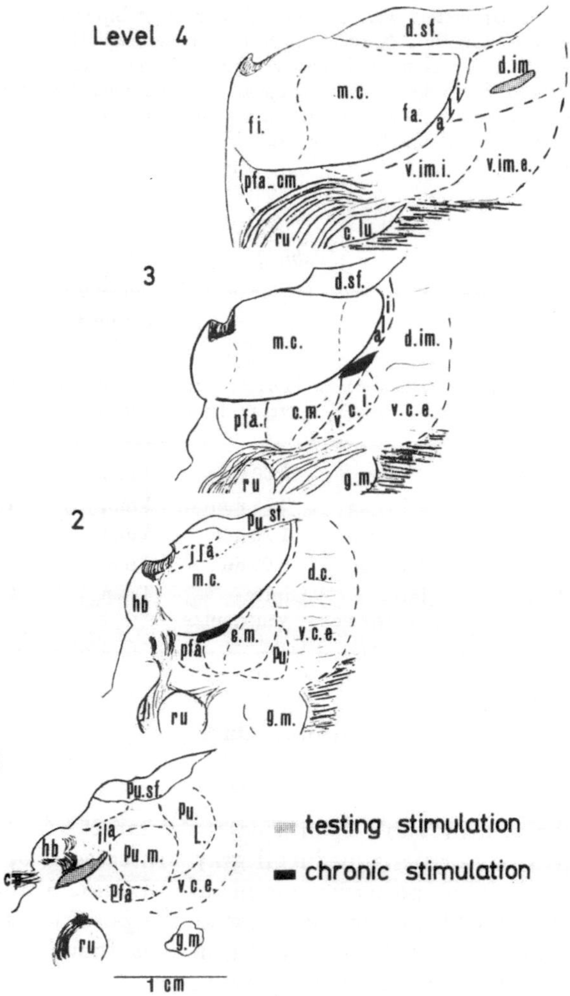

Fig. 1. Case 1 D. F. In this figure and the following ones, the nomenclature used is as in Bailey and Schaltenbrand's atlas (1959)

In case 2, 3, and 4 the trajectory crosses the medial thalamic nucleus (m.c.) and passes by the parafascicular nucleus (p.fa.) near the commissura posterior. In case 3, the trajectory ends at this level. In case 2 and 4, the trajectory continues medially from the red nucleus (ru) and ends in the periaqueductal gray matter at the upper pontine level.

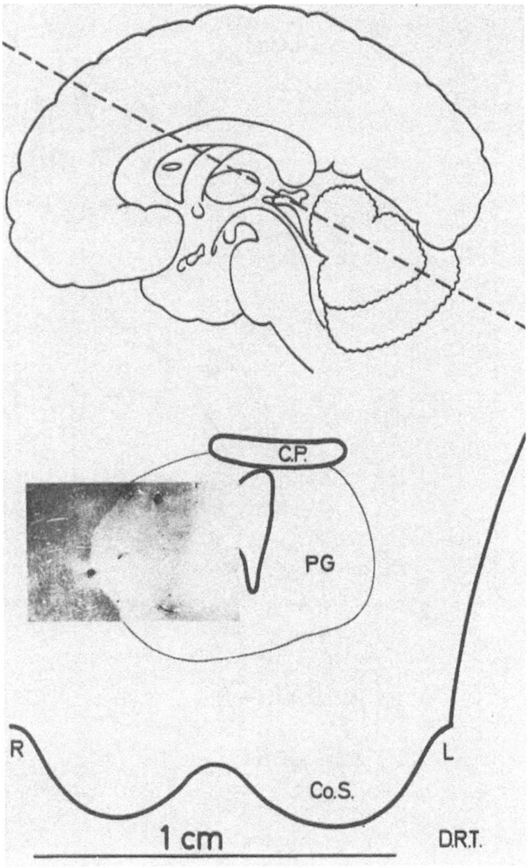

Fig. 2. Case 2 D. R. T. The upper part of the figure indicates the direction of the plane of section. The electrode trajectory near its end can be seen in the lower part of the figure at 9 o'clock at the border of the periaqueductal gray

In case 5, the trajectory passes just medial to the medial thalamic nucleus and ends into the third ventricle (Fig. 5).

3. Reaction of the Brain to the Presence of an Electrode

Table 3 summarizes the findings for all 5 cases. In cases 1, 4, and 5, a more extensive reaction is observed than in cases 2 and 3. In cases 2 and 3, PtIr electrodes were used, while in case 1 stainless steel and in cases 4 and 5 Pt electrodes were used. This might partly explain the different reaction. It should be noted that in cases 2

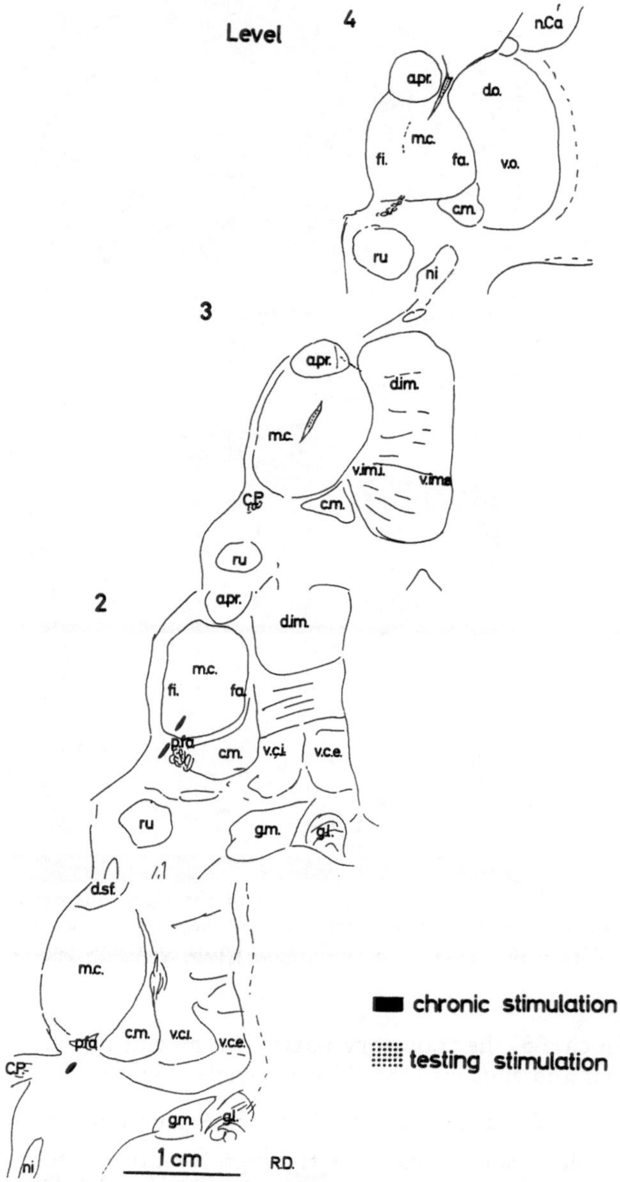

Fig. 3. Case 3 R. D.

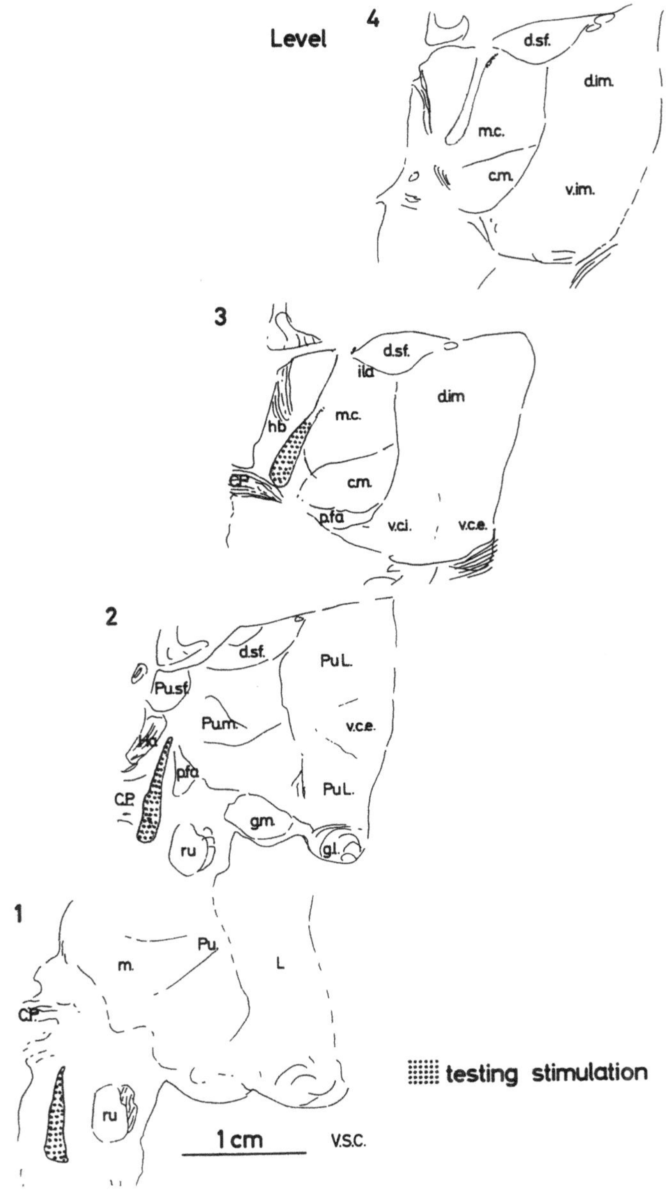

Fig. 4. Case 4 V. S. C.

and 3 no mesenchymal reaction was found in contrast to the other 3 cases. In case 1 and 4, brain oedema was observed. This might also explain a more extensive necrosis. In case 4 moreover, meningeal infection was found, complicating also the tissue reaction.

Table 3

Case	Electrode material	Maximal width trajectory	Histological reaction to electrode	Reaction to chronic stim.
1. D. F.	stainless steel	1,400 μ	— necrosis + — strong mesenchymal reaction + gitter cells — glial reaction	
2. D. R. T.	PtIr 90/10	300 μ	— spongiosis — microglial reaction	— mild chromatolysis of neurones
3. R. D.	PtIr 90/10	400 μ	— spongiosis — microglial reaction — minimal mesenchymal reaction	— mild gliosis
4. V. S. C.	Pt	1,700 μ	— necrosis ++ — strong mesenchymal reaction — glial reaction — inflammatory reaction + giant cells	
5. J. N.	Pt	800 μ	— necrosis + — mesenchymal reaction + gitter cells — glial reaction	

From these observations, we may conclude that PtIr electrodes, remaining for several months in the brain, cause little tissue reaction.

4. Reaction to Chronic Stimulation

Only in cases 1, 2, and 3, the electrodes were sufficiently long in the brain to evaluate chronic stimulation. In the brain areas where the stimulated contacts were situated, no specific tissue damage was observed. Only mild gliosis in the vicinity of the electrode was found. In case 1 and 3, mild chromatolysis of some thalamic neurones was seen in the parafascicular nucleus.

Discussion and Conclusions

From these 5 autopsy cases, in which electrical stimulation of the periventricular and periaqueductal gray for the treatment of chronic pain was performed, the following conclusion can be tentatively drawn:

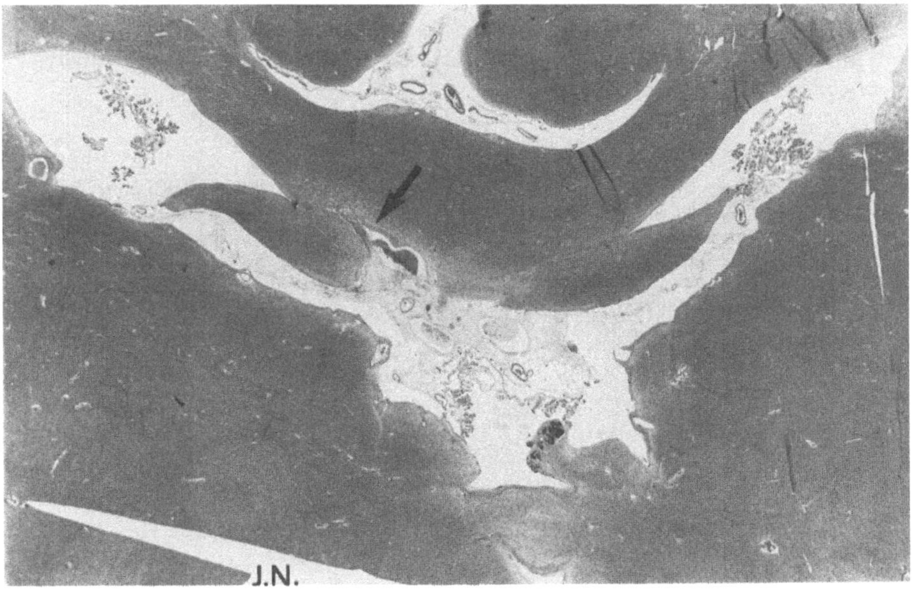

Fig. 5. Case 5 J. N. Vertico-frontal section. The arrow indicates the electrode trajectory

1. Stereotactic technique of recommended target and trajectory localization is satisfactory.
2. PtIr (90/10) electrodes cause little tissue reaction.
3. Chronic stimulation (biphasic, 10–120 csec, 200 μsec, 0.2–2 mA, 20 min, 4 × day) does not seem to provoke lesions observable by light-microscopy.
4. Cerebral oedema and meningitis seem to be contra-indications for electrode implantation.

Of immediate interest to the present discussion is the observation that the discrepancy between our "bad" results and the "good" results published in the literature is not to be explained by wrong electrode placement. In our opinion, the following questions have to be answered before periventricular and periaqueductal gray stimulation can be considered as a valuable therapeutic tool for the treatment of chronic pain: How well can central gray stimulation alleviate chronic pain? There are no data from animal studies; in human studies, evaluation of the results is an amply documented difficulty. What is the target to be reached? From animal studies, in which experimental pain was tested, it appears that the target areas are very critical indeed. And finally, how will we select the patients, suitable for implantation? It may be that besides acute testing stimulation, some pharmacological manipulations may be of help, but this certainly needs further investigation.

Acknowledgements

The authors are grateful to Mrs. Feytons-Heeren and Mrs. B. Wijnants, and Mr. P. De Sutter for their skillful technical assistance. They are indebted to Drs. M. Depierreux and J. Flament-Durand of the U.L.B. in Brussels, who performed the histopathological examination of case 2. The investigation was supported by the FGWO (grant 3.0045.79) of Belgium and the Onderzoeksfonds K.U. Leuven (grant OT/VII/34).

References

1. Cosyns, P., Gybels, J., Electrical central gray stimulation for pain in man. In: Advances in Pain Research and Therapy, Vol. 3, pp. 511—514 (Bonica, J. J., Liebeskind, J., Albe-Fessard, D., eds.). New York: Raven Press. 1979.
2. Gybels, J., Electrical stimulation of the central gray for pain relief in humans: a critical review. In: Advances in Pain Research and Therapy, Vol. 3, pp. 499—509 (Bonica, J. J., Liebeskind, J., Albe-Fessard, D., eds.). New York: Raven Press. 1979.
3. Richardson, D. E., Akil, H., Pain reduction by electrical brain stimulation in man. Part 2. Chronic self-administration in the periventricular gray matter. J. Neurosurg. *47* (1977), 184—194.
4. Schaltenbrand, G., Bailey, P., Introduction to stereotaxis with an atlas of the human brain. Stuttgart: G. Thieme. 1959.

Acta Neurochirurgica, Suppl. 30, 269—274 (1980)

Indications and Ethical Considerations of Deep Brain Stimulation

J. Siegfried*, Y. Lazorthes, and R. Sedan*****

Summary

Electrical impulses through chronically implanted electrodes in the human brain are used today in the relief of chronic crippling pain, motor movement disorders and behavior disturbances. A great number of reports from animal studies and several descriptions of the results produced by human stimulation seem to suggest that pain can often be adequately controlled. However, the perspectives of such methods raise many ethical problems and ask for caution. Nervous tissue damage after long-term stimulation, biochemical modifications, electrode migration and long-term follow-up of its clinical value are still under study and are the factors which might limit for the time being the indications. A restrictive role for this procedure is advocated for: 1. cases of chronic facial pain, 2. cases of chronic pain in other locations where other neurosurgical operations have failed and where the patient is not too young and is not suffering from pain of benign origin.

Therapeutic electrical neurostimulation is one of the most fascinating approaches in the treatment of functional disorders, is used more and more frequently, and will certainly continue to play an important role in the future course of the field of medicine. Electrical neurostimulation is one of the best examples of functional neurosurgery, permitting the resolution of one or more symptoms without destroying nervous structures. This really will be true, when the definitive innocuousness of a method in which electrodes within or in direct contact with nervous tissues will be proved. Implantation of chronic electrodes in the brain also raises other controversies, particularly since the brain is not only the organ of neural coordination, but also the organ of thought; deep brain stimulation can erroneously be interpretated as mind manipulation.

Electrical stimulation of the brain has been used since 1950 to treat a variety of intractable psychiatric and neurologic diseases [8]. The successful employment of septal stimulation as an analgesic tool

* Neurosurgical Department, University of Zürich, Rämistraße 100, CH-8091 Zürich, Switzerland.

** Neurosurgical Department, University of Toulouse, France.

*** Neurosurgical Department, University of Marseille, France.

0065-1419/80/Suppl. 30/0269/$ 01.20

by Heath and Mickle before 1960 can possibly be attributed to psychic interpretation since a number of emotional side effects resulted from stimulation of the septal area [9]. However, psychiatric neurosurgery using stimulation techniques seems to be accepted only in very few centres and publications on these topics are rather rare [6]. Deep brain stimulation in the treatment of motor disorders is a very recent approach and few statistics are yet available [22]. Pain reduction by electrical brain stimulation is much better known and relies on convincing animal studies [14, 19, 28]. This therapeutic method has become very attractive in the last few years and has been employed in over 500 cases throughout the world.

Since the introduction of stereotactic procedures, most surgical efforts to relieve pain have concentrated on localized destruction of various parts of the thalamus [3, 4, 10, 16, 30, 34] and mesencephalon [30, 33]. Since these pioneering efforts, stereotactic operations in the treatment of chronic pain were used frequently until a few years ago, when a large number of studies with long-term follow-up reported conflicting results. Practically all neurosurgeons familiar with stereotactic neurosurgery applied intracerebral stimulation before making a therapeutic lesion. Many sensations were reported, depending of the electrode site and the parameters of stimulation. However, the observation of disappearance of pain during electrical stimulation of different brain targets was very rarely mentioned. Mazars was one of the first to postulate that stimulation of pain pathways does not necessarily elicit pain sensation [17]; since 1962 (first published in 1973), he advocated intermittent stimulation with implanted electrodes in the sensory thalamic nuclei for pain relief [18], as did Hosobuchi and Adams [12] the same year. The internal capsule was also chosen as a target [12] and subsequently, Richardson and Akil [29] reported that pain could be reduced by electrical stimulation of the periventricular and periaqueductal gray matter in humans. Since then deep brain stimulation for persistent clinical pain states has been applied in a large number of cases. Analysing the overall results of more than 250 cases implanted by different neurosurgical groups prior to 1978, Sedan and Lazorthes report about 75% success rate [31]. Since then, the rate of success reported has varied considerably. At the recent 3rd European Workshop on Neurostimulation [20], Meyerson reviewed the results observed in 324 patients operated on in 13 different clinics, among them 11 in Europe. An overall analysis is quite difficult since many factors, including the selection of patients, the location of stimulating electrodes, the stimulation parameters and the method of evaluating results can account for the discrepancy between the groups who reported improvement varying from 20 to 80% of patients.

This uncertainty in the real and definite value of deep brain stimulation in the treatment of chronic pain, motor disorders and psychiatric disturbances, as well as the lack of information on the effect of repetitive stimulation on cell activity and the possibility of cell damage requires us to formulate some considerations for the use of this method, its actual limits, and its ethical implications.

Ethical Aspects

Ethics is that branch of philosophy relating to human conduct, to the rightness and wrongness of certain actions, and to the good and bad of the motives and ends of such actions [11]. By introducing a new procedure, the risk-benefit ratio has to be seriously considered. Any assessment of medical procedures that is carried out in order to establish standards of care reveals that the outcome of most procedures promise an almost certain benefit, which may not, however, come about in a particular application. Other procedures that will certainly benefit entail certain or probable concomitant harm [13].

Even if chronic deep brain stimulation has been demonstrated to be a safe method thus far some uncertainty remains.

a) Might long-term deep brain stimulation cause damage to the brain tissue?

Many factors must be considered, particularly the type of electrode (platinum, stainless steel, rhodium, tantalum pentoxide, capacitors electrodes, etc.) and the stimulus parameters (charge density, charge per phase, current density, pulse duration, pulse repetition rate, etc.). Extensive animal studies have been made [2, 5, 15, 21, 24, 26, 27]. A blood-brain barrier breakdown was reported [21], but seemed confined to the internal capsule and leptomeninges [26]. Various stages of neuronal damage were noted in both light and electron microscopic studies [24]. These studies were performed in cats after 36 hours of essentially continuous high-level stimulation of the brain. It has been demonstrated that lower level, but physiologically effective, stimulation produced negligible damage [25]. Pudenz reported encouraging data for safe stimulation [25]. However, we still need data on long-term stimulation of the human brain before being completely satisfied.

b) Might long-term deep brain stimulation cause biochemical modifications?

The effect of electrical stimulation on tissue pH, p 02, K^+, GABA and spermidine have been investigated [23]. The histofluorescence and the micro-electrophoresis of neurotransmitters at stimulated electrodes sites could also bring some important data. We certainly need information in this almost virgin research area.

c) Do chronically implanted deep brain electrodes move?

Fixation of the deep brain electrode outside the brain structures is soluble, but the possibility of migration of the tip of electrode by a few millimeters in time exists. Does the electrode move within or with the brain? Specific experiments to answer this question remain to be performed.

d) How clinically effective is therapeutic deep brain stimulation?

Deep brain stimulation was been used so far for chronic pain, movement disorders and psychiatric disturbances. Because this surgery is intended to improve the quality of life rather than to save life, measuring the improvement is important. For proper evaluation, we need to assess the patient's residual symptoms, state of restored health, feeling of well-being, limitations, new or restored capabilities, and responses to these advantages and disadvantages. We need long-term follow-up and both objective and subjective appraisals of the patient's quality of life [7]. Most of the clinical publications seem to be satisfied with the improvement of single symptoms without more information on the overall quality of life. More co-operative studies with the same method of evaluation could answer the question objectively.

Indications

At the 3rd European Workshop on Neurostimulation, the indications for 260 cases operated on for pain with deep brain electrodes in different clinics in Europe and one in South Africa were summarized [32] and will be discussed.

a) Location of pain. Only 14.2% of the cases had pain in the face and/or throat and 8.5% had thalamic pain on one side of the body with probably involvement of the face. This gives a total of 22.7% of the cases.

b) Cause of pain. Only 19.6% of the cases had pain due to malignant disease. Details of the primary diagnosis and location of pain are given in Table 1.

The uncertainty of deep brain stimulation mentioned under the ethical aspects must directly influence the indications. In this respect, we would like to propose limited indications for deep brain stimulation for chronic pain until some of the questions raised find their solutions:

1. Chronic pain in the face having almost no other neurosurgical alternatives seems to be a reasonable indication for deep brain stimulation.

2. Deep brain stimulation can certainly be considered for pain located elsewhere than the cephalic region, when other neurosurgical procedures have failed, especially dorsal cord stimulation. However, due to our incomplete knowledge, one cannot propose this indication to young people suffering from benign pain without reservations.

References

1. Adams, J. E., Hosobuchi, Y., Fields, H., Stimulation of internal capsule for relief of chronic pain. J. Neurosurg. *41* (1974), 740—744.
2. Agnew, W. F., Yuen, T. G. H., Pudenz, R. H., Bullara, L. A., Electrical stimulation of the brain. IV. Ultrastructural studies. Surg. Neurol. *4* (1975), 438—448.
3. Baudouin, A., Puech, P., Premiers essais d'intervention directe sur le thalamus (injections, électrocoagulations). Rev. Neurol. *81* (1949), 78—81.
4. Bettag, W., Yoshida, T., Über stereotaktische Schmerzoperationen. Acta Neurochir. (Wien) *8* (1960), 299—317.
5. Brummer, S. B., Turner, M. J., Electrochemical considerations for safe electrical stimulation of the neurons system with platinum electrodes. IEEE Trans. Biomed. Eng. BME *23* (1977), 59—63.
6. Dieckmann, G., Chronic mediothalamic stimulation for control of phobias. In: Modern Concepts in Psychiatric Surgery, pp. 85—93 (Hitchcock, E. R., Ballantine, H. T., Meyerson, B. A., eds.). Elsevier: North-Holland, publ. 1979.
7. Gilbert, J. P., McPeek, B., Mosteller, F., Statistics and ethics in surgery and anaesthesia. Science *198* (1977), 684—689.
8. Heath, R. G., Electrical self-stimulation of the brain in man. Amer. J. Psychiat. *120* (1963), 571—577.
9. Heath, R. G., Mickle, W. A., Evaluation of seven years' experience with depth electrodes studies in human patients. In: Electrical Studies on the Unanesthesized Brain, pp. 214—247 (Ramey, E. R., O'Doherty, D. S., eds.). New-York: P. B. Hoeber. 1960.
10. Hecaen, H., Talairach, J., David, M., Dell, M. B., Coagulations limitées du thalamus dans les algies du syndrome thalamique. Rev. Neurol. *81* (1949), 917—931.
11. Herbert, V., Acquiring new information while retaining old ethics. Science *198* (1977), 690—693.
12. Hosobuchi, Y., Adams, J. E., Rutkin, B., Chronic thalamic stimulation for the control of facial anesthesia dolorosa. Arch. Neurol. *29* (1973), 153—169.
13. Jonson, A. R., Do no harm. Ann. intern. Med. *88* (1978), 827—832.
14. Liebeskind, J. C., Guilbaud, G., Besson, J. M., Analgesia from electrical stimulation of the periaqueductal gray matter in the cat: behavioral observations and inhibitory effects on spinal cord interneurons. Brain Res. *50* (1973), 441—446.
15. Lilly, J. C., Injury and excitation by electric currents. In: Electrical stimulation of the brain, pp. 60—64 (Sheet, D. W., ed.). Austin: University of Texas Press. 1961.
16. Mark, V. H., Ervin, F. R., Hackett, T. P., Clinical aspects of stereotactic thalamotomy in the human. I. The treatment of chronic severe pain. Arch. Neurol. *3* (1960), 351—367.
17. Mazars, G., Ruge, R., Mazars, Y., Résultats de la stimulation du faisceau spino-thalamique et leur incidence sur la physiopathologie de la douleur. Rev. Neurol. *103* (1960), 136—138.

18. Mazars, G., Merienne, L., Cioloca, C., Stimulations thalamiques intermittentes antalgiques. Rev. Neurol. *128* (1973), 273—279.
19. Mayer, D. J., Wolfle, T. L., Akil, H., Analgesia from electrical stimulation in the brain stem of the rat. Science *174* (1971), 1351—1354.
20. Meyerson, B., Co-operative study on deep brain stimulation for pain. 3rd Workshop on Neurostimulation, Mégève, March 30–31, 1979 (not published).
21. Mortimer, J. T., Shealy, C. N., Wheeler, C., Experimental nondestructive stimulation of the brain and spinal cord. J. Neurosurg. *32* (1970), 553—559.
22. Mundinger, F., Neue stereotaktisch-funktionelle Behandlungsmethode des Torticollis spasmodicus mit Hirnstimulatoren. Med. Klin. *72* (1977), 1982—1986.
23. Pudenz, R. H., Report of the neural damage panel. In: Functional Electrical Stimulation, Vol. 1, pp. 479—482 (Hambrecht, F. T., Reswick, J. B., eds.). New York-Basel: Dekker. 1977.
24. Pudenz, R. H., Agnew, W. F., Bullara, L., Effects of electrical stimulation of the brain. Light and electron microscope studies. Brain, Behavior and Evol. *14* (1977), 103—124.
25. Pudenz, R. H., Agnew, W. F., Yuen, T. G. H., Bullara, L. A., Electrical stimulation of brain. In: Functional Electrical Stimulation, Vol. 1, pp. 437—457 (Hambrecht, F. T., Reswick, J. B., eds.). New York-Basel: Dekker. 1977.
26. Pudenz, R. H., Bullara, L. A., Dru, D., Talalla, A., Electrical stimulation of the brain. II. Effects on the blood-brain barrier. Surg. Neurol. *4* (1975), 265—270.
27. Pudenz, R. H., Bullara, L. A., Jacques, S., Hambrecht, F. T., Electrical stimulation of the brain. III. The neural damage model. Surg. Neurol. *4* (1975), 389—400.
28. Reynolds, D. V., Surgery in the rat during electrical analgesia induced by focal brain stimulation. Science *164* (1969), 444—445.
29. Richardson, D. E., Akil, H., Pain reduction by electrical brain stimulation in man. J. Neurosurg. *47* (1977), 178—194.
30. Riechert, T., Die chirurgische Behandlung der zentralen Schmerzzustände, einschließlich der stereotaktischen Operationen im Thalamus und Mesencephalon. Acta Neurochir. (Wien) *8* (1960), 136—152.
31. Sedan, R., Lazorthes, Y., La neurostimulation électrique thérapeutique. Neurochirurgie *24*, Suppl. 1, 138 pp. (1978).
32. Siegfried, J., Indications and ethical consideration on deep brain stimulation. 3rd European Workshop on Neurostimulation, Mégève, March 30–31, 1979 (not published).
33. Spiegel, E. A., Wycis, H. T., Mesencephalotomy for relief of pain. In: Anniversary Volume for O. Poetzl, Vienna, p. 438 (1948).
34. Talairach, H., Hecaen, H., David, M., Monnier, M., Ajuriaguerra, J. de, Recherches sur la coagulation thérapeutique des structures sous-corticales chez l'homme. Rev. Neurol. *81* (1949), 4—24.

Acta Neurochirurgica, Suppl. 30, 275—277 (1980)

Septal Stimulation on Painful and Symbolic Stress. Experimental Study

J. Broseta*, J. L. Barcia-Salorio, and J. Barberá

Summary

Based on the rewarding effect of septal area, therapeutic stimulation of this region has been applied to surgical management of chronic pain. However some basic problems of this technique remain unsolved. Thus the effect of septal stimulation was tested on an experimental model of painful and symbolic stress, comparing the variations in the pituitaryadrenal axis activity, the peripheral cathecolamine levels and the structural changes in gastric mucosa and adrenal glands, between the problem and different control groups. The bioelectrical activity of septal area and anterolateral hypothalamus during stimulation were recorded. A decrease in gastric ulceration and plasma cortisol were observed in the septal stimulation group. No direct influence on the cathecolaminic system was noted. A facilitation of septal activity and its influence on hypothalamic rythm were found. All these effects were mainly achieved in the posterior perifornical septal region.

Introduction

In cases in which the organism cannot be removed from a stressful situation, perhaps it might be possible to partially compensate this condition by adding some positive reinforcement to the situation. Thus based on the rewarding effect of septal area, therapeutic septal stimulation has been used in surgical management of chronic pain with diverse results [2–4]. However this technique still presents some unsolved problems: first, the distinct effects evoked by stimulation of different septal points; second, the possible spread of electric stimuli to other related areas giving spurious results; third, the possible role of other septal functions other than the rewarding one; and lastly, there is little known about the resistance or fatigability of the septum to electric stimulation.

With all this in mind, an experimental model to study the effect of electrical septal stimulation upon stress parameters has been

* Departamento de Neurocirugia, Hospital Clínico Universitario, P. Blasco Ibañez, 17, Valencia-10, Spain.

0065-1419/80/Suppl. 30/0275/$ 01.00

developed. This model is based on restraint stress because it generates pain-like stimuli and presents an important emotional load.

Material and Methods

One hundred and twenty Wistar male rats, weighing 250–300 g were used. The animals were distributed in a problem group (SS) subjected simultaneously to stress and septal stimulation and four control groups: normal (N), stress (NS), sham (SH) and neutral electric caudatum stimulation (SC).

The animals of the SS, SH and SC groups were chronically implanted with 0.5 mm epoxilited coated stainless steel bipolar electrode in their respective areas. Conventional animal stereotactic techniques were used for the implantation. The electrode was fixed to the skull with methyl-methacrilate. Two days after the implantation the animals were tested in a Skinner box to determine the self-stimulation threshold. The highest score of responses corresponded to 450–500 μa.

Three days later, following a fasting period of 24 hours, animals of all groups were immobilized during 24 hours in order to create the restraining stress. The 24 hours urine sample was collected by means of a plastic finger glove. During immobilization, the animals of the SS and SC groups were stimulated according to these parameters: square pulse train of 0.5 sec, 0.2 msec pulse duration, 100 Hz, *500 μa* intensity and 15 sec intertrain interval. The stimulation cadence was repeated every 20 minutes.

After the 24 hours period of immobilization/stimulation the animals were beheaded and blood collected for biochemical determinations. The stomach and adrenal glands were removed by laparotomy. Once the stomach was opened the stress ulcers were counted. First, gastric pathology was referred to a ranking scale according to Adami [1]. Because of the non parametric character of this method, the ulcerated areas were also measured comparing their surface in mm^2 per cm^2 of normal gastric mucosa.

Haematoxylin-eosin stain was used for histological examination of both organs and Sudan Black B was applied to evaluate the adrenal lipids. All stimulated brains were sectioned and stained by cresyl-violet method to determine the real position of the electrode tip.

Radiobioassay was employed for plasmatic cortisol determinations and thin layer chromatography was used for the VMA analysis.

Results

Gastric pathology was significantly decreased in the septal stimulation group (SS = 1.3 ± 0.7 rate and 1.07 ± 0.75 mm^2/cm^2; $p < 0.05$) when compared to all control groups ($\overline{NS}$ = 2.6 ± 1.5 rate and 4.1 ± 1.5 mm^2/cm^2; $p < 0.05$; $\overline{SH}$ = 2.4 ± 0.8 rate and 3.1 ± 1.5 mm^2/cm^2; $p < 0.05$; $\overline{SC}$ = 2.5 ± 0.9 rate and 4.4 ± 3.4 mm^2/cm^2; $p < 0.05$) in both measuring methods. The correlation coefficient between the non-parametric rating and the metric values was high significant (r = 0.7908).

The problem group had higher cortisol concentration ($\overline{SS}$ = 17.6 ± 5.8 μg/100 ml) when compared to normal levels ($\overline{N}$ =

12.3 ± 0.4 μg/100 ml) but consistently lower ones than all control groups ($\overline{NS}$ = 28.7 ± 8.18 μg/100 ml; $\overline{SH}$ = 27.2 ± 7.5 μg/100 ml; $\overline{SC}$ = 24.1 ± 5.3 μg/100 ml). These results are in accordance with these obtained in qualitative studies of lipid material in the adrenal cortex, in which the septal group was deficient occupying an intermediate position between the normal state and the total depletion of the stress control group.

The vanilylmandelic acid (VMA) concentrations confirmed the increase of cathecolamines in stress, manifested in the septal ($\overline{SS}$ = 33.1 ± 8.7 μg/24 hours) as well as in all control groups ($\overline{NS}$ = 33.3 ± 12.9 μg/24 hours; $\overline{SH}$ = 37.0 ± 13.8 μg/24 hours; $\overline{SC}$ = 35.3 ± 9.6 μg/24 hours) which are much higher than the normal values ($\overline{N}$ = 2.15 ± 5.2 μg/24 hours).

In a tridimensional mapping of the tip electrode localization in the septal group it was observed that all points that produced a decrease of stress parameters (ulcers or cortisol) were placed in the posterior septum and nearby the perifornical area.

During the 24 hours EEG recording of septal activity in enriching, facilitation and slowing of septal rhythm with some recruitment phenomena, which occasionally resembled a theta hippocampal activity, has been observed. Also, some synchronic recruitment in anterolateral hypothalamus during septal stimulation was found.

References

1. Adami, E., Pharmacological research on generfate, a new synthetic isoprenoid with antiulcer action. Arch. Intern. Pharmacodyn. *147* (1974), 113—117.
2. Gol, A., Relief of pain by electrical stimulation of the septal area. J. Neurol. Sci. *5* (1967), 115—120.
3. Heath, R. G., Mickle, W. A., Evaluation of seven years' experience with depth electrode studies in human patients. In: Electrical studies on the unanaesthetized brain (Ramey, E. R., O'Doherty, D. S., eds.). New York: Hoeber. 1960.
4. Obrador, S., Delgado, J. M. R., Martin-Rodriguez, J. G., Emotional areas of the human brain and their therapeutical stimulation. In: Cerebral localization, pp. 171—183 (Zülch, K. J., *et al.*, eds.). Berlin-Heidelberg-New York: Springer. 1975.

Acta Neurochirurgica, Suppl. 30, 279—287 (1980)

A Study on the Tridimensional Distribution of Somatosensory Evoked Responses in Human Thalamus to Aid the Placement of Stimulating Electrodes for Treatment of Pain

C. Giorgi*, P. J. Kelly*, D. C. Eaton*, G. Guiot, P. Derome****

With 4 Figures

Treatment of chronic pain by means of electrical stimulation of Ventralis Posterior (VP) has been carried out by several workers [6, 7, 9, 10, 11].

Best results are reported when the stimulating electrode is positioned in the subportion of VP which corresponds to the part of the body where the patient is having pain [9, 10].

Individual variability in VP in relationship to radiological landmarks has been demonstrated by several anatomical and clinical studies [1–3, 5, 8, 12, 13].

Therefore a neurophysiological control of the position of the chronic stimulating electrodes would improve the accuracy of the placement and thereby the results of chronic stimulation in the treatment of chronic pain.

In order to attain a clear understanding of the somatotopic arrangement of body parts within VP the following study was undertaken using neurophysiologic information derived from semimicroelectrode recording within VP during the course of stereotactic procedures.

Methods and Material

Semimicroelectrode recording has been employed at Hôpital Foch to aid the localization of lesions in the thalamus since 1962. The position of the target is determined with a geometrical construction on the outline of the third ventricle based on the position of the anterior and posterior commissures [4].

* University of Texas Medical Branch, Galveston, Texas, U.S.A.
** Hôpital Foch, Suresnes, France.

0065-1419/80/Suppl. 30/0279/$ 01.80

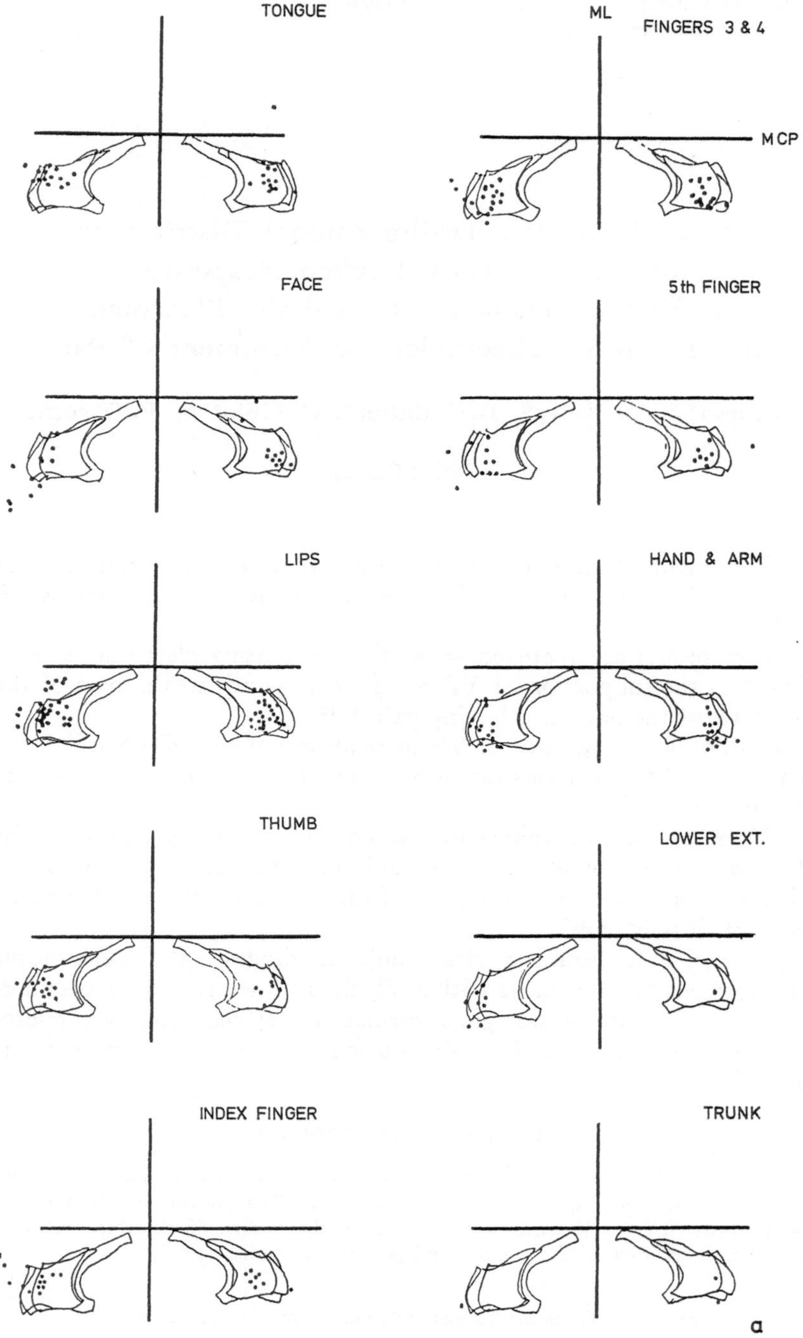

Fig. 1 a. Scatter of somatosensory evoked responses plotted with reference to radiologic landmarks in the horizontal plane

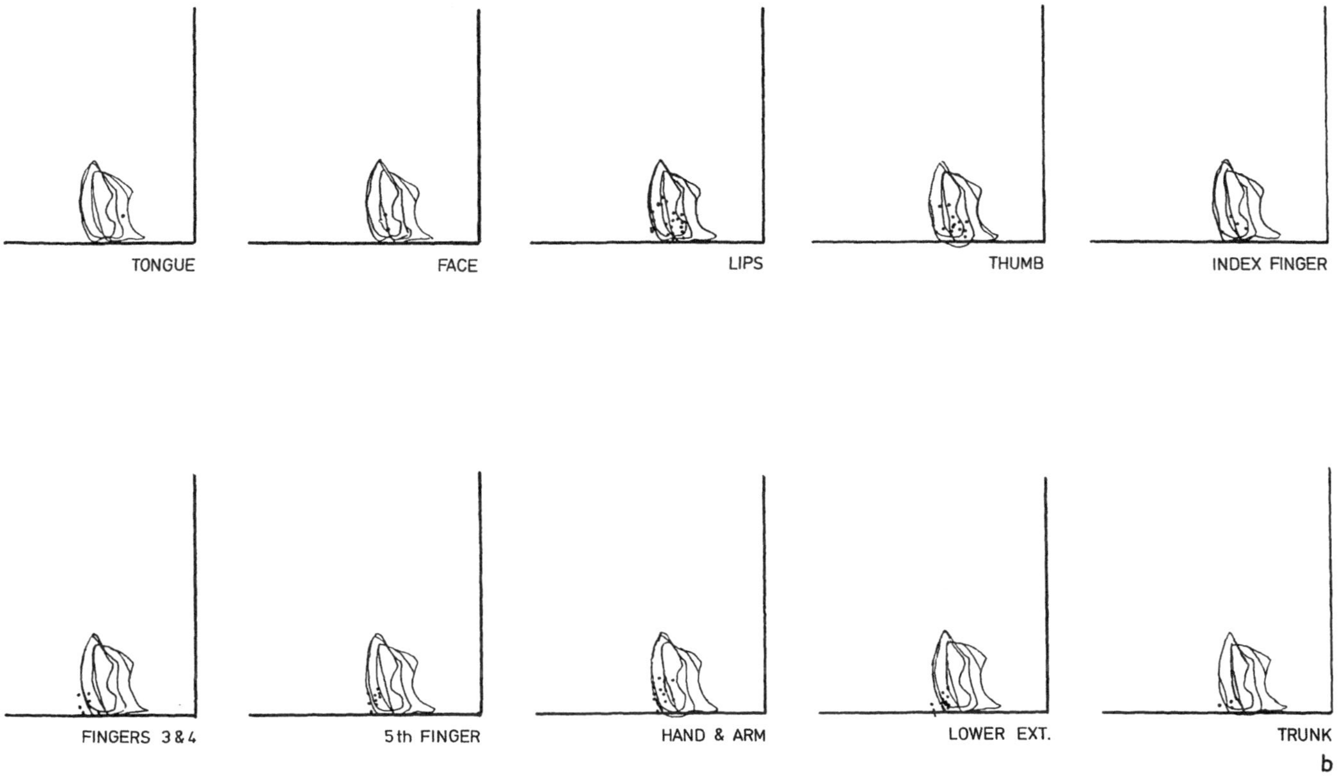

Fig. 1 b. Scatter of somatosensory evoked responses plotted with reference to radiologic landmarks in a frontal plane

The electrode is directed toward the target through an occipital burr-hole, and in a semihorizontal trajectory which transverses the Pulvinar, VP, Vim, VoP, VoA, and the internal capsule. Electrical activity recorded from the semimicroelectrode indicates the exact position of the anterior and posterior borders of VP and the internal capsule. Furthermore high amplitude evoked potentials may be recorded while the electrode transverses VP. These may be evoked by a variety of stimuli applied to the contralateral body, such as light touch, proprioception and pressure. Since the body is represented in a somatotopic fashion in VP, this information and the posteriority at which the internal capsule is encountered by a particular trajectory have been useful in establishing the neurophysiologic laterality of the probe. For example a trajectory from which evoked potentials are obtained from the face and lips in VP and from which the internal capsule is encountered at six millimeters posterior to the plane of the anterior commissure is more medial than a trajectory in which evoked potentials are obtained from the lower extremity and which encounters the internal capsule at sixteen millimeters posterior to the plane of the anterior commissure.

By these two pieces of information lesions may be more accurately placed in VL.

For the purpose of the present study we have selected data obtained from 104 recording trajectories performed at Hôpital Foch during the course of 67 stereotactic operations done for the treatment of Parkinson's or intention tremor between January 1968 and April 1977. These data gave information on the anterior to posterior arrangement of the body within VP.

At the University of Texas Medical Branch (Galveston) we have developed a similar technique for the localization of lesions in the treatment of movement disorders and for the placement of chronic stimulating electrodes in VP for treatment of chronic pain. This method differs from that at Hôpital Foch in that it utilizes a Todd-Wells frame and a coronal approach in which a superior to inferior recording trajectory is made through VP. The radiological position of VP is determined from a ventriculogram using the geometrical construction employed at the Hôpital Foch. Characteristic electrical activity from the white matter, caudate nucleus and dorsum of the thalamus is obtained from a bipolar concentric semimicroelectrode having a tip diameter of 10 μ, interpolar distance of 400 μ and outer diameter of 600 μ. The superior border of VP is recognized by the appearance of high amplitude background activity, as well as the appearance of evoked responses when specific areas of the contralateral body are stimulated. The dorsal to ventral somatotopic arrangement in VP is then demonstrated with this approach.

Thirteen patients underwent semimicroelectrode recording in VP between January 1978 and April 1978 with this technique and we have studied the data obtained from 26 trajectories from these patients.

Results

The responses recorders in VP from the Hôpital Foch and UTMB data were first plotted with reference to radiological landmarks, *i.e.*, the midline and the midcommissural planes. The position at which evoked responses were obtained from specific parts of the body were found to be widely scattered and the areas from different body parts were largely superimposed (Fig. 1 a and b).

Therefore, because of the individual spatial variability, specific somatotopic subportions of VP could not be accurately localized using radiological landmarks alone.

We next attempted to group the position of evoked responses for specific body parts in VP according to a physiologically determined

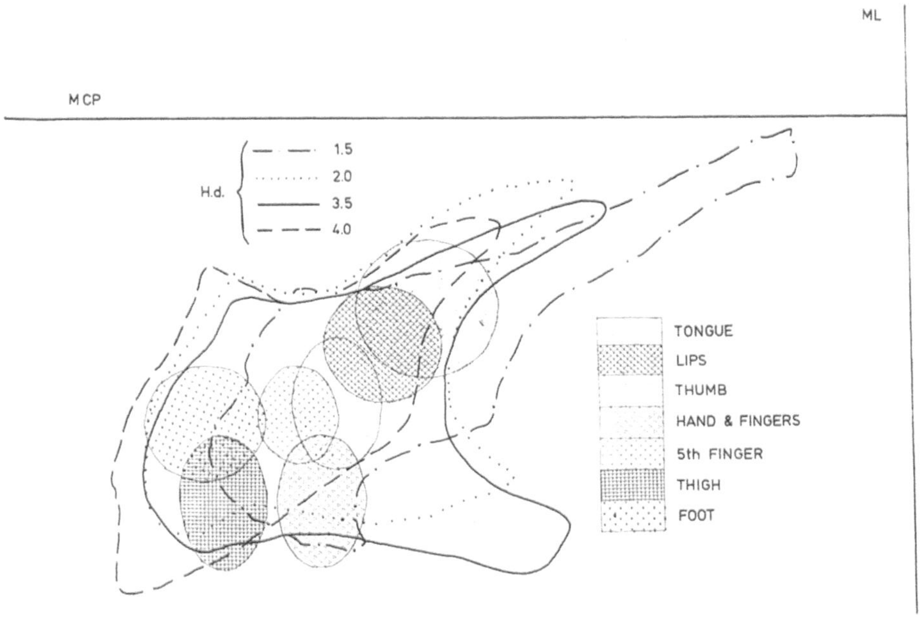

Fig. 2. Clusters of responses plotted with reference to the neurophysiologically determined laterality of the probe. The four outline of VP represent different hights from CA CP plane

landmark. Since the probe trajectories at Hôpital Foch were of a fixed obliquity and were oblique to the internal capsule, the posteriority at which the capsule was encountered could be used as an indication of the laterality of the probe as described above.

This was done with a computer program that set the laterality of the probe by the point at which the internal capsule was encountered on a three-dimensional computerized stereotactic atlas, and then plotted the points from different areas of the body within the limits of VP. This resulted in a clearer definition of somatotopic subportions of VP (Fig. 2).

In order to reconstruct in even more detail the tridimensional arrangement of the body within VP, we examined all the data

Table 1. *Average Distances Between Points at Which Evoked Responses Were Recorded in Patients in Which Two Recording Trajectories Were Made*

To	Lips	Face	Thumb	Index	Middle	Ring	Hand	Arm	Shoulder	5th	Hip	Leg	Foot
To													
Lips	2.5												
Face	2.5	—											
Thumb	3.2	0.7	0.7										
Index	3.5	1	1	0.3									
Middle	4.2	1.7	1.7	1	0.7								
Ring	5	2.5	2.5	1.8	1.5	0.8							
Hand	5	2.5	2.5	1.8	1.5	0.8	—						
Arm	5	2.5	2.5	1.8	1.5	0.8	—	—					
Shoulder	5	2.5	2.5	1.8	1.5	0.8	—	—	—				
5th	5.7	3.2	3.2	2.5	2.2	1.5	0.7	0.7	0.7	0.7			
Hip	6.5	4	4	3.3	3	2.3	1.5	1.5	1.5	1.5	0.8		
Leg	6.5	4	4	3.3	3	2.3	1.5	1.5	1.5	1.5	0.8	—	
Foot	6.5	4	4	3.3	3	2.3	1.5	1.5	1.5	1.5	0.8	—	—

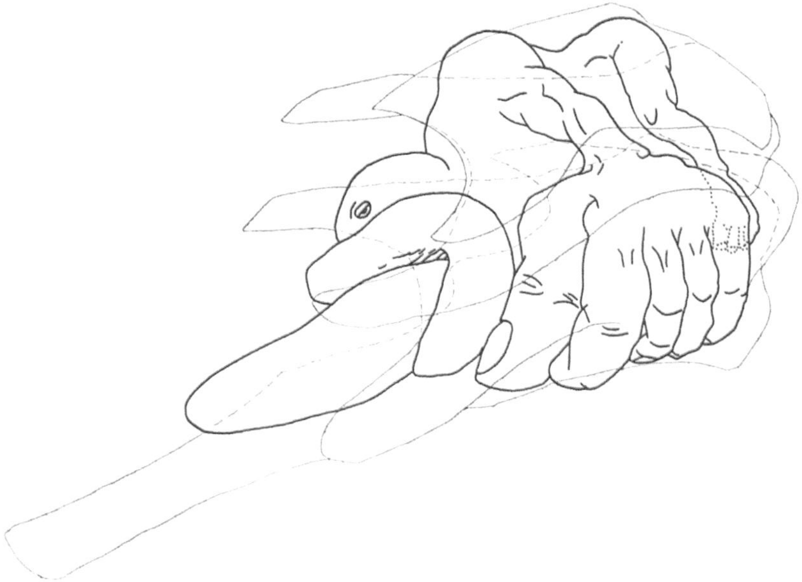

Fig. 3. Tridimensional arrangement of body parts within VP deducted by relative distances of evoked responses in patients explored with double trajectories

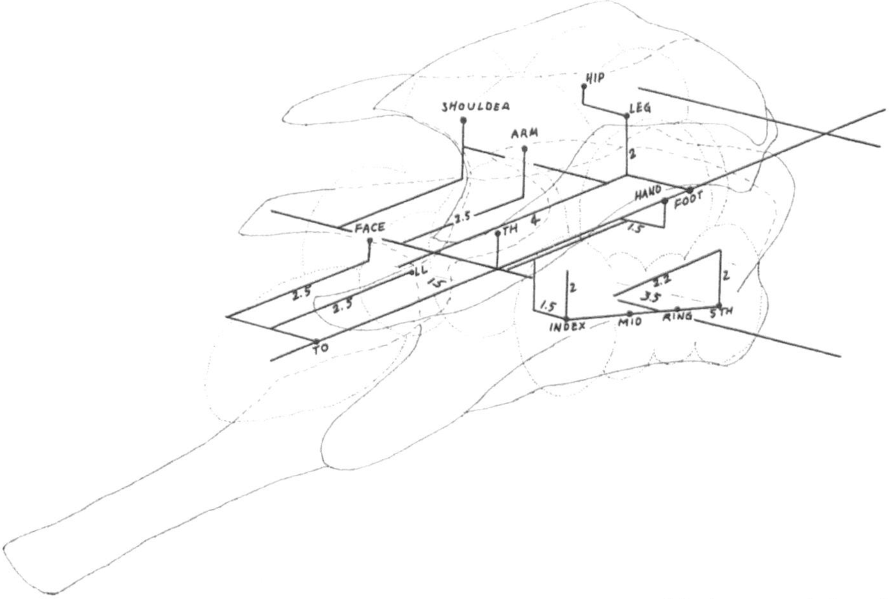

Fig. 4. Artist's drawing showing the relative volumes of body parts deducted by the spatial distribution of points shown in dotted lines in Fig. 3

obtained in cases in which two recording trajectories were made through the thalamus in individual patients.

There were 37 cases in whom 74 double trajectories were accomplished at Hôpital Foch, and 13 patients at UTMB, with 26 superior to inferior double trajectories.

Combining all of these data, the distance between points at which evoked responses were recorded in the same patient but on different trajectories were measured in millimeters in the medial, lateral, superior inferior and anterior posterior distances between somatotopic points.

An example of one of these tables is shown in Table 1.

With these values a map could be drawn, that indicated the spatial relationship of body parts within VP (Fig. 3).

The relative dimensions of various body parts within VP are ellipsoids described by one standard deviation from the center of the scatter of points.

The body, as shown in the map, is oriented along a medial-lateral axis. Its relevant features are, from medial to lateral: tongue, lips and face, thumb, close to the lips and hand, with the fingers directed caudally and slightly posteriorly. The shoulder and arm are located more superiorly and posteriorly, as it is the hip, which is located lateral to the shoulder. The thigh, leg and foot are less extensively represented and are the most laterally situated (Fig. 4).

This map is of value in guiding semimicroelectrode exploration of VP. In our experience we have found that the information derived from one or two semimicroelectrode recording trajectories has been helpful in the placement of chronic stimulating electrodes in the specific subportion of VP corresponding to the distribution of pain in individual patients.

Since January 1978 we have used this technique in the treatment of chronic pain and thus have been able to obtain paraesthesiae with VP stimulation within the part of the body where the patient is having pain.

This has resulted in excellent pain relief on a short term basis with the longest follow up of eighteen months.

References

1. Andrew, J., Watkins, E. S., A Stereotaxic Atlas of the Human Thalamus and Adjacent Structures. Baltimore: Williams and Wilkins Co. 1969.
2. Brierley, J., Beck, E., The significance in human stereotactic brain surgery of individual variation in the diencephalon and globus pallidus. J. Neurol. Neurosurg. Psychiat. *22* (1959), 287—298.
3. Guiot, G., Brion, S., Akerman, M., Anatomie stéréotaxique du pallidum interne du thalamus et de la capsule interne. Ann. Chir. *15* (1961), 557—586.

4. Guiot, G., Derome, P., Arfel, G., Walter, S., Electrophysiological recordings in stereotaxic thalamotomy for Parkinsonism. Prog. neurol. Surg. *5* (1973), 189—221.
5. Hanieh, A., Maloney, A., Localization of stereotaxic lesions in the treatment of Parkinsonism. A clinico-pathological comparison. J. Neurosurg. *31* (1969), 393—399.
6. Hosobuchi, Y., Adams, J. E., Rutkin, B., Chronic thalamic stimulation for the control of facial anesthesia dolorosa. Arch. Neurol. *29* (1973), 158—161.
7. Hosobuchi, Y., Adams, J. E., Rutkin, B., Chronic thalamic and internal capsule stimulation for the control of central pain. Surg. Neurol. *31* (1975), 91—92.
8. Kelly, P. J., Derome, P., Guiot, G., Thalamic spatial variability and the surgical results of lesions placed with neurophysiologic control. Surg. Neurol. *9* (1978), 307—315.
9. Mazars, G., Mérienne, L., Cioloca, C., Stimulation thalamiques intermittentes antalgiques. Rev. neurol. *128* (1973), 273—279.
10. Mazars, G. J., Intermittent stimulation of nucleus ventralis posterolateralis for intractable pain. Surg. Neurol. *4* (1975), 93—94.
11. Mundinger, F., Die Behandlung chronischer Schmerzen mit Hirnstimulatoren. Dtsch. med. Wschr. *102* (1977), 1724—1729.
12. Smith, M. C., Location of stereotactic lesions confirmed at necropsy. Brit. Med. J. *1* (1962), 900—906.
13. Van Buren, J., Maccubbin, D., An outline atlas of human basal ganglia with estimation of anatomical variants. J. Neurosurg. *19* (1962), 811—839.

Acta Neurochirurgica, Suppl. 30, 289—293 (1980)

Deep Brain Stimulation for Severe, Chronic Pain

Ch. D. Ray* and **Ch. V. Burton***

Summary

Deep brain electrodes placed in the parafasicularis-centre-median area (pf-CM) can reliably relieve severe chronic pain of long duration by simple electrical stimulation, in selected cases. Twenty-eight patients are presented here who had one or more electrodes placed for periods ranging from a few days to several months. Overall results rated good-to-excellent (having 50% or more relief of the prestimulation pain) were seen in 76% of the cases. Intraoperative test stimulation has been very useful in predicting future effectiveness. Also presented are a new disposable ventricular catheter and a burr hole plug and cap for anchoring the electrode wires in the skull.

Keywords: Stereotaxic surgery; deep brain electrodes; neurostimulation; chronic pain control.

Acute and chronic electrical stimulation of deep structures of the brain has been used for several years in the course of the study of pain. The practical clinical use of deep stimulation in humans dates back to the early 1970's with the first investigators being Mazars, Richardson, Delgado, and a few others [3, 6]. There shortly followed the work of Adams, Hosobuchi, Long, Mundinger, the present authors, and others [1, 2, 4]. The majority of patients on whom deep stimulation of the brain has been used in clinical practice for the control of severe, chronic pain have been implanted within the last three years. Several targets have been investigated but the two most commonly utilized are: 1. the region of the periventricular gray, near the wall of the posterior third ventricle, and 2. regions in or around the specific sensory thalamus. The caudate nucleus has occasionally been used, especially in animal studies. Some implantations, in animals, have been made in the deep periaqueductal gray and even in the dorsal raphé nucleus. The majority of the clinical cases reported thus far have been those utilizing the periventricular (or

* Department of Neuroaugmentive Surgery, Sister Kenny Institute, 2727 Chicago Ave., Minneapolis, MN 55407, U.S.A.

0065-1419/80/Suppl. 30/0289/$ 01.00

parafasicularis centre-median) or specific thalamic nuclei. With the advent of the discovery of endogenous opiate compounds [5], which on electrical stimulation in the periventricular region, are activated or released, thus having a profound influence on chronic pain, these targets have been particularly utilized.

Table 1. *Depth Brain Stimulator Implants, Sister Kenny Institute, June 1979*

Cases:	28
Ages:	range 22 to 70 years; median 47 years
Sex:	15 male, 13 female
Duration of pain:	range ½ to 49 years; median 14 years
Follow-up period:	range 1 to 33 months; median 14 months
Deaths:	3 (1 to 7 months, due to carcinoma): 1 operative mortality
Stimulation paraesthesias:	21 had warmth after 8 to 20 minutes stimulation
	23 had visual effects (higher stimulation voltage, frequency below 30 second)
	6 had adversive effects (deeper periaqueductal gray only)
	[17 required adjunctive medication—Elavil (amitriptyline)]

Methods and Material

The present study reports results in 28 cases suffering from severe, chronic, intractable pain of multiple etiologies. The principal target utilized was the parafasicularis-centremedian (pf-CM). Stimulation was used intraoperatively to localize the paleospinothalamic tract producing a reduction in the deep-seated, agonizing, mechanical pain and generally the production of a paraesthesia of warmth enveloping most of the body but particularly on the contralateral side.

The target point used is 1.5 millimeters anterior to the posterior commissure, on the AC—PC line, 1.5 to 2.5 millimeters lateral to the wall of the posterior third ventricle. The electrode utilized is a 4-contact, Schreiver-type (Medtronic, Inc. **) deep brain electrode system. The electrode contacts are 1 millimeter long and separated by spacing of 2 millimeters. During the period of trial stimulation, it was determined that the majority of patients preferred a bipolar stimulation pair of electrodes which was 4–8 millimeters above the target point mentioned above. A number of them were 8–10 millimeters above. It was therefore our conclusion that utilizing the trajectory angle (burr hole placed 3 cm lateral to the sagittal suture) of about 28 degrees lateral and about 60 degrees forward above the AC—PC line would place the preferred zone of stimulation approximately in the centre-median or median nucleus of the thalamus (see Table 1). Deeper stimulations into the region of the periaqueductal gray (4–6 millimeters anterior to the posterior commissure) usually produced adversive responses. The patients simply did not like the stimulation even though it was a non-specific form of distress. A few cases stimulated somewhat more anterior to the target showed

** Medtronic, Inc., Box 1453, Minneapolis, MN 55440 U.S.A.

sympathetic responses similar to those reported by Sano during stimulations in the posterior hypothalamus. Because of the proximity of our deeper target to the nucleus of Edinger-Westphal and also the third nerve nucleus, most patients will show eye signs, first as subjective and then objective nystagmus.

Tests in the intraoperative period, generally produced pain relief and paraesthesias of warmth as were seen during the trial stimulation period and after

Table 2. *Depth Brain Stimulator Implants, Sister Kenny Institute, June 1979*

Diagnoses	No. of cases	Failures *
1. "Failed back", multiple operations	11	4 (1 death)
2. Carcinoma (breast, rectum, lung, bone)	6	0
3. Post-traumatic cord/roots	5	1
4. Atypical facial, multiple operations	2	1
5. Thalamic stroke	1	0
6. Meningioma of cord, postoperative	1	0
7. Post-fusion, cord irradiation	1	0
8. Phantom limb, central pain	1	1
	28	7 (1 op. death, 2 screened out)

* Less than 50% reduction in prestimulation pain level.

internalization of the receiver system, even extending into years. It is important to note that in humans, pf-CM stimulation produces hypalgesia (particularly of paleospinothalamic type) and never analgesia, in contrast with animal studies. It was our conclusion, therefore, that the intraoperative testing was quite promonotory of the ultimate results.

Patients who did not show adequate response on the operating table were screened out; that is, the electrodes were simply removed. Two other cases were screened out during the trial stimulation phase due to persistent ineffectiveness. Trial stimulation, using the percutaneous extension wires emerging from the scalp, usually lasted from 5 to 12 days. During this time, most combinations of the four electrodes were tried (with forward and reverse polarity), searching for bipolar pairs yielding the best pain relief and least side effects. A few patients showed mild euphoria, perhaps implicating the activation of superior connections into the medial limbic system. Two recent cases had an additional set of electrodes placed in the medial head of the caudate; one had good results (case of visceral spasms and pain associated with a cord injury), but in the other (metastatic bone cancer) it was ineffective. Both cases showed good results using pf-CM stimulation, however. One additional patient had implanted a second electrode in the anterior cingulum. Stimulation produced a mild awareness and minor involuntary movements in the contralateral hand. On one occasion the patient used the stimulator at an unauthorized high level; "kindling" occurred, followed by a major motor seizure. No effect on behavior was noted. No pain relief occurred. This electrode was removed at time of internalization of the receiver. Somatosensory evoked responses (contralateral median nerve stimulation) were recorded in the pf-CM in each case so tested; latencies were 19 ms (± 1 ms). Simultaneous stimulation of the medial caudate reduced or abolished the pf-CM responses, presumably by a collision effect, in two cases.

Results

Eighty-two percent of patients reported good-to-excellent relief (more than 50% reduction in the prestimulation pain) during the testing and trial stimulation. However, this number fell to 76% over the next months. Longer-term results (median 14 months) indicate that the 50%-or-better result level remains at about 75%. After long periods of stimulation, the effectiveness may suddenly decline. This is apparently due to local exhaustion of available endogenous opiate materials since resting (increasing the time between stimulations) restores the effectiveness in most cases. Adjunctive medications (tricyclic antidepressants or levo-tryptophan) have been used in most cases and will sometimes significantly increase the pain-relieving effectiveness of the stimulation (by augmenting serotonin production or sparing) (see Table 2).

A new disposable, flexible plastic ventricular catheter has been developed to facilitate ventriculography and permit removal of cerebrospinal fluid for analysis during the stereotaxic procedure. The catheter is 1.5 mm in diameter, has a removable stylet and is equipped with simple fittings that may be connected with a syringe. There is a radio-opaque stripe on the cathether to aid in localization; the lateral hole, 5 mm from the tip, is drilled through the stripe so that it may be seen as a gap on X-ray films. A special burr hole plug and cap have been developed to retain and protect the leads as they pass through the calvarium and beneath the scalp.

In spite of earlier criticisms and uncertainty, this technique and the target used (pf-CM) have proved to be a major, reliable means for the treatment of chronic, severe pain principally involving the paleospinothalamic system (deep, agonal, visceral, mechanical or weight-bearing pain as opposed to the neospinothalamic system, passing nociceptive information of sharp, highly localizing, acute and surface pain). We continue to search for secondary or ancillary targets that will further improve the overall results, especially for central and deafferentation pain states.

Included in this group of patients are four cases operated on by one of us (CDR) together with the following colleagues: E. S. Watkins (London), J. G. Martin-Rodrigues (Madrid), and O. Schrottner (Graz). Appreciation is extended to them for their participation and cooperation.

Addendum

Addendum: Since June, 1979, four additional cases have been implanted with results that continue to be supportive of those reported here.

References

1. Burton, C. V., Ray, C. D., Nashold, B. S. (eds.), Symposium on the safety and clinical efficacy of implanted neuroaugmentive devices. Neurosurgery *1* (1977), 185—232.
2. Hosobuchi, Y., Adams, J., Linchitz, R., Pain relief by electrical stimulation of the central gray matter in humans and its reversal by Naloxone. Science *197* (1977), 183—186.
3. Mazars, G., Merienne, L., Ciolocca, C., Stimulations thalamiques intermittentes antalgiques: Note préliminaire. Rev. Neurol. *128* (1973), 273—279.
4. Ray, C. D., New electrical stimulation methods for therapy and rehabilitation. Orthop. Rev. *6* (1977), 29—39.
5. Ray, C. D., editorial, On opiates, pain and the nervous system. Neurosurgery *1* (1977), 188—189.
6. Richardson, D. E., Akil, H., Long term results of periventricular gray self-stimulation. Neurosurgery *1* (1977), 199—202.

Acta Neurochirurgica, Suppl. 30, 295—301 (1980)

Chronic Self-Stimulation of the Medial Posterior Inferior Thalamus for the Alleviation of Deafferentation Pain

J. R. Schvarcz*

With 1 Figure

Summary

Since current techniques yield uncertain results on deafferentation pain, chronic brain stimulation may presumably be a valuable alternative method, without deterrent side-effects. Disappointing results with stimulation of the somato-sensory structures prompted the selection of the medial posterior inferior thalamus and adjascent brain stem for chronic stimulation in pain states of central origin. Six such cases are reported. Abolition of the hyperpathia and marked reduction in the deep background pain was achieved in 2 cases, and disappearance of the hyperpathia and moderate reduction in the deep pain was obtained in another 2, but *none* had complete alleviation of pain. The follow-up time ranged between 6 and 42 months. Reversal of analgesia by naloxone was not observed. Acute experimentally-induced pain was not modified by stimulation.

Keywords: Brain stimulation; central pain; periaqueductal gray; paraventricular thalamus; stereotaxis.

Central pain phenomena are elusive problems to deal with. So far, conventional techniques have either failed or yielded uncertain results on dysaesthesic pain, but chronic brain stimulation via indwelling electrodes may well be a specially suitable method for pain of central origin, at least as an initial non-destructive approach.

There is, for the time being, a definite trend toward stimulation in two different systems, viz. the periaqueductal-periventricular gray region or the somato-sensory structures. On theoretical grounds, the latter are presumably better targets for deafferentation pain, but our results at either the thalamic ventralis posterioris or the posterior limb of the internal capsule have nevertheless been disappointing. Hence, the medial posterior inferior thalamus was tentatively selected

* Institute of Neurosurgery, School of Medicine, University of Buenos Aires, Beruti 2926, Buenos Aires 1425, Argentina.

0065-1419/80/Suppl. 30/0295/$ 01.40

for chronic stimulation in a small but clinically homogeneous group of intensely studied patients. Six such cases, with a long-standing history of pain of central origin, are reported.

Material and Methods

Patients were operated upon under slight sedation, in the sitting position, with a modified Hitchcock stereotactic apparatus. The ventricular system was outlined by water soluble positive contrast, and a Schriver type multipolar platinum electrode (Medtronic®) was implanted in the contralateral periaqueductal-paraventricular region.

The electrode tip was aimed at the posterior commissure in the coronal and horizontal planes, 2 mm lateral to the wall of the third ventricle (Fig. 1 a–b), but its definite location depended on the results elicited by acute stimulation. It was usually placed in such a way as to have at least one contact at, and another below, the site of maximum clinical effect. If satisfactory relief was induced, particularly for acute exacerbation of the patients pain, if feasible, or on hyperpathia, a less reliable criterion, or rarely with changes of pin-prick appreciation, the electrode was externalized for a period of percutaneous trial stimulation, during which different electrode combinations and parameters of stimulation were evaluated.

The results on clinical pain were assessed from the patient's own estimate of pain reduction, by visual analogue scales and from self-administered questionnaires, but additional data from staff and family were also taken into account. Thus, the initiation and duration of each period of stimulation, the onset of analgesia, the latency of maximum relief and its persistance beyond the actual stimulation were plotted, in respect to both the hyperpathia and the deep background pain. A daily pain profile was then obtained, whereby changes in the intensity and in the duration, or eventually, in the pattern of spontaneous pain could be sequentially evaluated re stimulation variables. Since self-stimulation was below the threshold to subjective sensation, placebo sham stimulation was easily performed.

Most of the patients who achieved definite relief had a naloxone reversal test, given in doses from 0.4 to 1.2 mg, on a double blind basis.

The effect of stimulation on acute experimentally-induced pain was evaluated by a radiant heat test, measuring the latency of the withdrawal reflex, and by the maximum effort tourniquet test, measuring the time of tolerance to ischemic pain.

If the clinical result was satisfactory, usually after 4 weeks of in- and out-patient percutaneous stimulation, the system was revised and permanently implanted. Under general anaesthesia, the percutaneous extension was removed and the chronic electrode was connected to a radiofrequency receiver, subcutaneously placed in the infraclavicular region, where it is transdermally activated by an inductively coupled portable radiofrequency transmitter. Throughout this process, *i.e.* before, during and after percutaneous stimulation, repeated radiographic and computerized tomography controls were made to confirm that no electrode displacement has occurred.

All the patients had a meticulous psychiatric screening prior to surgery, and psychological testing was carried out before and serially repeated after the second stage of surgery.

After evaluation of their suitability for implantation, 6 patients with pain of central origin were selected for medial posterior inferior thalamic chronic

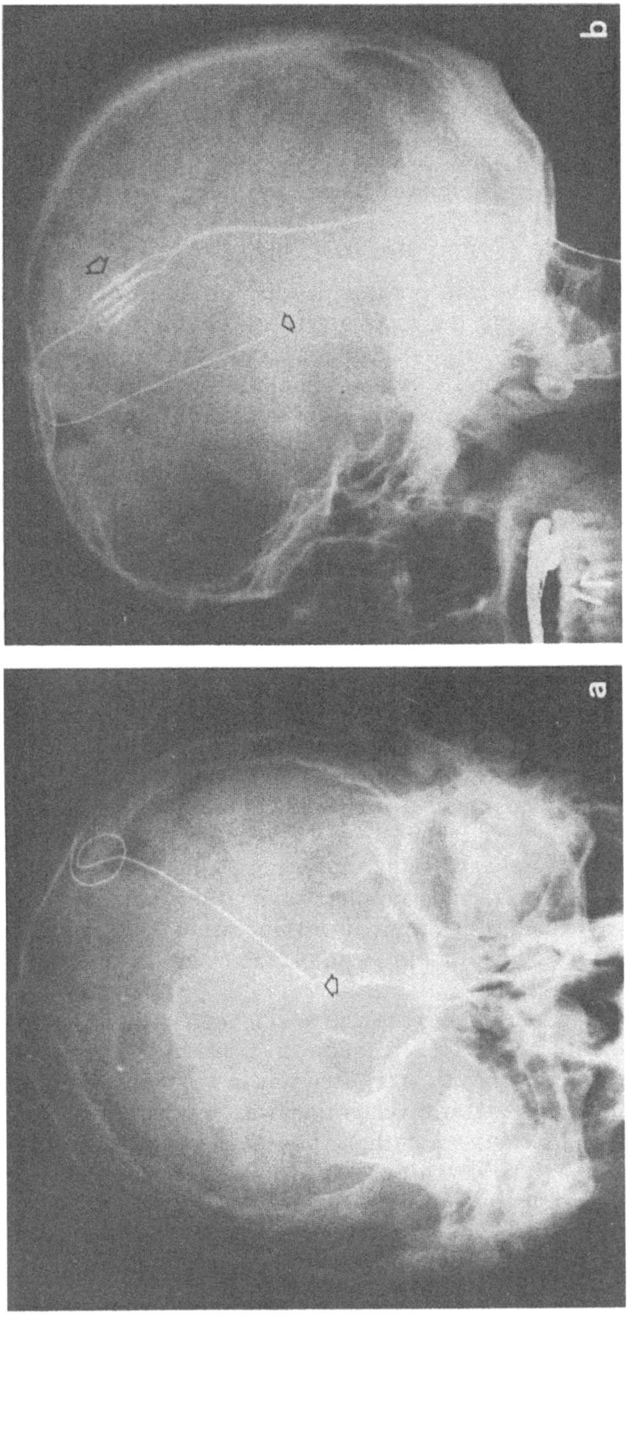

Fig. 1 a–b. Anteroposterior and lateral radiographs demonstrating the implanted system (small arrow: indwelling electrode; large arrow: extracranial connector)

stimulation. The clinical diagnoses were 2 thalamic syndromes, 1 post-cordotomy dysaesthesia and 3 partial spinal cord injuries. All had severe, disabling dysaesthesia, with both hyperpathia and deep background pain. They had high IQ's, were highly motivated to surgery, and agreed to undergo a series of pre- and post-operative assessments. None but the post-cordotomy dysaesthesia patient had previous pain surgery, although they all have had extensive medical treatment, including carbamazepine, amitriptyline and fluphenazine, which have failed. None of them was on narcotic medication. Their pain history ranged from 1.5 to 8.5 years.

Results

The results on clinical pain depended critically on electrode coupling as well as on the parameters of stimulation. The best responses were typically produced by capacitatively coupled 0.25 ms pulses, at 20 Hz and 0.5 mA, with a cyclic ramp-type output. As a rule, stimulation of the posterior paraventricular thalamus yielded clinical analgesia without subjective concomitant sensations. The onset of analgesia was felt about 10 minutes after the initiation of stimulation, but the maximum effect was only produced about 20 minutes later. However, it then persisted beyond the actual stimulation, often up to 3 hours. The hyperpathia was typically modulated before the deep pain.

The clinical assessment reflects the patient's own estimate of pain reduction, expressed with the aid of visual analogue scales and by self-administered questionnaires. Results re hyperpathia and deep burning pain are considered together. To be meaningful, the results should analize both the trial and the definitive periods of stimulation.

Thus, 2 patients were tested out by percutaneous stimulation, *i.e.*, they failed to obtained a useful pain alleviation; 2 patients obtained a moderate pain relief, *i.e.*, from 50 to 75% reduction; and 2 patients achieved a significant pain relief, *i.e.*, more than 75% reduction. None of them, however, had complete alleviation of pain. A slight residual pain remained, but required only occasional analgesics. The follow up period ranged from 6 to 42 months. There were no permanent side-effects.

Stimulation at thalamic paraventricular loci produced clinical analgesia below the threshold to subjective sensations. Just above threshold a feeling of warmth was often felt in the contralateral face. A sensation of well being and relaxation was frequently mentioned. Lower electrode locations, near the raphé nuclei complex, produced undesirable side-effects that usually precluded their use, such as oscillopsia, nystagmus, dizziness or vertigo. However, to induce emotional reactions of unpleasant fearful quality [16, 21] a definitely higher intensity is required. High frequency stimulation usually enhanced the spontaneous pain.

Unequivocal reversal of analgesia by naloxone was not observed. Acute experimentally-induced pain was not modified by stimulation.

There were no mayor changes in the degree of relief re time of follow up. Curiously enough, if the immediate results are excluded, *i.e.*, the 2 tested out cases and certain progressive improvement following surgery, there was no significant difference between delayed and long-term assessments, but longer observation is required. Current requirements have not changed either.

Discussion

Pain states of central origin are notoriously difficult to treat. In most of them, current techniques yield erratic results, and protracted relief is seldom secured, though rare but specific exceptions seemingly exist [22]. However, chronic brain stimulation presumably offers a rational functional approach to dysaesthesic pain, yet devoid of the deletereous side-effects often entailed by conventional procedures.

Two different anatomical systems have been primarily implanted for the control of chronic intractable pain, namely the somato-sensory structures in the thalamic relay nucleus ventralis posterioris or in the posterior limb of the internal capsule [2, 7, 13], and the periaqueductal-periventricular region and adjacent paraventricular thalamus [2, 6, 8, 10, 15, 19]. Although the former have been electively indicated for pain of central origin [2, 8, 13], the available data are contradictory, whereas our results with both somato-sensory targets have been rather poor [20].

Since the initial report of Reynolds [17], stimulus produced analgesia (SPA) from the central gray has been demonstrated in the rat [11], cat [9], monkey [4] and also in man [18]. However, despite the elapsed time, few clinical reports are as yet available [15, 16]. The material is also clinically heterogenous, with pain of different origins, types and locations, and often difficult to evaluate, also as regards effective electrode sites or vis-à-vis multiple implants.

An intrinsic pain suppressing system has been demonstrated, activated by either narcotic drugs or stimulation, producing a specific antinociceptive effect, related to the release of endorphins, the endogenous ligands of the opiate receptor system (*cf.*, [3, 12]). However, if clinical SPA is an exclusive endorphin-mediated phenomenon, there is no reason whatsoever to expect pain alleviation in central pain states, as they are refractory to opiates. Nevertheless, many complex interactions may occur and several systems may be implied. Furthermore, puzzling differences between SPA in man and animals do exist.

Adams, Hosobuchi and Linchitz [2] and Hosobuchi [8] have stated that periaqueductal-periventricular stimulation is not indicated in pain of central origin, but Richardson and Akil [19] have reviewed 10 such cases, followed up to 46 months, that achieved a significant relief in 4, a minor relief in 2, and no effect in 4 cases. Martin-Rodriguez [10] has also reported good results in patients with deafferentation pain, and Gybels' [5] case is conceivably of the same type.

In this series, clinical alleviation of pain was not achieved in 2, was only moderate in 2, and was significant in 2 cases, followed for up to 42 months. Analgesia was induced from a fairly large area, that presumably involved the periventricular gray and the endymalis, parafascicularis and centromedianum nuclei. However, Meyerson *et al.* [15] have elegantly demonstrated, by placing parallel electrodes in the same saggital or coronal plane, that the lateral distance is crucial.

Although often conflictive, the available data seemingly suggest that chronic self-stimulation of the medial posterior inferior thalamus may well be a useful method to induce protracted alleviation in selected cases with central pain phenomena, but further analysis is as yet required.

References

1. Adams, J. E., Naloxone reversal of analgesia produced by brain stimulation in the human. Pain *2* (1976), 161—166.
2. Adams, J. E., Hosobuchi, Y., Linchitz, R., The present status of implantable intracranial stimulators for pain. In: Clinical Neurosurgery, Vol. 24, pp. 247—261. Baltimore: Williams and Wilkins. 1977.
3. Fields, H., Basbaum, A., Brain-stem control of spinal pain transmission neurons. Ann. Rev. Physiol. *40* (1978), 217—248.
4. Goodman, S. J., Holcomb, V., Selective and prolonged analgesia in monkeys resulting from brain stimulation. In: Advances in Pain Research and Therapy, Vol. 1., pp. 495—502 (Bonica, J., Fessard, D., eds.). New York: Raven Press. 1976.
5. Gybels, J., Cosyns, P., Modulation of clinical and experimental pain in man by electrical stimulation of thalamic periventricular gray. In: Sensory functions of the skin, pp. 521—530 (Zotterman, Y., ed.). Oxford: Pergamon Press. 1976.
6. Gybels, J., Electrical Stimulation of the central gray for pain relief in humans: A critical review. In: Advances in Pain Research and Therapy, Vol. 3, in press (Bonica, J., Liebeskind, J., Fessard, D., eds.). New York: Raven Press. 1979.
7. Hosobuchi, Y., Adams, J. E., Rutkin, B., Chronic thalamic and internal capsule stimulation for the control of central pain. Surg. Neurol. *4* (1975), 91—93.
8. Hosobuchi, Y., Central gray stimulation for pain suppression in humans. In: Advances in Pain Research and Therapy, Vol. 3, in press (Bonica, J., Liebeskind, J., Fessard, D., eds.). New York: Raven Press. 1979.
9. Liebeskind, J. C., Guilbrand, G., Besson, J. M., Oliveras, J. L., Analgesia from electrical stimulation of the periaqueductal gray matter in the cat: behavioral observations and inhibitory effects on spinal cord interneurons. Brain Res. *50* (1973), 441—446.

10. Martín Rodriguez, J. G., Obrador, S., Therapeutic electrical stimulation of the brain. Biochemical changes induced in the ventricular cerebrospinal fluid with regard to opiate-like substances. In: Modern Concepts in Psychiatric Surgery, pp. 47—56 (Hitchcock, E. R., Ballantine, H. T., Meyerson, B. A., eds.). Amsterdam: Elsevier. 1979.
11. Mayer, D. J., Wolfle, T. L., Akil, H., Carder, B., Liebeskind, J. C., Analgesia from electrical stimulation in the brainstem of the rat. Science *174* (1971), 1351—1354.
12. Mayer, D. J., Prince, D. D., Central nervous mechanisms of analgesia. Pain *2* (1976), 379—404.
13. Mazars, G. L., Intermittent stimulation of nucleus ventralis posterolateralis for intractable pain. Surg. Neurol. *4* (1975), 93—95.
14. Meyerson, B. A., Boëthius, J., Carlsson, A. M., Percutaneous central gray stimulation for cancer pain. Appl. Neurophysiol. *41* (1978), 57—65.
15. Meyerson, B. A., Boëthius, J., Carlsson, A. M., Alleviation of malignant pain by electrical stimulation in the periventricular-periaqueductal region. Pain relief as related to stimulation sites. In: Advances in Pain Research and Therapy, Vol. 3, in press (Bonica, J., Liebeskind, J., Fessard, D., eds.). New York: Raven Press. 1979.
16. Nashold, B. S., Wilson, W. P., Slaughter, D., Sensations evoked by stimulation in the midbrain of man. J. Neurosurg. *30* (1969), 14—24.
17. Reynolds, D. V., Surgery in the rat during electrical analgesia induced by focal brain stimulation. Science *164* (1969), 444—445.
18. Richardson, D. E., Akil, H., Pain reduction by electrical brain stimulation in man. Chronic self-administration in the periventricular gray matter. J. Neurosurg. *47* (1977), 184—194.
19. Richardson, D. E., Akil, H., Long term results of periventricular gray self-stimulation. Neurosurg. *1* (1977), 199—202.
20. Schvarcz, J. R., Estimulacion cerebral crónica. Bol. Asoc. Argent. Neurocir. *20* (1976), 60.
21. Schvarcz, J. R., Para-aqueductal mesencephalotomy for facial central pain. In: Neurosurgical Treatment in Psychiatry, Pain and Epilepsy, pp. 661—667 (Sweet, W. H., Obrador, S., Martín, J., eds.). Baltimore: University Park Press. 1977.
22. Schvarcz, J. R., Postherpetic craneofacial dysaesthesiae. Their management by stereotactic trigeminal nucleotomy. Acta Neurochir. (Wien) *39* (1977), 65—72.

Acta Neurochirurgica, Suppl. 30, 303—309 (1980)

Alleviation of Atypical Trigeminal Pain by Stimulation of the Gasserian Ganglion via an Implanted Electrode

B. A. Meyerson* and **S. Håkansson**

With 2 Figures

Summary

Facial pain associated with disturbances of sensitivity as a sign of injury of the trigeminal nerve is difficult to treat. Drug therapy as well as blocking procedures are generally ineffective. Transcutaneous nerve stimulation offers a new possibility for pain alleviation but is inconvenient for the patient. A method for stimulation of the gasserian ganglion via an implanted electrode has been developed. Five cases are reported on and they all experienced excellent or good pain relief. Follow-up is 6–21 months.

Keywords: Pain; trigeminus; stimulation.

Introduction

Atypical trigeminal neuralgia is generally used to denote facial pain other than tic douloureux. It is characterized by a continuous aching pain that may be dull or burning and is confined to the trigeminal region. Often there is a marked disturbance of sensory functions with a distribution that respects the boundaries of the trigeminal divisions. The aetiology varies. Frequently, there is an injury of the peripheral part of the trigeminal neurone or the ganglion. An obvious cause is facial trauma but more common is a history of pain following tooth extraction or surgery of the maxillary sinus. Not infrequently, treatment of tic douloureux with repeated peripheral alcohol blocks or neurotomy may create a continuous burning type of pain with hyperaesthesia and hyperalgesia in the area corresponding to the

* Department of Neurosurgery, Karolinska sjukhuset, S-104 01 Stockholm-60, Sweden.

0065-1419/80/Suppl. 30/0303/$ 01.40

injured nerve branch. If marked hypaesthesia is present the condition is suggestive of anaesthesia dolorosa.

Atypical trigeminal neuralgia is notoriously difficult to treat, and Sweet [9] in one of his extensive reviews on trigeminal pain refers to this condition as the "bête noir". Contrary to what is the case in tic douloureux this condition rarely responds to carbamazepine or phenytoin, and analgesics also generally fail. Lesioning procedures such as neurolytic blocks of the peripheral nerve or the ganglion is not only ineffective but may also worsen the pain. For treatment of the typical trigeminal neuralgia differential thermocoagulation is presently considered to be the method of choice. However, for other types of trigeminal pain the results are poor [6, 9]. The characteristic features of atypical trigeminal neuralgia suggest that the pain could be controlled with transcutaneous nerve stimulation (TNS). In a series of 25 patients suffering from facial pain and classified as atypical trigeminal neuralgia of various aetiology 14 were found to have excellent to moderate alleviation of pain with TNS (unpublished). In spite of the effective relief of pain many of the patients were annoyed with having a black rubber electrode taped to their face, and they felt socially handicapped. In order to overcome this inconvenience, and with the idea to be able to produce more effectively paraesthesias in the area of pain, the possibility of implanting an electrode for direct stimulation of the gasserian ganglion was considered. This report gives the preliminary results obtained with this treatment in a small series of patients.

Patient Material and Technique

Six patients have been implanted. They were all females. The duration and probable origin of the pain and previous treatment are listed in Table 1. In one patient (case 1) the pain covered most of the trigeminal area whereas the others had one or two divisions involved. The facial sensitivity was tested bilaterally using a battery of semiquantitative methods developed by Lindblom [8]. Sensory functions were disturbed in all patients and the pattern of disturbance was complex comprising quantitative and qualitative changes in both coarse and thin fibre functions. It should be noted that all patients, except case 6, had experienced a good or moderate reduction of pain with TNS. Only one of the patients had pain relief, although slight, with carbamazepine.

The electrode, designed by Medtronic according to our specifications, is bipolar and consists of two platinum discs, 3 mm in diameter, and embedded 6 mm apart in silicon rubber (Fig. 1). The electrode leads have connections that permit percutaneous test stimulation. The leads are similar to those of a deep brain stimulating electrode (Medtronic) and may be exchanged for a subcutaneous connecting cable to a receiver for external stimulation. The gasserian ganglion and the trigeminal rootlets are exposed via an extradural, subtemporal approach. The electrode plate is sutured to the dura (cf. Fig. 2). The electrode plate is

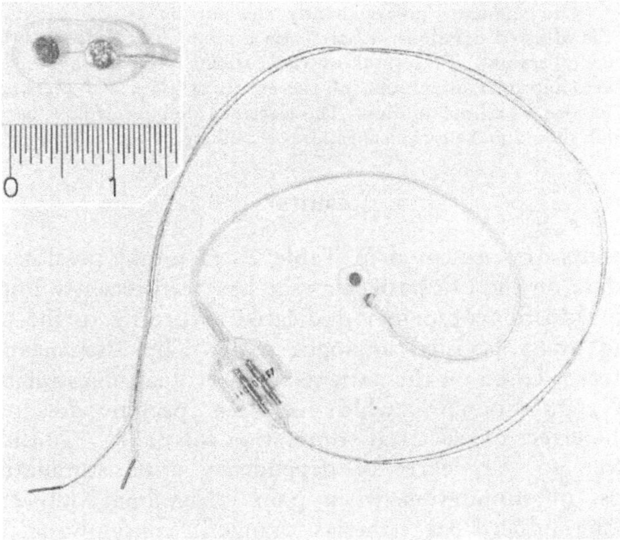

Fig. 1. Electrode for gasserian stimulation with percutaneous extension leads

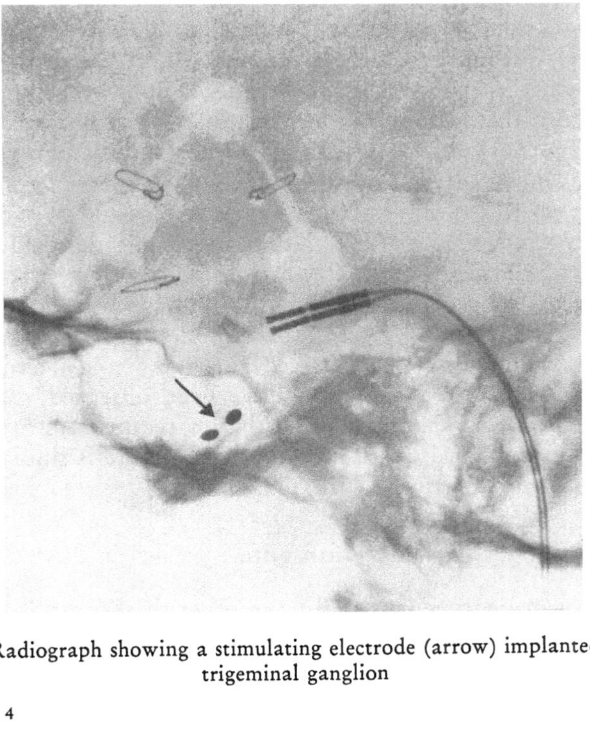

Fig. 2. Radiograph showing a stimulating electrode (arrow) implanted on the trigeminal ganglion

orientated so as to stimulate predominantly the portion of the ganglion corresponding to the affected devisions. Apart from a minor local infection there were no surgical complications. In several of the patients there have been technical problems due to inproper orientation of the electrode plate and breakage of the leads which has led to reimplantation. The electrode design has now been slightly modified which should make technical failures less likely to occur.

Results

The results are presented in Table 2. It is not possible to give complete data on the 6th patient as she has been recently implanted. Percentage reduction of pain is indicated according to the patients' own rating using a visual analogue scale. The assessment of the clinical effect is based on the patients' own evaluation estimated with the aid of a questionnaire, which has been specially developed for assessing the effect of electrical stimulation for pain [4]. Consideration is also given to the degree of dependency upon stimulation, the effectiveness of stimulation when pain is maximal, subjective reactions to the induced paraesthesias, change in consumption of drugs etc. [1]. Regardless of the degree of pain reduction all patients reported that ganglion stimulation was more effective than TNS and that the induced paraesthesias had a smoother and more pleasant character.

The production of paraesthesias that entirely covers the area of pain is a prerequisite for relief. It appeared that the distribution of these paraesthesias was highly dependent upon the polarity of stimulation and the pulse duration. In general, the patient preferred to use a frequency of 50–100 Hz. The poststimulatory relief was 2–4 hours except in case 1 who still can enjoy pain free periods sometimes lasting up to 1–2 days after a very short period of stimulation. On the other hand, most patients report that when the pain is exceptionally severe, during "bad days", in cold weather etc., they have to stimulate during long periods of time in order to obtain relief. Thus, one of the patients, case 5, uses the stimulator a couple of times during the morning but continuously during the whole afternoon. No signs of habituation to stimulation have been observed. As a rule, induction time, *i.e.*, the time of stimulation required until the pain is felt to be influenced, is 5–10 minutes. This figure is similar to that generally given for treatment with TNS.

Comments

Treatment of neurogenic facial pain, other than typical trigeminal neuralgia, offers considerable problems. Medication is generally ineffective and lesioning procedures carry a high risk of aggravating

Table 1. *Stimulation of the Gasserian Ganglion for Atypical Trigeminal Pain*

Case/age	Duration of pain (years)	Origin of pain	Trig. sens. disturb.	Previous treatment	Pain relief with TNS
1/22	4	facial trauma	hyperaesth dysaesth	—	+
2/52	2	unknown	hyperaesth hyperalg	—	+
3/48	11	labyrinth surg	slight hyperaesth	ganglion block	+
4/53	8	tooth extract	hyperaesth dysaesth	periph and ganglion block. Neurotomy VPM stim	(+)
5/54	11	tooth extract	hypaesth hyperalg (cold)	periph block	+
6/53	8	maxil sinus surg	hypaesth	periph and ganglion block. VPM stim	—

Table 2. *Stimulation of the Gasserian Ganglion for Atypical Trigeminal Pain*

Case	Reduction of pain at stim. (%)	Assessment of clinical effect	Follow-up (months)	Poststim. duration (hours)	Induction time (min)	Stim. time (min)
1	100	excellent	21	24	1–5	1–5
2	75–100	excellent	17	2–4	5–15	15–45
3	75–100	excellent	16	3–8	10	30–60
4	50–75	good	23	2–4	10	30
5	100	good	6	½–1	5	> 30
6	50	—	0	—	—	—

the pain. Also the results of selective thermocoagulation is discouraging in these conditions and is actually warned against [7]. TNS has proven to be a valuable method for the alleviation of pain in some of these patients [2]. The inconvenience of transcutaneous facial stimulation and the difficulty of producing paraesthesias covering the whole of the pain area have prompted the development of an implantable gasserian electrode. This approach to facial pain has actually been tried previously. Already in 1966 Shelden [5] described an implantable device for ganglion stimulation which was used on three patients with tic douloureux. It should be noted that this was performed before the era of electric nerve stimulation for pain. Sweet [9] also mentions a patient with postherpetic facial neuralgia who had pain relief during stimulation of the second trigeminal devision behind the foramen rotundum. Recently, it was reported that trigeminal pain due to herpes infection and neoplasm could be relieved by stimulation in the region of the trigeminal tract [8]. The stimulating electrode was introduced with a technique similar to that used for percutaneous cordotomy. In three of the patients the electrode was permanently connected to a subcutaneous receiver. In essence, this approach to treating atypical trigeminal pain is very similar to ours. However, with the percutaneous method difficulties in directing the electrode to the appropriate position and to ensure that it remains in place may be anticipated.

In the first five cases in our series some pain relief with TNS was considered a prerequisite for implantation. The last patient, case 6, was implanted in spite of being a non-responder to TNS. A comparison may be made with dorsal column stimulation (DCS) which in experimental cases may work regardless of the fact that TNS has been totally ineffective. Similarly to DCS, direct gasserian stimulation activates the retroganglionic portions of the primary afferent fibres. It is of relevance to note that one of the patients (case 4) who is now doing fairly well with the gasserian stimulation previously had been treated with intracerebral stimulation within the specific thalamic nuclei. This stimulation was effective during about a year but than failed although it was still possible to produce paraesthesias covering the painful area. This observation indicates that the production of paraesthesias per se is not a sufficient condition for obtaining relief, and that stimulation at different levels of the afferent system may have different effects with regard to pain.

Facial pain, with the exception of the typical tic douloureux, is often difficult to diagnose and is badly understood. Subtle changes of sensitivity is often overlooked and difficult to interpret. Most of these patients are under the care of otologists, anaesthesiologists and dentists and are not referred to neurosurgeons. Alcohol blocks and other lesioning procedures are often performed with worsening of the pain as result. Presumably, these conditions are not uncommon and the method of direct stimulation of the trigeminal ganglion and rootlets may be a possible treatment for the future.

References

1. Carlsson, A. M., Development of a schedule for the assessment of chronic pain patients. (In manuscript.)
2. Gregg, J. M., Post-traumatic trigeminal neuralgia: response to physiologic, surgical and pharmacologic therapies. Int. Dent. J. *28* (1978), 43—51.
3. Lindblom, U., Verrillo, R. T., Sensory functions in chronic neuralgia. J. Neurol. Neurosurg. Psychiat. *42* (1979), 422—435.
4. Meyerson, B. A., Boëthius, J., Carlsson, A. M., Alleviation of malignant pain by electrical stimulation in the periventricular-periaqueductal region. Pain relief as related to stimulation sites. In: Advances in Pain Research and Therapy, Vol. 3, pp. 525—533 (Bonica, J., *et al.*, eds.). New York: Raven Press. 1979.
5. Shelden, C. H., Depolarization in the treatment of trigeminal neuralgia. In: Pain. Henry Ford Hospital International Symposium, pp. 373—386 (Knighton, R. S., Dumke, P. R., eds.). Boston, Mass.: Little, Brown and Co. 1966.
6. Siegfried, J., Neurochirurgische Behandlung der symptomatischen und atypischen Gesichtsschmerzen. Münch. med. Wschr. *120* (1978), 675—678.
7. Siegfried, J., 500 percutaneous thermocoagulations of the Gasserian ganglion for trigeminal pain. Surg. Neurol. *8* (1977), 126—131.
8. Steude, U., Percutaneous electro-stimulation of the trigeminal nerve in patients with atypical trigeminal neuralgia. Neurochirurgia *21* (1978), 66—69.
9. Sweet, W. H., Controlled thermocoagulation of trigeminal ganglion and rootlets for differential destruction of pain fibers: Facial pain other than trigeminal neuralgia. Clin. Neurosurg. *237* (1976), 96—102.

Acta Neurochirurgica, Suppl. 30, 311—316 (1980)

Stimulation of Conus-Epiconus with Pisces

Further Indications

K. Nittner*

With 2 Figures

Summary

Stimulation by epidurally implanted bipolar electrodes placed upon the conus and epiconus, not only reduces pain, but also sensitive and vegetative sensations. Seven patients suffered from pain in the sacral and coccygeal region as in coccygodynia, also from sensitive and vegetative discomforts in the perineum, anus, rectum, bladder and vagina.

Introduced between L 2/3, the tips of the electrodes were placed between the levels of D 10 and L 1 (6 patients) and between D 7 and D 8 (1 patient), the optimal location was found by stimulation.

The stimulation was tested in procumbent standing or sitting positions before fixing the electrodes. In all 7 patients there was a reduction of symptoms.

Keywords: Epidural electrostimulation; incurable pain; vegetative disorders; causalgia.

Electro-stimulation of the spinal cord by means of bipolar electrodes is not only indicated in cases of severe pain, but may also be helpful with sensory and vegetative malsensations, especially of the causalgia type. So far we implanted epidural electrodes into the spinal canal of 12 patients, 7 of whom also had those above mentioned symptoms (Table 1).

Material and Methods

These 7 patients consisted of 4 cases with malignant processes which had been treated some time ago and which at the time of implantation had no sign of metastasis, and of 3 patients with benign disorders. These patients did not show any relation between (subjective) symptoms and (objective) neurological disorders. Except for pain, patients complained about very unpleasant sensory and vegetative disturbances concerning the bladder, the reproductive system or the large intestine, which failed to respond to treatment.

---

* Prof. Dr. K. Nittner, Neurochirurgische Universitätsklinik, D-5000 Köln, Federal Republic of Germany.

0065-1419/80/Suppl. 30/0311/$ 01.20

Table 1

Patients, Age Date of Op.	Malig.	Benig.	Diagnosis	Symptoms	Op.	Radio-therapy	Pisces loc.	Catamnesis Time	Catamnesis Results	Improvement %
♂ Br. J. 76 yrs Op. 5-XII-77	O		ca of rectum 10 yrs	pain: perianal veget.: anus, rectum	proctectomy preternatural anus (pr.an.)	x-ray	D 10 L 1	4 months	satisfic + recidivation	50 % 100 %
♀ Be. I 68 yrs. Op 8-VI-78	-	O	clitoris crisis	pain. clitoris vagina veget. vagina	leucotomy		D 7 D 8	1 year	good	80 % 80 %
♀ Ka A. 51 yrs. Op 21-VIII-78	O		ca of rectum 3 yrs	pain perineum, coxa veget · vagina causalgia	proctectomy pr. an	x-ray	D 11/12 D 12	4 months	satisfic. + recidivation	70 % 70 %
♀ St. A 67 yrs Op 3-XI-78	O		ca of ureter 1 3/4 yrs	pain · gluteal muscle veget abdom. crises urin. bladder	nephrectomy	x-ray	D 11 D 11/12	4 months	satisfic + recidivation	70 % 100 %
♀ Po A. 61 yrs. Op 29-I-79		O	coccygodynia	pain perineum veget urin bladder causalgia	sacrococcyg. resect		D 12 L 1	5 months	satisfic	30 % 70 % 70 %
♀ Ro H 72 yrs. Op 30-IV-79	O		ca of rectum 11 yrs	pain: coccygodynia veget anus	proctectomy pr. an. coccyg. resect.	x-ray cobalt	D 12 L 1	2 months	good	70 % 70 %
♂ Tr. P 67 yrs. Op 10-V-79		O	traumatic spinal fracture	pain. ischialgia perineum veget. perianal causalgia	spinal operation lumb. vertebr. col, coccyg. resect.		D 10 D 11	2 months	very good	70 % 100 % 100 %

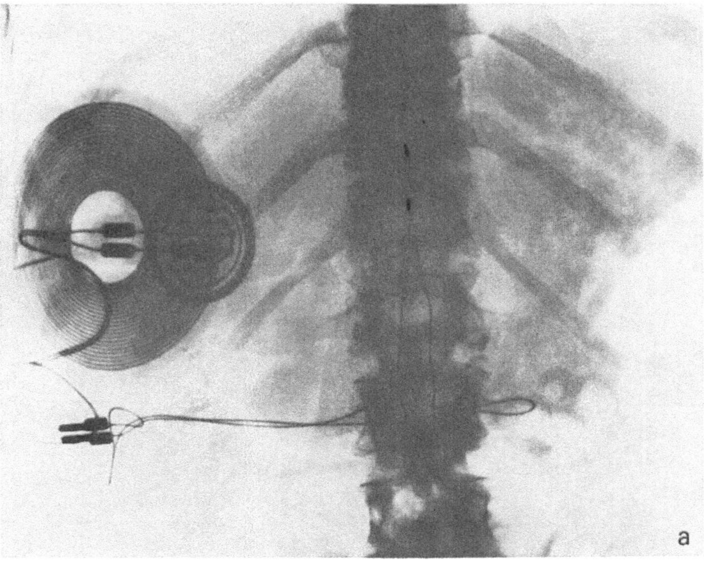

Fig. 1 a

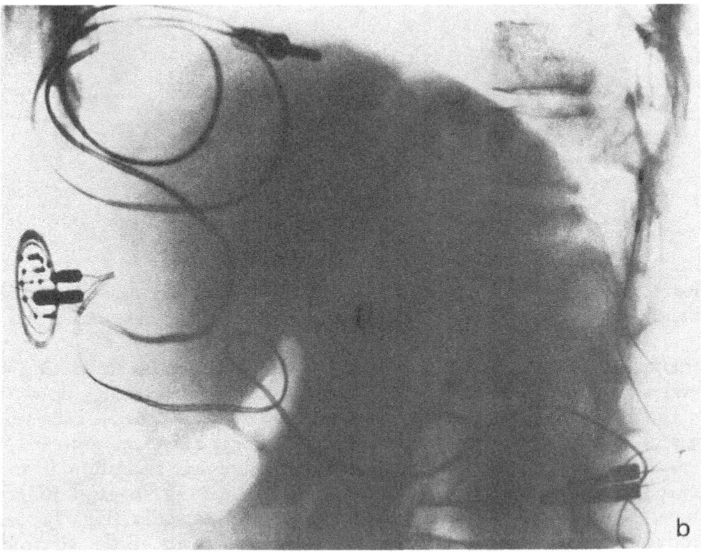

Fig. 1 b

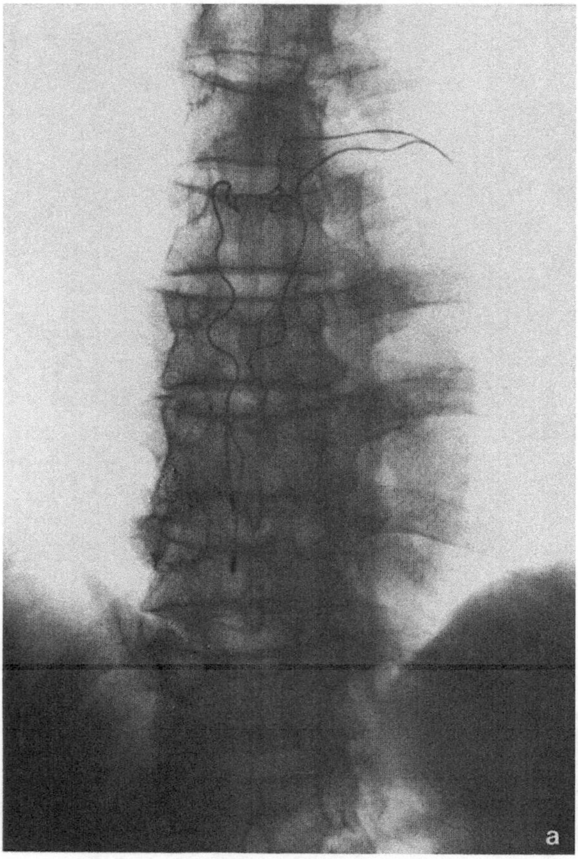

Fig. 2 a

Prior to implantation, in all patients surgery had been performed for their basic disease or for pain. The 4 cases with malignomas had also undergone radiation.

Introduction of the electrodes epidurally was done as usual starting with a horizontal skin incision between two spinal processes, penetrating down to the fascia. The level of the puncture depends on the local situation: Routinely it was done at L 2/3 (Fig. 1). If in this region epidural adhesions or scars are expected as for example after preceding laminectomy, our procedure is to insert the electrodes in the middle thoracical spine—between D 7/8—and to go from there under X-ray supervision and stimulation slowly caudally (Fig. 2). Stimulation produced optimal results in all patients when the tip of the electrode was placed between D 10 and L 1, that is at the level of the conus and epiconus. We always stimulate up to the point where the patient feels tingling sensations in the

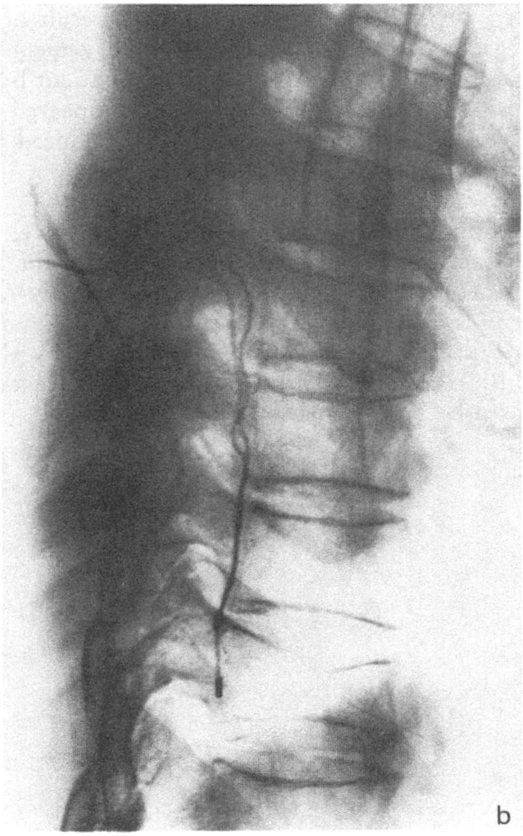

Fig. 2 b

area of his pain, malsensations, vegetative disorders or causalgia. In order to prevent failure due to the patients *positioning*, stimulation was tested not only in the prone and side positions but also while sitting and standing, before the final fixation.

Results

Our study covers observation periods from two months up to one year. The results are shown on the table.

Stimulation has the following effects upon the different pain, sensory and vegetative disturbances. The neurological symptoms were not affected.

Six of the patients were satisfied with the result of the stimulation. With regards to pain 5 stated 70% improvement or more, one patient had improved by about 50% and one patient by about 30%.

The vegetative disturbances completely, disappeared in 3 patients, while in the remaining 4 patients, they were reduced by 70% and more.

In short this study shows:

Epidurally implanted bipolar electrodes at the level of conus and epiconus, are beneficial not only in cases of severe pain, but also have a positive effect on sensory, vegetative and especially causalgia-type malsensations in the perineum, anus, rectum, bladder and vagina.

Causalgia-type of pain can only be ameliorated by electrostimulation and not by chordotomy, which usually is the method of choice with pain caused by malignomas or metastases.

Acta Neurochirurgica, Suppl. 30, 317—332 (1980)

B. Spasticity

Chronic Cerebellar Stimulation for Cerebral Palsy—Five-Year Study

R. Davis*, G. Barolat-Romana*, and H. Engle**

With 3 Figures

Summary

Two hundred sixty-two patients were implanted with cerebellar stimulator systems since February 1974. Cerebral Palsy (CP) patients constituted 88% (230) of this series. The age range was 3 to 53 years with 70% under 20 years of age. Half the CP series were severely affected with the rest being moderately to mildly involved. Athetosis was present in 50%. The primary effect of CCS has been a lowering of spastic muscle tone in 90% of the patients. Improvements in control of immature reflexes such as startle response, head control, scissoring, balance and sitting occur in the first month. Athetosis progressively decreases to a 50% level. In the moderate mild CP group abilities improve over the first six months leading to better feeding, dressing, and ambulation with clearer speech and less drooling. After six months, 25 of 48 patients were out of wheelchairs, walking. A further 47 patients were ambulating better.

No deaths from surgery. Five have died during the 5 years from other causes. Eleven patients (4%) have had infected systems. Equipment problems especially with malfunctioning radio receivers (40%) have served as blind controls—spasticity returning and abilities decreasing. Replacements with another receiver or with a totally implantable lithium powered pacemaker (May 1979) have lead to a return of benefits. Post-mortum findings indicate the low current levels (0.8 uC/sqcm) applied intermittently produced no appreciable damage to the cerebellar cortex.

Keywords: Cerebellar stimulation; cerebral palsy.

---

* Department Neurological Surgery, Mt. Sinai Medical Center, 4300 Alton Road (Suite 221), Miami Beach, FL 33140, U.S.A.

** Department Pediatrics and Adolescent Medicine, Mt. Sinai Medical Center, 4300 Alton Road, Miami Beach, FL 33140, U.S.A.

0065-1419/80/Suppl. 30/0317/$ 03.20

Introduction

In 1972, I. S. Cooper initiated the technique of chronic stimulation to the superior surface of the cerebellum in humans for the reduction of intractable muscle hypertonia and the modification of some forms of epilepsy [1, 2, 7]. As early as 1897, Lowenthal and Horsley [27] and Sherrington [34] showed in decerebrate animals a decrease in extensor hypertonia following stimulation of the anterior lobe cerebellar cortex.

Table 1. *Chronic Cerebellar Stimulation 1972—July 1979*

Clinicians series—North America	Patients
Cooper, I. S.	325 (40)
Davis, R.	262 (4)
Larson, S. J.	75
Heath, R. G.	38
Heimburger, R. F.	30 (2)
Penn, R.	18 (2)
Hoffman, H.	8
Van Buren, J.	5 (5)
Medtronic report (17 clinicians)	71 (21)
Collected cases (10 clinicians)	71 (8)
Patient total	903
Epilepsy patients	(82)

During the past 6–7 years, clinics in North America have implanted approximately 900 patients for chronic cerebellar stimulation (CCS; Table 1). About 90% of the cases have cerebral palsy (CP), CCS has been used to reduce the various forms of spasticity and athetosis [1, 2, 5–9, 11–17, 24–26, 28–30, 32, 36]. Less than 2% of the patients implanted have brain damage with spasticity secondary to cerebrovascular accidents, head injuries and asphyxia [7, 14, 15, 17, 24]. A few cases of dystonia, torticollis, Huntington's Chorea, Parkinsonism and multiple sclerosis have been implanted with varied results [12, 14, 15, 24]. 82 cases (9%) of intractable epilepsy have been implanted and are under follow-up studies [1–7, 24, 38]. CCS has been used in 38 cases of behaviour disorders [21].

The following report covers generally our results of 262 cases (Table 2) implanted over a five-year-period (February 1974–July 1979) and specifically the results of the 230 cerebral palsy patients (88%) following CCS.

Methods and Material

Patient Selection: The 262 patients selected for CCS, had disabling, intractable neurological diseases (Table 2), and had been treated by neurologists, paediatrician's, and in many cases, orthopaedists. Many had received some success through medication, physical therapy and corrective surgery but wanted to achieve more through the effects of CCS.

The usefulness of CCS has been shown in the CP series [1, 2, 5–9, 11–17, 24–26, 28–30] to reduce muscle hypertonus, decrease the excitable "immature" reflexes and athetoid movements when present. As a result, the patients' abilities, however limited can be more effective. When evaluating a CP patient for CCS, we explain this carefully to the parents and patient, then try to project realistically, the improvements in each part of the body if the spastic processes were reduced by 25 to 30%.

Table 2. *Chronic Cerebellar Stimulation—262 Patients—July 1979*

Aetiological factors	Patients implanted	%
Cerebral palsy	230	87.8
Head trauma	11	4
CVA	5	2
Asphyia	4	1.5
Anaesthetic arrest (2)		
Drowning (1)		
Carbon monoxide (1)		
Encephalitis	2	0.8
CNS degenerative disease	1	0.4
Huntington's chorea	2	0.8
Dystonia		
Retrocollis	1	0.4
Torticollis	2	0.8
Epilepsy	4	1.5

Our series of 230 CP patients consisted of a) *Very Severely Affected Patients* (10%): Generally they were either bed-ridden or able to be strapped into a wheelchair, always under the care of a family member who had to expend considerable energy and time to dress, feed, and attend to their elimination problems. b) *Moderate-Severely Affected Group* (45%): These patients were wheelchair bound with some control of their upper extremities, and needed some assistance in feeding, dressing, and bathroom activities. Head control and speech were usually moderately to severely affected. Athetoid components to their movements often made simple, important movements of the arms impossible. c) *Moderately Affected Group* (40%): These patients could generally walk awkwardly with or without aids. They were independent in regards to feeding, the bathroom, and some did need assistance with dressing. Head control and speech was moderately affected in some. Half of the group had athetoid movements. d) *Mildly Affected Patients* (5%): These patients usually had only one side of the body or one limb (especially dominant upper limb) involved. Speech, was usually moderately involved so making their life difficult in work or school activities.

The goals for each group are therefore very different even though CCS works on the same basic mechanisms in every patient. The clinical results of CCS of course, depend upon the equipment working, the degree of decrease in spasticity and the improvements in the patient's disabilities.

In the CP series, the patients' ages ranged from 3 years to 53 years with (37%) below the age of 10 years, and another (34%) in the 11–20 year age group. *Hospitalization and Evaluations:* Usually 6 to 12 weeks elapsed between the initial office evaluation and hospitalization, so allowing the parents and patients time to consider all the aspects of CCS, its surgery and risks before deciding. Hospitalization was usually 10 days. Pre-operative evaluations were tabulated separately by a paediatric neurologist, paediatrian, physical and speech therapists, and a neurosurgeon. Biomedical photography, including audio-visual taping, was

Table 3. *CCS—Equipment Complications—262 Patients (February 1974–July 1979)*

		%
Broken leads		16 (6)
Radio receiver malfunction		90 (34)
Radio receiver changed	51	
Changed to "Neurolith"	3	
Awaiting change	36	
Uncertain whether working (awaiting testing)		44 (18)
Electrode repositioning		4 (2)
Patients requesting removal		2 (1)

used to record pre-operative status and later the effects of CCS. Clinical evaluations with tabulation were made at 6-month intervals, yearly in some cases. Some data have been collected from either the patient or the family by telephone enquiries, because of the distances involved. Pre-operatively tests included skull X-rays, EEG's and computer tomography. In the CP series about a half had abnormal scans, indicating ventricular enlargement and/or cortical atrophy. A biomedical engineering laboratory has been built to measure spastic muscle resistance and activity, athetoid movements, head control, balance and gait.

Cerebellar Stimulating Equipment: In all but two patients, bilateral superior cerebellar cortical stimulation was used through the two electrode pads placed in parallel, 2–3 cm apart [13–15]. The other two patients had unilateral right-sided placements of the electrode pads; with one of these two patients, also having a set of posterior surface electrodes [17]. Unilateral superior stimulation produced bilateral lessening of spasticity; whereas superior surface stimulation was far more effective than that to the posterior surface [14, 15, 17].

The two electrode pads are wafer thin (Fig. 1) and each has four platinum buttons; the total stimulating area of the eight buttons is 0.64 cm^2. The pulse energy was supplied by two different stimulators (Fig. 1), each producing a pulse of 0.5 msec duration at a frequency of 150–180 per second. The "ON-OFF" timing was in the range of 4–7 minute periods. Whether the generator was of the alterphasic-pulse type [14, 15], having an external transmitter with antenna and an internally placed radio receiver (Avery Laboratories, Farmingdale, NY; Fig. 1 A), or was of the monophasic type, having a lithium battery-powered totally implantable unit (Pacesetter Systems Inc., Sylmar, California; Fig. 1 B)

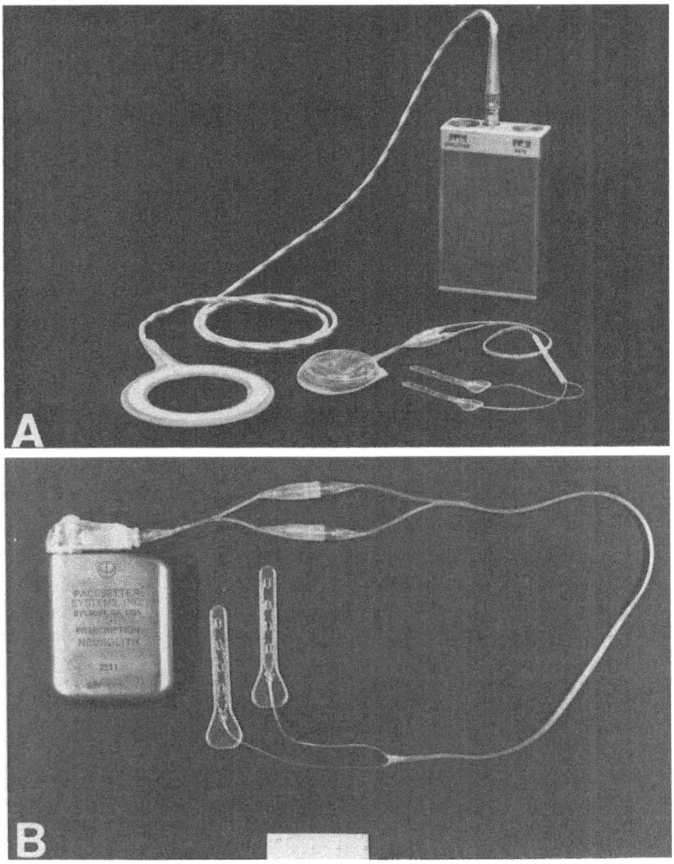

Fig. 1. Cerebellar stimulation equipment. A) Radio-frequency linked generator system; external transmitter with antenna, internally placed radio receiver (I108) with cerebellar electrodes. B) Totally implantable lithium powered "Neurolith" generator attached to cerebellar leads

the pulse energy was set at 0.8 μCoulombs per cm^2 per phase. In this latter, fully implanted unit, "Neurolith" (Fig. 1 B) the cathodal pulses go to the eight electrode buttons on the cortex, while the anode is connected to the case surface. The lithium battery is calculated to last 4½ years, and can be turned off with a magnet.

Of considerable concern was the failure rate of the radio receiver (I 108), determined definitely in 90 cases with possibly another 44 cases affected (more than 40% of the series, Table 3). Indications of failure were lack of muscle relaxation and loss of gained abilities; after of course, the external transmitter and antenna were checked. The important test has been to record on an oscilloscope, the pulse shape and amplitude from the scalp between the forehead and mastoid regions. The I 108 receiver should give an alternating pulse train of about 200 microvolts. When a drop in amplitude was recorded, adjustments were made to the amplitude knob on the transmitter, usually resulting in return of effectiveness. If the amplitude could not be brought to these levels and the pulse shape was not of equal amplitude above and below the baseline, the radio receiver was diagnosed as malfunctioning.

With this failure of the I 108 receiver, 44 replacements in the past nine months have been with the monophasic I 110 receivers; the cathodal side was connected to the eight buttons, and the anodal lead was connected to a ground plate placed in the same pocket. The total "Neurolith" implant was used (May, 1979) in three patients whose radio receivers had failed after 2–3½ years of useful results.

Table 4. *CCS—Post-Operative Complications—262 Patients (February 1974–July 1979)*

		%
Death—post-op. in hospital	0	0
Infected systems (all removed, 5 re-implanted)	11	4
C.S.F. into pocket	42	16
Post-op. ventr.-perit. shunt	2	0.8
Hematoma in pocket	5	2
Post-op. mid. cerebr. art. thromb.	1	0.4

Benefits from CCS were noticeable again after 1–2 days (Fig. 2), with continuing improvements over the following four weeks.

Using the impedance meter (50 KHz, Radionics Corp., Mass.), impedance measurements of the four (button) electrodes-cerebellar cortex-four electrodes pathway in 85 patients at the initial surgery was averaged at 390 ohms. Eight to 16 months after the implantation, seven patients had their radio receiver changed, so allowing impedance to be measured again: at initial surgery—314 ohms, at replacement of receiver—330 ohms. The lack of significant change indicated little or no build up of tissue reaction which could have caused an increase in impedance. This has been confirmed, as a result of replacing 12 broken cerebellar leads (Table 3), the electrode pads on removal had shown no fibrous encapsulation [11, 16, 20, 22] except in 2 cases, one pad of each pair was coated on both sides.

Operative Techniques and Complications: Following induction of general anaesthesia, the patient has a central venous catheter placed in the right atrium before being positioned into the sitting position. Doppler cardiac monitoring has been essential and has recorded micro-air embolisms in 60% of the patients, plus signs of hypotension and arrthymias in 10–15% [14]. After discontinuing nitrous oxide and changing to 100% oxygen mixed with the anaesthetic agent, this incidence has been reduced by half. After a right occipital twist-drill hole was made and closed, the surgeon fashioned an infra-clavicular subcutaneous pocket for the radio receiver or "Neurolith". Then a midline suboccipital exposure allowed bilateral burr holes to be placed 1 cm lateral and below the occipital protuberance. The two openings were enlarged to expose the lateral sinuses. After the electrode lead had been passed inside an Argyle 20 G plastic tube, down to the clavicular opening, 5 mm horizontal dural incisions were made bilaterally.

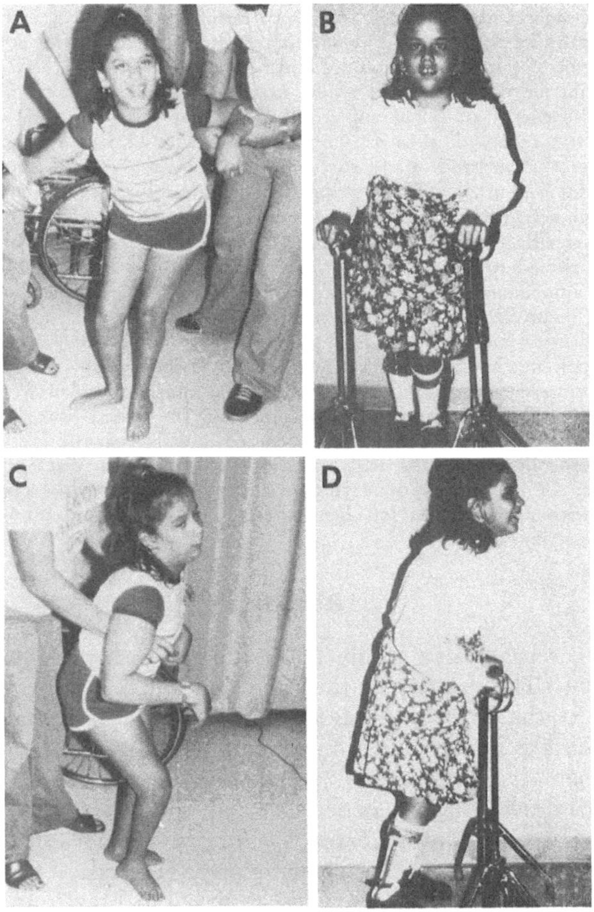

Fig. 2. Cerebral palsy patient, 11 year old female with spastic paraparesis. A) and C) Pre-operative status. B) and D) two days after replacement of malfunctioning radio receiver with the "Neurolith" generator

Hyperventilation produced a shrinkage of the cerebellum so an adequate space was obtained below the tentorium, so allowing the 2 electrode pads to be gently positioned over the paramedian surfaces about 2–3 cms apart. Radiographic evidence confirmed the placements. The electrode pads are flexible and have doubled or been diverted by a blood vessel.

No posterior fossa haematoma has occurred in this series (Table 4), although five patients did have pocket haematomata. The most common problem (16%) has been CSF leaking down along the lead to the pocket; purse-string sutures placed around the tissues at the upper and lower ends of the lead during the initial surgery, have definitely reduced this problem. However, when it does occur, a supraclavicular incision with sutures placed around the tract usually stops this leak; in two cases, a ventriculo-peritoneal shunt was used. Patients are advised not to exercise the shoulder and neck regions for 2–3 weeks.

Calibration of the system, electrodes and pulse generator, were performed to ensure a pulse energy of 0.8 μCoul./cm² [11, 14, 15]. The impedance of the electrode and cortex was recorded, then a 10 ohm resistor was inserted in series with the radio receiver and electrode pads, so current flowing in the circuit could be measured and then adjusted. When using the I 108 receiver which sends alternate pulses to each set of 4 buttons, the pulse current was set at 0.5 mA by the transmitter via a sterilized antenna. With the I 110 monophasic receiver whose cathode side was connected to the 8 buttons, the current was therefore doubled to 1 mA. Because the impedance and resistance of the system was relatively constant (see above), the "Neurolith" was designed to produce a constant pulse current of 1 mA. The charge density is $1.0\ mA \times 0.5\ msec \div 0.64\ cm^2 = 0.8\ \mu C/cm^2/phase$.

Eleven patients had infected systems (Table 4) mostly due to staphylococcus aureus. In most cases, the infection entered the supraclavicular wound used in repairing CSF leaks to the pocket. Once infected the system was removed. The only severe post-operative complication occurred in a 63-year-old lady with severe disabling retrocollis secondary to advanced cerebrovascular disease. In the recovery room, she became hypotensive and suffered a right middle cerebral artery thrombosis with a subsequent left hemiparesis. There has been no postoperative deaths in the series (Table 4).

Results

In the cerebral palsy group (230 patients), each patient acts as his own control. The severity of the condition and the patient's abilities are stable at the time of implantation. *Primary improvements* following CCS are in the reduction of muscle hypertonus and lessening of hyperexcitable "immature" reflexes. As much as 20–40% reduction in muscle tone are experienced by over 90% of the patients during the first 6 months (Table 5). Improvements experienced by the patient range from feeling of being more relaxed, of not "fighting myself", finding it easier to use his abilities, to breath and swallow easier, less drooling, not being so tired and having more energy. Objective improvements following the reductions in spasticity (primary effect of CCS), are seen in the first 6 months as: 20–30% improvement in forearm supernation, steadier head and neck control, with better posture of sitting and standing, 20–30% improvement in voluntary hip flexion, diminished startle response, decrease in the dysarthric component of speech (Table 5). Over the ensuing weeks, the athetoid component in movements were decreased allowing better control of the movements (Table 5).

If progress ceases and muscle stiffness returns, the equipment both external and internal are checked. In almost all the cases when malfunction occurred and was corrected, the spasticity process was reduced within hours of reinstituting CCS. Because of the gradual changes that occur over the weeks and months following CCS, a prospective double blind study is very difficult to manage. However, a retrospective double blind study is essentially in effect at all times, as the patient and physician does not know when the equipment may fail leading to this loss of effects.

Table 5. *Summary Table: CCS—Cerebral Palsy Patients. 226 Patients—November 1974–November 1978*

	Relaxation		Athetosis		Drooling		Speech	
	imp.	no	imp.	no	imp.	no	imp.	no
1st week	214	3	79	18	78	29	140	37
6 months	103	5	35	3	34	9	65	7
1 year	89	12	32	4	36	13	58	21
2 years	56	7	25	8	16	13	28	15
3 years	19	1	5	3	4	2	7	6

Mode of Independent Mobility

Mode (95 patients)	Pre-op.		Post-op. *	
	#pts.	%	#pts.	%
Normal—mild gait impairment	3	3	10	10
Moderate gait impairment	15	16	16	17
Walks with aids	19	20	30	32
Crawling	10	10.5	14	15
Wheelchair	48	50.5	25	26

* Post-operative category is a summary of patients' progress 6 months onwards following CCS.

Following the above improvements, *secondary effects* occur in co-ordinating movements. As muscle tone has been decreased, agonist and antagonist muscle groups do less "jamming" with better range of movement in joints. Complicated movements can now be co-ordinated better with improvements in the functional status of the individual. Usually these secondary effects, likened to a learning experience, take 3–9 months to reach near maximum benefits. Improvements in feeding, dressing, grooming and independent mobility (Table 5) follow in those patients that have the neurological circuits capable of functioning in these areas, especially in group C and D of the above classification. Physical therapy, encouragement, determination and in some cases orthopaedic correction, are all important in reaching the full potential, however limited (Fig. 3).

Patients in category A and many in B, are severely disabled and do not have the neurological mechanisms to achieve much in the area of *secondary effects* from CCS. However, the patients are more relaxed can sit in chairs without restraints, do not drool as much,

Table 6. *Patient Report. CCS—July 1979*

	Patients	%
Implanted (since February, 1974)	262	
Information not available	12	
Information available	250	100
1. Benefiting from CCS	152	61
2. Benefited from CCS—not using	5	2
3. Tested, mal-funct. radio receiver	36	14
4. Tested, broken leads	2	1
5. Infected system, removed and not replaced	6	2
6. No benefit from CCS, awaiting testing	44	18
7. Deaths from other causes	5	2

scissoring is less, allowing better dressing and grooming. Swallowing and respiratory function definitely improve leading to a better nutritional status with less illness (especially recurrent pneumonia) [14, 15, 28]. Parents or attendents of these severely affected patients, have found them much easier to care for and even take them out of the home for excursions. The goals of this group are obviously different from the more capable patients.

In reviewing the upper part of Table 5, the patients that show no improvement after 1 year and onwards, have achieved and reached their own plateau. The improvements in the mode of independent mobility (Table 5) is a summary of the patients reviewed following 6 months of CCS. These patients are from group B, C, and D.

During May–July 1979, a survey of the 262 patients implanted was completed (Table 6). Twelve patients could not be contacted due to change of address or being out of the country. Information as to the status of the remaining 250 patients is shown in Table 6. One hundred fifty-two patients (61%) are benefiting from CCS use, another 5 (2%) patients have or do benefit from occasional use of CCS. A further 44 patients (18%) claim no benefit from CCS, how-

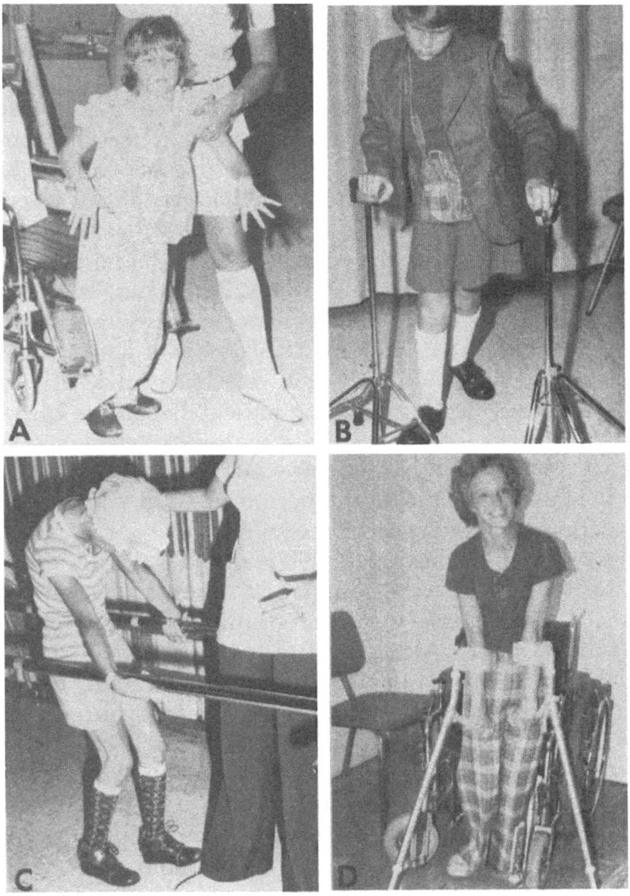

Fig. 3. Two female cerebral palsy patients with spastic paraparesis, unable to ambulate without constant support. A) and C) pre-operative status. B) and D) 7–12 months post-implant CCS

ever, most want their systems checked for malfunction and if found, repaired. A group of 38 patients (15%) are awaiting repair.

Autopsy Findings: In the series, 5 patients had died from other causes, 2 with gastric haemorrhage, 2 with respiratory complications and 1 from suicide (the stimulator had been removed on request 2 years prior to death). Two brains have been examined for the effects of stimulation on the cerebellar cortex [11, 20]. Only slight indentation of the electrode pads with no evidence of arachnoid reaction was seen macroscopically. The cerebellar cortex of the patient, where CCS was kept to our standard charge density level of 0.8 μCoul/cm²/phase, showed no histological changes under the buttons as compared to control areas lateral to the pads. The broad flange at the posterior edge of the electrode pad (Fig. 1) protects the cerebellar surface from the emerging wires. The other patient had used, against our warnings and without our control, higher charge densities ranging from 9–31 μCoul/cm²/phase. This caused atrophy in only the underlying superficial folia, where focal loss of Purkinje and granule cells were found with reactive Bergmann gliosis [11, 20].

Seizure Activity: A survey showed 29 patients (16%) of the first 176 CP patients implanted had a history of seizures at some time in their life. Of these, 15 patients (8.5%) had seizures within 1 year prior to implantation. With CCS, 13 reported fewer seizures, 1 had the same frequency while the other patient had more of a different type-occurring when the patient was hypoglycemic. There were 14 patients (8%) who had seizure activity at an earlier age or detected in the EEG. During the period of CCS, 13 patients had no seizures while 1 patient reported a seizure.

Anticonvulsant medication, during the period of CCS, has been reduced in 10 patients, the same in 8, more in 1 and changed in 2 patients. The decrease was seen primarily in hydantoin, phenobarbital and mysoline. Although detailed information and analysis is not available here, the majority of the seizures were of the grand-mal type. In a patient who normally had a strong history of seizures (2–3/day, 40 per year) before CCS, malfunction of the equipment would often be seen as a sudden increase in the number or a return of seizures. An interesting case has been a 14 year old CP female with 50–100 myoclonic jerks or seizures a day with drug-controlled grandmal and petit-mal seizures. After 24 hours of CCS, she had almost stopped having the myoclonic jerks or seizures. After 3½ years of CCS, these myoclonic jerks and associated seizures have remained under control. Medication has been reduced.

Discussion

There are many factors influencing the results of CCS in CP patients. Firstly, the equipment must be functioning at the adjusted levels; patients do not know how nor can they adequately check every part of their system. They certainly know when they are suddenly not obtaining muscle relaxation and its secondary effects. However, when the equipment fails gradually, it is difficult for the patient to realize this loss. Regular or as necessary, checks should be done to test the pulses emitted from the electrodes by recording them with an amplifier and oscilloscope. Equipment design and reliability testing should be improved especially in regard to any implanted equipment. Wires and insulation are being made stronger to resist breakage; encapsulation of the pulse generator circuit with a lithium battery "Neurolith" for total implantation should reduce some of the problems in the radio frequency linkage systems, and adds further convenience to the patient.

There is much discussion as to the parameters of stimulation used in CCS. Cooper's group [4, 8] used charge density in the range of 20–30 μCoul/cm²/phase. Larson's parameters are in the range of 13–16 μCoul/cm²/phase [25, 26]. These are 10–30 times more than our level of stimulation. When the strength of stimulation is increased 4–5 times in our equipment, the effects of CCS are lost—paradoxical effect of stimulation level [14].

There is general agreement as to the frequency of stimulation (100–200 Hz) and the pulse width (0.2–1.0 msec). The intermittent stimulation of from 1–10 minutes (ON and OFF) are all agreed on and used. Gilman's monkey showed less damage when intermittent stimulation was used [10].

There appears to be a damage factor from CCS to the surface of the cerebellum however, which is dependent upon the level of the charge density. Gilman's results from the monkey, cerebellar stimulation (30 μCoul/cm²/phase [10, 35]) showed more damage than has been seen in any of the human material reported [3, 11, 16, 20, 22, 26, 33, 37]. T. L. Babb (personal communication) has repeated Gilman's experiments of CCS effects in monkey with minimal to no damage to the cerebellar surface. In the human material, charge densities at levels over 7–10 μCoul/cm²/phase, can cause local folia damage under the electrode buttons, but not beyond. According to Robertson *et al.* [33], the damage is in the range of 1–3% of the entire cerebellar surface using the higher levels of stimulation [8, 18, 37]. Another factor causing damage to the cerebellar cortex is the electrode characteristics. If rigid, thick and large, the electrode presents more chance of indenting the surface and damaging bridging veins. Connecting wires to the buttons must be protected from cutting into the posterior edge of the cortex.

Clinical effects of CCS in the CP patients depends considerably on the degree of spasticity and under-lying abilities. The primary effect of cerebellar stimulation as Lowenthal and Horsley [27] and Sherrington [34] indicated, are to reduce muscle hypertonus. Then the secondary effects of self feeding, dressing and walking can only be achieved if these abilities are adequate and allowed to function better with the lessening in spasticity.

Until the clinics categorize patients as to their under-lying abilities, comparison of results will be difficult. If a clinic decides to assist severely affected patients on behalf of their parents, knowing full well that little functional improvements will occur, but that caring for the patient will be easier, this is an end point in itself. However, children with certain potentials can be selected for CCS in order to achieve walking and other independent modalities.

Acknowledgements

We gratefully acknowledge the excellent assistance of Ms. Alice Dusnak in preparing the data. We thank Drs. M. Flitter, R. Cullen, D. Duenas and O. Papazian as well as Messrs. Ed Gray and Bruce Ennis, Ms. Bonita Weis and Lyndell Jenkins for their assistance. Our sincere thanks to Bio-medical photographer, Mr. Gary Lustgarten.

References

1. Cooper, I. S., Chronic stimulation of paleocerebellar cortex in man. Lancet *1* (1973), 206.
2. Cooper, I. S., Effect of chronic stimulation of anterior cerebellum on neurological disease. Lancet *1* (1973), 1321.
3. Cooper, I. S., Amin, I., Gilman, S., Waltz, J. M., The effect of chronic stimulation of cerebellar cortex on epilepsy in man. In: The Cerebellum, Epilepsy, and Behaviour, pp. 119—171 (Cooper, I. S., *et al.*, eds.). New York: Plenum Press. 1974.
4. Cooper, I. S., Amin, I., Riklan, M., Waltz, J. M., Poon, T. P., Chronic cerebellar stimulation in epilepsy. Clinical and anatomical studies. Arch. Neurol. *33* (1976), 559—570.
5. Cooper, I. S., Amin, I., Upton, A., Riklan, M., Watkins, S., McLellan, D. L., Safety and efficacy of chronic cerebellar stimulation. Neurosurgery *1* (1977), 203—205.
6. Cooper, I. S., Amin, I., Upton, A., Riklan, M., Watkins, S., McLellan, L., Safety and efficacy of chronic cerebellar stimulation. Appl. Neurophysiol. *40* (1977/78), 124—134.
7. Cooper, I. S., Crighel, E., Amin, I., Clinical and physiological effects of stimulation of the paleocerebellum in humans. J. Amer. Geriatr. Soc. *21* (1973), 40—43.
8. Cooper, I. S., Riklan, M., Amin, I., Waltz, J. M., Cullinan, T., Chronic cerebellar stimulation in cerebral palsy. Neurology (Minneap.) *26* (1976), 744—753.
9. Cooper, I. S., Riklan, M., Tabaddor, K., Cullinan, T., Amin, I., Watkins, E. S., A Long term follow-up study of chronic stimulation for cerebral palsy. In: Cerebellar Stimulation in Man, pp. 59—99 (Cooper, I. S., ed.). New York: Raven Press. 1978.
10. Dauth, G. W., Defendini, R., Gilman, S., Tennyson, V. M., Kremzner, L. T., Long-term surface stimulation of the cerebellum in the monkey. I. Light microscopic electrophysiologic and clinical observation. Surg. Neurol. 7 (1977), 377—384.
11. Davis, R., Chronic cerebellar stimulation: the effect of low charge density stimulation on the human cortex and clinical functions. Proc. Ass. Adv. Med. INSTR. (14 Ann Meet) (1979), 55.

12. Davis, R., Cullen, R. F., Duenas, D., Engle, H., Cerebellar stimulation for cerebral palsy. J. Fla. Med. Assoc. *63* (1976), 910—912.
13. Davis, R., Cullen, R. F., Duenas, D., Flitter, M., The effects of chronic cerebellar stimulation on cerebral palsy patients. Amer. Assoc. Neurol. Surg. (1977).
14. Davis, R., Cullen, R. F., Flitter, M., Duenas, D., Engle, H., Ennis, B., Control of spasticity and involuntary movements. Neurosurgery *1* (1977), 205—207.
15. Davis, R., Cullen, R. F., Flitter, M., Duenas, D., Engle, H., Papazian, O., Weis, B., Control of spasticity and involuntary movements—cerebellar stimulation. Appl. Neurophysiol. *40* (1977/78), 135—140.
16. Davis, R., Flitter, M., Cerebellar Stimulation (letter). Surg. Neurol. *9* (1978), 115.
17. Davis, R., Gesink, J. W., Evaluation of electrical stimulation as a treatment for the reduction of spasticity. Bull. Proseth. Res. (Fall 1974), 302—309.
18. Dow, R. S., Historical perspective and a physiological overview of chronic cerebellar stimulation. Proc. Ass. Adv. Med. Instr. 14th Ann. Meet (1979), 63.
19. Eccles, J. C., Ito, M., Szentagothai, J., The cerebellum as a neuronal machine. Berlin-Heidelberg-New York: Springer. 1967.
20. Gyori, E., Davis, R., Chronic cerebellar stimulation and its relationship to subsequent histological changes in the surface of the cerebellar cortex. (In preparation.)
21. Heath, R. G., Dempsey, C. W., Fontana, C. J., Cerebellar stimulation for behavioral pathology: clinical results and possible neural mechanisms. Proc. Assoc. Adv. Med. Instr. 14th Ann. Meet. (1979), 115.
22. Heimburger, R. F., Damage from cerebellar stimulation (letter). Surg. Neurol. *8* (1977), 248.
23. Hemmy, D. C., Larson, S. J., Sances, A., Jr., *et al.*, The effect of cerebellar stimulation on focal seizure activity and spasticity in monkeys. J. Neurosurg. *46* (1977), 648—653.
24. Hirsch, R., Medtronic cerebellar stimulation system, single and dual channel. Preliminary clinical status report, February 1974 through November 1977. Medtronic, Inc. Minn. (1978).
25. Larson, S. J., Quantitative evaluation of cerebellar stimulation. Proc. Ass. Adv. Med. Instr. 14th Ann. Meet. (1979), 158.
26. Larson, S. J., Sances, A., Jr., Hemmy, D. C., Miller, E. A., Walsh, P. R., Physiological and histological effects of cerebellar stimulation. Appl. Neurophysiol. *40* (1977/78), 160—174.
27. Lowenthal, M., Horsley, V., On the relations between the cerebellar and other centers. Proc. R. Soc. Lond. *61* (1897), 20—25.
28. Miyasaka, K., Hoffman, H. J., Froese, A. B., Influence of chronic cerebellar stimulation on respiratory muscle co-ordination in a patient with cerebral palsy. Neurosurg. *2* (1978), 262—265.
29. Penn, R. D., Etzel, M. L., Chronic cerebellar stimulation and developmental reflexes. J. Neurosurg. *46* (1977), 506—511.
30. Penn, R. D., Gottlieb, G. L., Agarwal, G. C., Cerebellar stimulation in man. Quantitative changes in spasticity. J. Neurosurg. *48* (1978), 779—786.
31. Pudenz, R. H., Bullara, L. A., Jacques, S., Hambrecht, F. T., Electrical stimulation of the brain. III. The neural damage model. Surg. Neurol. *4* (1975), 389—400.
32. Ratusnik, D. C., Wolfe, V. I., Penn, R. D., *et al.*, Effects on speech of chronic cerebellar stimulation in cerebral palsy. J. Neurosurg. *48* (1978), 876—882.
33. Robertson, L. T., Dow, R. S., Cooper, I. S., Levy, L. F., Morphological changes associated with chronic cerebellar stimulation in the human. J. Neurosurg. *51* (1979), 510—520.

34. Sherrington, C. S., Double (antidrome) conduction in the central nervous system. Proc. R. Soc. Lond. *61* (1897), 243—246.
35. Tennyson, V. M., Kremzner, L. T., Dauth, G. W., Defendini, R., Gilman, S., Long-term surface stimulation of the cerebellum in the monkey. II. Electron microscopic and bio-chemical observation. Surg. Neurol. *8* (1977), 17—29.
36. Upton, A. F. M., Cooper, I. S., Some neurophysiological effects of cerebellar stimulation in man. Can. J. Neurol. Sci. *3* (1976), 237—254.
37. Urich, H., Watkins, E. S., Amin, I., Cooper, I. S., Neuropathologic observations on cerebellar cortical lesions in patients with epilepsy and motor disorders. In: Cerebellar Stimulation in Man, pp. 145—159 (Cooper, I. S., ed.). New York: Raven Press. 1978.
38. Van Buren, J. M., Wood, J. H., Oakley, J., Hambrecht, F., Preliminary evaluation of cerebellar stimulation by double-blind stimulation and biological criteria in the treatment of epilepsy. J. Neurosurg. *48* (1978), 407—416.

Acta Neurochirurgica, Suppl. 30, 333—338 (1980)

Side Effects and Long-Term Results of Chronic Cerebellar Stimulation in Man

M. Manrique*, J. Vaquero, S. Oya, A. P. Lozano, and **G. Bravo**

With 2 Figures

Keywords: Cerebellum; electrical stimulation; side effects; long-term results.

Chronic cerebellar electrical stimulation has been one of the most controversial problems in the literature since Cooper *et al.* [3] first reported the clinical and physiological effects of stimulation of the paleocerebellum in man.

Some side effects have been reported as being rare and of no major importance [5–7, 9]. Some of them are due to surgical technique [6, 7, 13] and several to the effects of acute and chronic electrical stimulation in animals [8, 11, 14] and man [10].

Nevertheless good results have been reported by several authors [5–7, 9, 12, 13] and the potential dangers of the procedure are not high when weighed against the benefits [2].

This report summarizes our clinical and histological observations of the effects of chronic stimulation of the cerebellar cortex in 7 patients with movement disorders and intractable epilepsy.

Clinical Material and Method

From January 1976 to December 1977, seven patients underwent paleocerebellar electrode implantation through small suboccipital craniectomies.

One patient suffering intractable epilepsy (case 7) was studied by two stereo-electroencephalographic [1] explorations and revealed bilateral frontal epilepsy, corticectomy was therefore contraindicated, and chronic cerebellar stimulation indicated. The other six patients had severe neuromuscular diseases: one patient complained of paraplegic spasticity (case 1), one had a familial cerebellospinal atrophic disease (case 2), and 4 suffered from cerebral palsy (case 3, 4, 5, 6).

The chronic stimulating system was installed as described by Cooper *et al.* [3, 4]. The electrode plate was plotted following the method of electrode localization as

* Departement of Neurosurgery, Clinica Puerta de Hierro, Madrid, Spain.

0065-1419/80/Suppl. 30/0333/$ 01.20

described by Cooper *et al.* [4, 10], in all cases. Cerebellar biopsies were performed in all patients at the time of electrode implantation.

In two patients, 3 posterior fossa explorations were necessary for revision of the stimulation apparatus. During the operation cerebellar tissue was taken and prepared for light and electron microscopy study with the method described in a previous paper [10].

Electrode implantation was performed bilaterally in 6 patients and on the right side in 1 patient. 5 Dual cerebellar stimulators and 2 single cerebellar stimulators (Avery Lab. Inc. systems) were used.

The patient with intractable epilepsy (case 7) was stimulated 24 hours daily for two years, and 12 hours daily, during the day, for one year at 10 cps, 6 volts and a schedule of 15 minutes ON, 15 minutes OFF.

In four patients (cases 1, 2, 3, 4) stimulation was applied 90 minutes to 7 hours daily with a rate of 20—180 cps and 6–10 V with a schedule of 15 minutes ON, 15 minutes OFF.

Two patients (cases 5, 6) were stimulated for 6 hours daily with a rate of 200 cps using a single channel stimulator with a schedule of 2 minutes ON, 2 minutes OFF from 6 to 8 volts.

Five patients were observed postoperatively with a follow up of 3 years. In one of those patients the electrodes were removed after three months of chronic stimulation (case 1). The other four patients were chronically stimulated during all the observation time (case 2, 3, 4, 7). Two patients were studied with a follow up of fifteen months (cases 5, 6).

Results

Surgical Complications

There were no deaths, infection, or morbidity related to the surgical technique in the 10 posterior fossa operations. Postoperatively two patients (cases 2 and 3) presented fluid accumulation in the infraclavicular pocket. A compressive pack was fixed on the area, and in 7 to 10 days the accumulation disappeared.

Side Effects Related to Acute Electrical Stimulation

Four patients noted a suboccipital headache which was proportional to the intensity of stimulation. Three patients (case 1, 6, 7) could clearly identify the stimulated side and one noted only a diffuse headache (case 4) (Fig. 1). In two cases irradiation to the ear on the stimulated side was noted and one patient also reported difuse slight pain in the ipsilateral eye (cases 6 and 7) (Fig. 2). The dull headache appeared between 4 to 6 volts and was only reported during the first minute of each cycle. In all cases headache and irradiation abated after two to three months of chronic stimulation.

After two minutes of stimulation from the first session two patients described a "peacefull" (cases 1 and 2) and "feeling good" (case 3) sensation. One of them also reported a clear improvement in sight (case 2).

Side Effect Related to Chronic Stimulation

One patient (case 1) presented seizures during two days, after 3 months of chronic stimulation, characterized by extension of the extremities with hands pronated and stiffness of the trunk and neck. The EEG preformed during the fit did not show paroxysmal activity [10]. The seizures did not stop either with interruption of stimulation neither changing the frequency from 180 to 10 cps. Only barbiturate coma controlled the fits. One patient complaining of

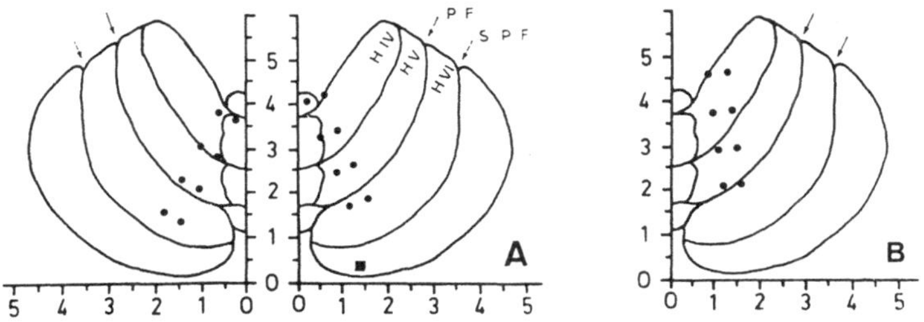

Fig. 1. Schematic diagram of the cortex of the anterior lobe of the cerebellum showing the electrode localization (●) in cases 1 (A) and 4 (B). The position of the electrode did not explain the headache without irradiation reported by the patients. *PF* primary fissure, *SPF* superior posterior fissure. ■ Biopsy in case 1

dystonia (case 3) with choreoathetosic component underwent electrode implantation in the right side and was stimulated for 12 months.

As the result was satisfactory electrode implantation was performed on the left side. After 6 months of bilateral stimulation he presented Parkinsonian tremor and violent jerks in the right extremities. These effects ceased after one month interruption of stimulation and did not reappear on reapplying stimulation. In two cases (cases 1 and 2), three posterior fossa reexplorations were performed for revision of the stimulation apparatus. A marked meningeal proliferation was observed surrounding the electrodes. The study of the biopsies taken at reoperation has been described in detail elsewhere [10], showing loss of Purkinje cell and gliofibrillar reaction. Alterations were found mostly with electron microscope. Nevertheless no clinical cerebellar sequelae resulted from chronic cerebellar stimulation.

Long-Term Results

The patient suffering intractable epilepsy did not show any change in the rate or intensity of the seizures after 3 years of chronic cerebellar stimulation (Table 1). The results of the patient with paraplegic spasticity (case 1) has been presented in detail elsewhere [10]. After removing the electrodes the seizures did not reappear and the follow up observation for two and half years showed an improvement in spasticity.

Table 1. *Long-Term Results of Our Cases.* Case 7, operated between cases 1 and 2 has been placed at the end of the table in order to follow the data of our previous paper [10]

	Diagnosis	3 months	6 months	1 year	2 years	3 years
Case 1	paraplegic spasticity	moderate (seizures)	—	—	—	—
Case 2	cerebello-spinal disease	moderate	moderate	mild	unchanged	unchanged
Case 3	cerebral palsy athetosis	mild	mild	mild	mild	mild
Case 4	cerebral palsy spasticity	unchanged	id.	id.	id.	id.
Case 5	cerebral palsy athetosis	unchanged	id.	id.	—	—
Case 6	cerebral palsy spasticity	unchanged	id.	id.	—	—
Case 7	epilepsy	unchanged	id.	id.	id.	id.

After a moderate improvement during 6 months of chronical stimulation the patient with familiar cerebellospinal atrophic disease did not show further improvement and has been stable for 2 years.

In the group of cerebral palsy only one patient improved slightly during the first six months and then stabilized. This patient had a right electrode installed for one year and then bilateral implantation was performed. After two years of bilateral stimulation improvement is mild (case 3). The other 3 patients of this group did not show any improvement after a follow up of 3 years or 15 months.

Discussion

In our small series we had no major surgical complications, and most side effects were related to electrical chronical stimulation.

Location of the electrodes has no relation to the appearance of headache (cases 1, 4, 6, 7), but in patients with irradiation to ear and eye on the right side, the electrode was placed very laterally, near the petrous bone (cases 6 and 7); the spread of current to the angle may be an explanation for this side-effect. Nevertheless, case 2 has an electrode in a similar position and did not complain of headache.

The appearance of "fits" has been discussed elsewhere [10]. We have no explanation for the tremor and jerks that presented case 3. Our

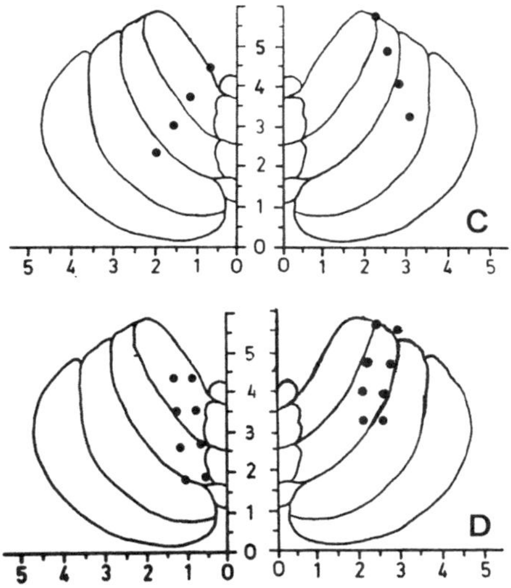

Fig. 2. Plotting of the electrodes on cases 6 (C) and 7 (D). Headache with irradiation to ear and eye on the right side was reported by the patients. Note that the electrodes on the right side are laterally placed near the petrous bone

parameters are similar to those used by Cooper *et al.* [5, 6] but the intensity of current delivered (1–1.5 mA) is higher than that used by others [7, 9].

The anatomopathological lesions could be related to the relatively high intensity applied [10], but experimental studies show that the electrode acting as a foreign body can produce a lesion similar to that ascribed to stimulation [14]. Our poor results could be attributed to the sometimes, incorrect and asymmetrical location of the electrodes. Nevertheless in case 2, the electrodes were not ideally placed and the improvement was moderate, and in cases 4 and 5 the electrodes were near the midline and there was no improvement. The best results were obtained with patients suffering diseases other than cerebral palsy which seemed, according the literature [3, 6, 7, 9, 12, 13] to be the major indication for this type of treatment. Our best results were obtained during the first six months of stimulation.

Although most of our patients reported a subjective improvement, the poor objective long-term results and the several side effects observed, forced us to reconsider our position and to postpone any further cerebellar stimulation procedures.

Acknowledgement

This study was supported in part by a Grant from the Spanish Instituto Nacional de Previsión (INP. 13.351.75).

References

1. Bancaud, J., Talairach, J., Bonis, A., Schaub, C., Szikla, G., Morel, P., Bordas-Ferrer, M., La stéréoélectroencéphalographie dans l'épilepsie, pp. 321. Paris: Masson et Cie. 1965.
2. Bensman, A. S., Szegho, M., Ban proposed on cerebellar electrical stimulation. Neurology (1977), 996.
3. Cooper, I. S., Crighel, E., Amin, I., Clinical and physiological effects of stimulation of the paleocerebellum in humans. J. Amer. Geriatr. Soc. *21* (1973), 40—43.
4. Cooper, I. S., Amin, I., Gilman, S., Waltz, J. M., The effects of chronic stimulation of the cerebellar cortex upon epilepsy in man. In: The cerebellum, epilepsy, and behaviour, pp. 119—171 (Cooper, Riklan, Snider, eds.). New-York: Plenum Press. 1974.
5. Cooper, I. S., Amin, I., Riklan, M., Waltz, J. M., Poon, T. P., Chronic cerebellar stimulation in epilepsy. Arch. Neurol. *33* (1976), 559—570.
6. Cooper, I. S., Riklan, M., Amin, I., Waltz, J., Cullinan, J., Chronic cerebellar stimulation in cerebral palsy. Neurology *26* (1976), 744—753.
7. Davis, R. M., Cullen, R. F., Flitter, M. A., Duenas, D., Engle, M., Ennis, B., Control of spasticity and involuntary movements. Neurosurgery *1, 2* (1977), 205—206.
8. Gilman, S., Dauth, G. W., Tennyson, V. M., Kremzner, L. T., Chronic cerebellar stimulation in the monkey. Preliminary observations. Arch. Neurol. *32* (1975), 474—477.
9. Larson, S. J., Sances, A., Hemmy, D. C., Millar, E. A., Physiological and histological effects of chronic cerebellar stimulation. Neurosurgery *1, 2* (1977), 212—213.
10. Manrique, M., Oya, S., Vaquero, J., Lozano, A. P., Herrero, J., Bravo, G., Chronic paleocerebellar stimulation for the treatment of neuromuscular disorders. Four cases report. Appl. Neurophysiol. *41* (1978), 237—247.
11. Manrique, M., Lozano, A. P., Vaquero, J., Oya, S., Bravo, G., Estimulacion electrica cronica del cerebelo (estudio clinico y experimental). Progressi in Epilettologia. Lega contro l'epilessia. Boll. No. 22—23 (1978), 281—284.
12. Penn, R. D., Etzel, M. L., Chronic cerebellar stimulation and developmental reflexes. J. Neurosurg. *46* (1977), 506—511.
13. Vaernet, K., Chronic cerebellar stimulation in spastic choreo-athetosis. Acta Neurochir. (Wien) Suppl. 24 (1977), 59—63.
14. Vaquero, J., Lozano, A. P., Oya, S., Manrique, M., Bravo, G., Chronic implanting of electrodes in the cerebellar vermis of the cat. Morfological findings. Acta Neurochir. (Wien) *46* (1979), 259—266.

Acta Neurochirurgica, Suppl. 30, 339—344 (1980)

Correlation of Clinical and Physiological Effects of Cerebellar Stimulation

I. S. Cooper*, A. R. M. Upton, Z. H. Rappaport, and **I. Amin**

With 1 Figure

Summary

The value of clinical assessment in patients undergoing chronic cerebellar stimulation (CCS) is limited by lack of objective measures but neurophysiological tests can be used to "biocalibrate" the stimulator and may be used to predict effects of CCS. Eighty-seven patients undergoing CCS have been assessed clinically and neurophysiologically over the last 4 years. Somatosensory evoked responses were significantly ($p < 0.05$) reduced in amplitude in 35 patients, cortical somatosensory evoked responses in 44 patients and one or both responses were reduced in 55 patients. There were no clinical or physiological changes in 16 patients. Evoked responses showed significant changes in only 3 patients who did not show clinical improvement. The mean voltage settings were 5.2 volts and most patients were stimulated at 200 herz. These results indicate that significant changes in those somatosensory evoked potentials are a good indication of clinical benefits from CCS but clinical improvement may occur in the absence of any acute effect on evoked responses.

Keywords: Cerebellar stimulation; somatosensory evoked potentials.

Based on animal studies showing that low rates (10 cycles per second) stimulation of the cerebellar cortex could inhibit seizures [3] and that higher rates of stimulation (100–200 cycles per second) would reduce spasticity [12, 14] chronic cerebellar stimulation (CCS) in humans was introduced by Cooper in 1973 [4, 5]. The precise mechanism of the action of cerebellar stimulation has not as yet been fully understood. It is likely that CCS acts on brain stem structures with activation of the reticular formation and inhibition of the thalamus inducing upstream inhibition of cerebral cortex and downstream inhibition of spinal cord reflexes [2, 8]. The clinical efficacy of CCS has also been somewhat difficult to assess due to the lack of properly

* Center for Physiologic Neurosurgery, Westchester County Medical Center, Valhalla, New York, U.S.A.

0065-1419/80/Suppl. 30/0339/$ 01.20

controlled studies [5, 9]. This is especially true when trying to estimate clinical benefits in patients with cerebral palsy where observers may disagree in the same patient [13]. We are presently setting up a movement analysis laboratory in order to provide some objective quantification of improvement in spastic disorders [11]. In order to establish effective parameters of stimulation for individual patients we have evaluated them neurophysiologically and correlated the neurophysiological changes with the clinical results of CCS.

Material and Methods

Eighty-seven patients were seen over the past 4 years, the majority of which had cerebral palsy, underwent recordings of somatosensory evoked responses. Sixty-four potentials produced by median nerve stimulation were averaged with a Nicolet CA 1000 recorder for cortical evoked responses. There was a 10 millisecond delay in responses which were recorded over the following 190 milliseconds. An artifact rejection device was used. Two average responses were superimposed before CCS and after at least 1 minute of CCS at varying voltages. The responses of the right and left cerebral cortexes were recorded simultaneously. Subcortical somatosensory evoked responses (SCSSEP) were recorded for 25 milliseconds after electrical stimulation of median nerve. Recording electrodes were surface silver chloride buttons over the vertex (C_z) and contralateral supraclavicular region with a ground electrode over the supraclavicular region on the side of stimulation. All electrode impedances were adjusted to less than 3 kiloohms. An average of 2,000 potentials were used in conjunction with artifact rejection. SCSSEPs were compared before and after CCS and all results were plotted on a Hewlett Packard X-Y recorder, Type 9862 A.

The implanted cerebellar stimulators consisted of 8 platinum disc electrodes imbedded in a siliconized mesh. The electrode array measured 32 mm^2 and each array was implanted beneath the tentorium over both anterior and posterior lobes bilaterally. Stimulation was carried out in a crossed fashion, alternating the two sides every one minute. Clinical assessment in epileptics was based on reduction in seizure frequency or in an improvement on EEG. Clinical assessment in patients with cerebral palsy was based on a composite of evaluations from psychologists, physical therapists, physicians, parents and the patient, him or herself.

Quantitative gait analysis was attempted in a preliminary fashion only [11].

Results

The 87 patients consisted of 33 females and 54 males. Mean age was 25 ± 9 years. Sixty-nine patients suffered from cerebral palsy and 18 patients had a variety of epileptic disorders. Two pairs of SCSSEP were assessed by t-test ($P < 0.05$) for changes before and after CCS. SCSSEPs were significantly reduced in amplitude in 35 patients, CSSEPs in 44 patients and one or both responses were reduced in 55 patients (Table 1). There were no clinical or physiological change in 16 patients. Evoked responses showed signif-

Table 1

CCS	No.	Age (years)	Diag-nosis	SCSSEP	CSSEP	SCSSEP +CSSEP	No clinical (+) and EVP (0)	Clinical (0) and EVP (+)
200 Hz 5.2 ± 3.5 V	87	25 ± 9 33 F, 54 M	CP 69 EP 18	↓ 35	↓ 44	↓ 55	16	3

Key: *CCS* Chronic stimulation at mean voltage necessary to produce maximal inhibition, *CP* cerebral palsy, *EP* epilepsy, *SCSSEP + CSSEP* subcortical and cortical somatosensory evoked potentials, (+) = presence of clinical improvement or evoked potential inhibition.

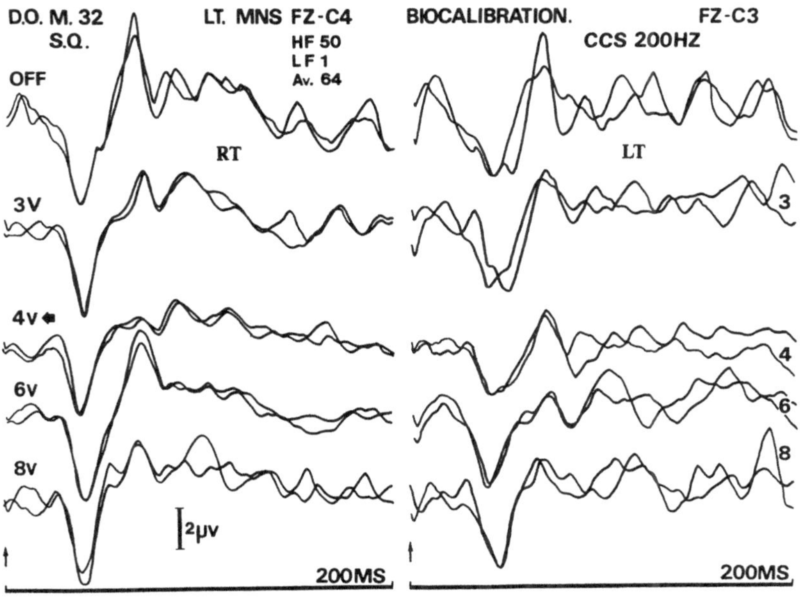

Fig. 1. Cortical somatosensory evoked potential responses following left median nerve stimulation (average of 64 stimulations) in a 32-year-old man with spastic quadriparesis. The top tracing shows the precerebellar stimulation evoked response, the second to fifth tracings showing the effect of increasing cerebellar stimulation (200 Hz, 3–8 "volts" as per stimulator dial). F_2–C_4 is the recording system over the right hemisphere, F_2–C_3 over the left hemisphere. Maximal inhibition of the evoked response is achieved at 4 V. Note the tendency for rebound of the evoked response at higher settings

icant changes in only 3 patients who did not show clinical improvement but 13 patients showed clinical effects of CCS without significant effects on evoked responses. In 16 patients a clinical response was evident although no physiologic changes could be demonstrated. The mean voltage settings to achieve suppression in somatosensory evoked potentials were 5.2 ± 3.5 volts (Fig. 1).

Discussion

In previous reports we have shown that cerebellar stimulation reduces the amplitude of H-reflexes, blink reflexes and V_1 and V_2 responses to supramaximal stimulation of a peripheral nerve [15]. This effect is predominantly ipsilateral. Auditory brain stem evoked potentials sometimes show an elevation of waves 4 and 5 (upper pons and midbrain) with depression of the late waves which are correlated with thalamic potentials. This parallels the predominantly contralateral reduction in potential at approximately 15 milliseconds seen in the SCSSEP [7].

Cryothalamotomy patients display a similar reduction in the SCSSEP between 15 and 19 milliseconds illustrating the overlap between clinical effects of cryothalamotomy and CCS which may to a limited extent be producing a "functional thalamotomy" [16].

Deep brain recordings tend to confirm that the wave at 15–18 milliseconds is related to the thalamus [10] and we have seen reduction in amplitude of the potential evoked by deep electrodes in VL during CCS [16]. This predominantly inhibitory effect of CCS on the neurophysiological responses may show its potential as a general therapy for diseases of disinhibition [8]. It provides a rationale for selecting those parameters of CCS that will produce inhibition of evoked responses and, judging from the clinical correlation, biocalibration does appear to have some predictive value. The paradoxical increase in the somatosensory evoked potentials that occurs with higher voltage settings correlates with a deterimental clinical effect at these settings. This could account for differences when comparing uncontrolled clinical series of CCS, particularly when voltage of CCS are adjusted to produce headache [17].

The major challenge in the evaluation of chronic cerebellar stimulatory work still remains in arriving at control trials with appropriate quantification. Implantable, rechargeable, programmable electrodes are at the animal testing phase and should prevent nonmedical manipulation of the stimulator; increase patient acceptance, and allow assessment of electrode impedance or stimulating charge at any time after implantation. Double blind studies will be possible and quantitative analysis of movement will provide objective measurement of clinical effects. Implantable units which are not programmable, are not presently ready for clinical application. Although our clinical and physiologic studies have been confirmed by Penn [13], Davis [9] and others, we cannot confirm the statistics of clinical improvement nor the implications for cerebellar stimulation reported by Davis. We have consistently reported that selection of patients is exceedingly important and that clinical improvement, although useful, is modest. This procedure is considered by us to be a first step, not a definitive treatment.

The concept of biocalibration can be applied to patients undergoing deep brain stimulation for movement disorders with electrodes implanted in the parathalmic internal capsule [1]. On SCSSEP recordings the thalamic potential depressed at settings ranging from 4 to 8 "volts" (50 Hz) and elevated again beyond that. One patient with pontocerebellar degeneration and dysarthria showed remarkable improvement in strength, clarity and tone of speech during right thalami (VL) stimulation at 6 "volts", while at 8 "volts" he deteriorated again and experienced paraesthesae in the left hand and face. The beneficial clinical effect could be reachieved by lowering the stimulation to 6 "volts".

It thus appears that the monitoring of neurophysiologic parameters can play an important role in understanding the mechanism and optimizing the function of neuroaugmentative devices.

References

1. Adams, J. E., Hosobuchi, Y., Session on deep brain stimulation: Techniques and technical problems. Neurosurgery *1* (1977), 196—199.
2. Bantli, H., Bloedel, J. R., Tolbert, D., Activation of neurons in the cerebellar nuclei and ascending reticular formation by stimulation of the cerebellar surface. J. Neurosurg. *45* (1976), 539—554.
3. Cooper, I. S., Snider, R. S., The effect of varying the frequency of cerebellar stimulation upon epilepsy. In: The cerebellum, epilepsy and behavior, pp. 245—256 (Cooper, I. S., *et al.*, eds.). New York: Plenum Press. 1974.
4. Cooper, I. S., Riklan, M., Amin, I., Waltz, J. M., Cullinan, T., Chronic cerebellar stimulation in cerebral palsy. Neurology (Minn.) *26* (1976), 744—753.
5. Cooper, I. S., Amin, I., Riklan, M., Waltz, J. M., Poon, T. P., Chronic cerebellar stimulation in epilepsy. Arch. Neurol. (Chic.) *33* (1976), 559—570.
6. Cooper, I. S., Amin, I., Upton, A. R. M., Riklan, M., Watkins, E. S., McLellan, L., Safety and efficacy of chronic stimulation. Neurosurgery *1* (1977), 203—205.
7. Cooper, I. S., Upton, A. R. M., Effects of cerebellar stimulation on epilepsy, the EEG, and cerebral palsy in man. In: Contemporary Clinical Neurophysiology (EEG suppl. 34), pp. 349—353 (Cobb, W. A., Van Duijn, H., eds.). Amsterdam: Elsevier. 1978.

8. Cooper, I. S., Upton, A. R. M., Use of chronic cerebellar stimulation for disorders of disinhibition. Lancet (1978), 595—600.
9. Davis, R. M., Cullen, R. F., Jr., Flitter, M. A., Duenos, D., Engle, H., Ennis, B., Control of spasticity and involuntary movements. Neurosurgery *1* (1977), 205—207.
10. Ervin, F., Mark, V., Studies of the human thalamus: IV. Evoked responses. Ann. N.Y. Acad. Sci. *112* (1964), 81—92.
11. Milner, M., Hershler, C., de Bruin, H., Baker, R. S., Upton, A. R. M., Cooper, I. S., Preliminary investigation of influence of cerebellar stimulation on gait by analyzing angle-angle diagrams. In: Cerebellar stimulation in man, pp. 123—144 (Cooper, I. S., ed.). New York: Raven Press. 1978.
12. Moruzzi, G., Problems in cerebellar physiology. Springfield, Ill.: Ch. C Thomas. 1950.
13. Penn, R., Gottlieb, G. L., Agarwal, G. C., Cerebellar stimulation in men. Quantitative changes in spasticity. J. Neurosurg. *48* (1978), 779—786.
14. Sherrington, C. S., Double (antidromic) conduction in the central nervous system. Proc. Roy. Soc. (London) *61* (1897), 243—246.
15. Upton, A. R. M., Cooper, I. S., Some neurophysiological effects of cerebellar stimulation in man. Canad. J. Neurol. Sci. *3* (1976), 237—254.
16. Upton, A. R. M., Rappaport, Z. H., Amin, I., Cooper, I. S., Evoked potential recordings following thalamectomy. 1979. Submitted for publication.
17. Van Buren, J. M., Wood, J. H., Oakley, J., Hambrecht, F., Preliminary evaluation of cerebellar stimulation by double-blind stimulation and biological criteria in the treatment of epilepsy. J. Neurosurg. *48* (1978), 407—416.

Acta Neurochirurgica, Suppl. 30, 345—349 (1980)

Stereotactic Approach to Therapeutic Stimulation of Cerebellum for Spasticity

M. Galanda*, P. Nádvorník, and **S. Fodor**

With 4 Figures

Summary

A Stereotactic approach for transtentorial implantation of deep wire electrodes directly into the anterior lobe of cerebellum has been shown as a beneficial method for the treatment of cerebral palsy in 9 patients. Proper placement of the electrodes especially into the central lobule were checked by evoked potentials and by choosing an optimal program of therapeutic stimulation which appears to be essential. With its favourable effect particularly on axial musculature stimulation seems to promote physiologic maturation of functional mechanisms in the brain, which were delayed in the course of development.

Keywords: Stereotaxy; cerebellar stimulation; cerebral palsy; evoked potentials.

Chronic cerebellar stimulation is achieved by electrodes placed on the surface of the cerebellum via a classical infratentorial craniotomy. In our stereotactic laboratory we have used a stereotactic approach for therapeutic stimulation of children with cerebral palsy. According to anatomical studies (Noback 1975) 85% of the cerebellar cortex faces the sulcal surfaces deep between the cerebellar folia. Because of this wire electrodes were directly implanted into the anterior lobe of cerebellum—into the central lobule and the anterior quadrangular lobule respectively—through a unilateral transtentorial approach.

Selection of Targets and Stimulating Program

Burr hole was located over the nondominant hemisphere close to the lambdoid suture. Initially four or three electrodes (Fig. 1) were implanted, but after more experience, only two electrodes each with

* Research Laboratory of Clinical Stereotaxy VUHB and Neurosurgical Department, Comenius University, Limbova cesta, Bratislava, Kramáre, Czechoslovakia.

0065-1419/80/Suppl. 30/0345/$ 01.00

three contacts were implanted. One was placed in the midline and the other into the paravermal region 15 mm laterally. After PEG examination in the lateral projection, targets points were chosen 1/4 respectively and 1/8 from the fastigium on the line between the fastigium and the posterior commissure. This line also represented safety border to avoid introducing electrodes into brain stem.

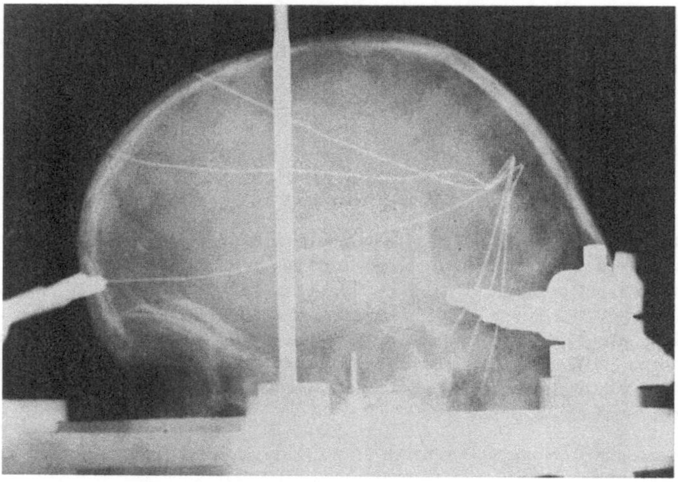

Fig. 1. X-ray control of electrode position implanted transtentorially into the cerebellum; lateral view

About the fourth day after implanting the electrodes, when the patient was in good condition, parameters for the stimulating program were chosen. At first currents of low rates were applied to eliminate responses from brain stem structures. For therapeutic bipolar stimulation the rate was set at 100–200 alternating pulses per second applied between the electrodes. The pulse width was 1 millisecond, optimal intensity of stimulating current was selected according to tonic muscle response (usually 1–1.3 mA). Parameters were considered suitable if stimulation suddenly increased muscle tonus, resembling the natural pattern of movement disorder of the patient, which was immediately replaced by distinct successive reduction in spasticity, reported by the patient as similar to gradual relaxation. This response was usually increased for approximately 7 minutes and if in that time the rate of stimulation was slightly changed, the whole effect was repeated, but shortened. Because of this we decided to use 10 minutes stimulating sessions. Stimulation was repeated 2–3 times daily. We applied stimulation together with physical therapy to use the decreased spasticity and try to set neuro-

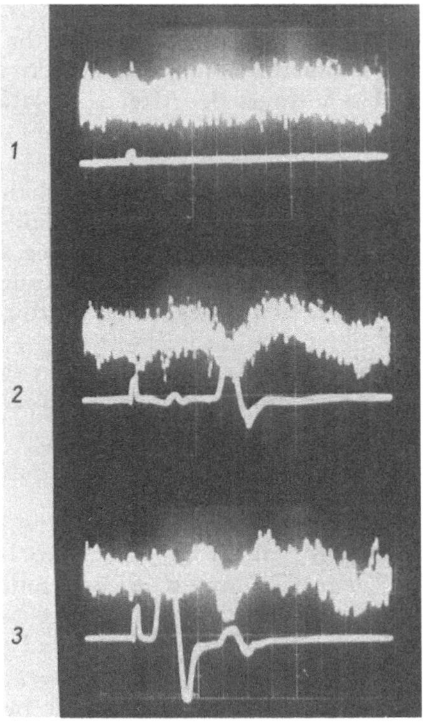

Fig. 2. Superimposed recordings from the central lobule of cerebellum (upper traces) and from soleus muscle (lower traces). DISA *1* The records of subthreshold stimulus applied to the tibial nerve. Small deflection on the lower traces indicates the stimulus artifact. *2* A submaximal stimulus applied to the tibial nerve. Elicitation of H wave in the muscle of lower extremity simultaneously accompanied by evoked potential in the central lobule of cerebellum. *3* The response to supramaximal stimulation to the tibial nerve

physiological conditioning between the relaxation of muscles induced by stimulation and rehabilitation.

As well as this physiological control of the selection of targets, we used recording of evoked potentials from stimulation of the tibial nerve (Fig. 2). Simultaneously with the stimulation of the tibial nerve we recorded the EMG from soleus muscle and SEEG from the cerebellum. The criteria for the proper position of electrode in the regulating system for muscle tonus in the cerebellum was the eliciting of M and H reflexes in competent muscle together with evoked responses in SEEG recorded from selected cerebellar structures.

The electrodes were left free outside the scalp. This externalized stimulation allowed us to check SEEG recordings from the cerebellum during therapeutic stimulation. In SEEG from the central lobule we sometimes recorded modulated, high voltage activity, during movement of the limb desynchronized. After stimulation of the central lobule this activity was reinforced with prompt recurrence after disruption by movement.

Recorded activities from central lobule and the dentate nucleus can be modified by i.v. application of ethylalcohol. After administration of ethylalcohol we observed the appearance of groups of symmetrical waves of high frequency in the dentate nucleus and the same time regulation of muscle action was deteriorating. Activity in the central lobule was desynchronized. Following stimulation of the central lobule activity in the dentate nucleus was changed (desynchronized) but the regulation of muscle action was improved.

Application of Method and Results

By this type of stimulation we treated without complication nine patients with cerebral palsy at the age from 4 to 18 years, clinically with rigidospasticity involving usually all extremities, but sometimes with prevalency on lower extremities. Dyskinesias were present in about half of these patients. Three of them had previously undergone destructive stereotactic surgery before therapeutic stimulation of the cerebellum. One are occasion bilateral pulvinarotomy was performed and two patients underwent thalamotomy in the region of VIM-VCP nuclei. The average application of therapeutic stimulation varied between one to two months. During that time it was possible to notice evident reduction of spasticity, associated with distinct improvement during stimulation followed again with slight return of spasticity, although in general, the effect was progressive. Dyskinesias showed improvement only after a longer period of time. Patients become more relaxed and their interest of surrounding was enhanced.

During the period of reduction of spasticity and dyskinesias, stability of the axial muscles increased. Patients could better sit or stand more safely walk and keep the head up (Figs. 3 and 4). The results of stimulation persisted after completing the program and were supported by physical therapy. From this point of view especially, the influence on the axial musculature seems to promote physiologic maturation of functional mechanisms in the brain, which were delayed in the course of development. Patients have been followed up to two years.

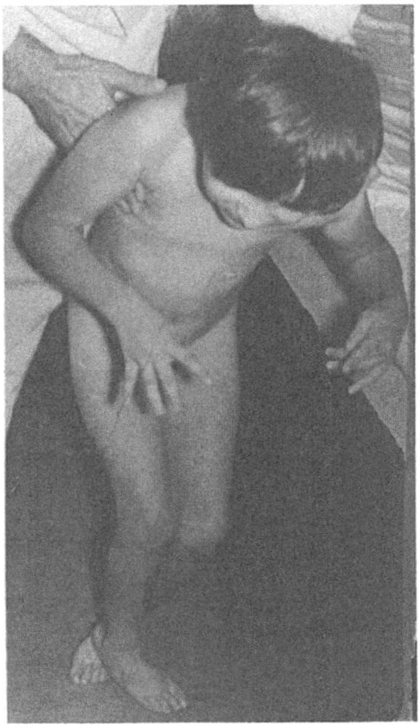

Fig. 3

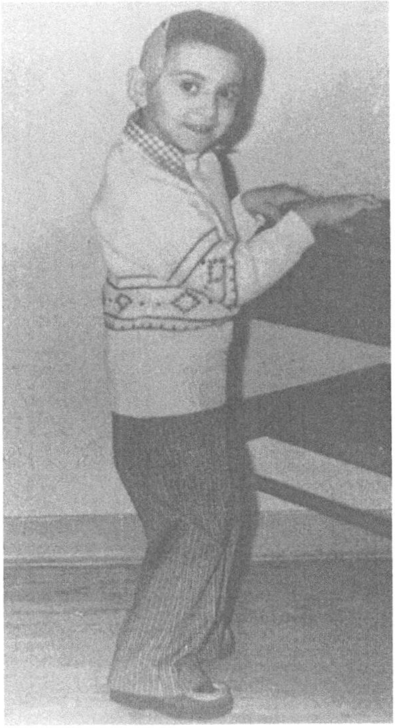

Fig. 4

Fig. 3. Complete inability to stand before stimulation

Fig. 4. Marked reduction of spasticity and increasing of stability of axial musculature permit ambulation with support 2 months after operation

References

Cooper, I. S., Crighel, E., Amin, I., Clinical and physiological effects of stimulation of the paleocerebellum in humans. J. Amer. Geriatr. Soc. *21* (1973), 40—43.

Galanda, M., Fodor, S., Nádvorník, P., Paleocerebelárna stimulácia v liečbe detskej mozgovej obrny. Bratisl. lek. Listy *70*, 1 (1978), 99—105.

Noback, Ch. R., Demarest, R. J., The Human Nervous System, 2nd ed., pp. 289—304. New York: McGraw—Hill Book Comp. 1975.

Penn, R. D., Etzel, M. L., Chronic cerebellar stimulation and developmental reflexes. J. Neurosurg. *46* (1977), 506—511.

Acta Neurochirurgica, Suppl. 30, 351—359 (1980)

Chronic Self-Stimulation of the Dentate Nucleus for the Relief of Spasticity

J. R. Schvarcz*, R. E. Sica, and **E. Morita**

With 4 Figures

Summary

It has been assumed but not yet proved that cerebellar cortical stimulation activates the Purkinje cells, with subsequent inhibition of the deep cerebellar nuclei. However, the relatively crude, widespread excitation induced by several surface electrode arrays and the parameters of stimulation currently used, may produce other effects than selective activation of only one specific cellular type which, furthermore, seems to be rarely present in these particular patients, as demonstrated by biopsy studies prior to electrode placement.

The dentate nucleus was chronically implanted with a stimulating system in a patient with spasticity due to cerebral palsy. Chronic self-stimulation induced a significant improvement in motor function, with relief of spasticity and improvement in speech, posture, balance and gait. Electrophysiological studies demonstrated a decrease in the amplitude of V_1 and V_2 responses and in the H/M and T/M ratios, an increase in the silent period, and marked effects in the H reflex recovery curve, as well as diminished contralateral cortical somato-sensory evoked potentials. This result seems to indicate that the clinical effects of cerebellar cortical stimulation are not due to prosthetically induced inhibition of the dentate nucleus.

Keywords: Cerebellar stimulation; dentate nucleus; spasticity; cerebral palsy; stereotaxis.

In 1972, Copper[8, 9] introduced chronic stimulation of the cerebellar cortex for the relief of spasticity, thereby presumably activating the Purkinje cells and inhibiting the deep cerebellar nuclei. Nevertheless, the effectiveness and safety of cerebellar cortical stimulation are still questionable, and its rationale has not yet been fully proved.

---

* Institute of Neurosurgery, School of Medicine, University of Buenos Aires, Beruti 2926, Buenos Aires 1425, Argentina.

0065-1419/80/Suppl. 30/0351/$ 01.80

Indeed, when the several surface electrode arrays currently implanted as well as the parameters of stimulation clinically used are considered, other more likely phenomena than the assumed selective activation of Purkinje cells may occur, such as antidromic and/or synaptic and/or transsynaptic activation of neurons of the dentate nucleus and of the reticular formation. Furthermore, the preexisting loss of Purkinje cells usually demonstrated in biopsy material should also be accounted for.

These possibilities as well as certain responses induced by acute stimulation during dentatotomy, led one of us to implant, in November 1978, the first deep chronic self-stimulation system in the dentate nucleus of a patient with cerebral palsy.

Material and Methods

A 25-year-old patient with cerebral palsy, whose main symptom was unilateral disabling spasticity, was chronically implanted in the ipsilateral dentate nucleus. He has a high IQ, and was highly motivated to surgery. There was a definite history of perinatal hypoxia. A severe spasticity, which interfered with voluntary movements, affected predominantly the right upper extremity. He was unable to voluntarily flex the arm or to open that hand. When attempting to do so, he developed a spasmodic contralateral deviation of the head. The right lower extremity was moderately affected, and he could walk with only mild impairment. He also had a marked dysarthria. His left hand had slight athetoid features as well as difficulties in relaxation.

The patient was operated on under slight sedation, in the sitting position, with the head flexed within a modified Hitchcock apparatus, which was rigidly fixed to the operating table. The ventricular system was then outlined by water soluble positive contrast, and a Schriver type multipolar platinum electrode array (Medtronic®) was stereotactically implanted in the ipsilateral dentate nucleus through a directionally drilled burr hole. The electrode tip was aimed at the fastigium of the fourth ventricle in the coronal and horizontal planes, 6 mm lateral to the mid-sagittal plane, along a trajectory that followed the main axis of the nucleus (Fig. 1 a–b). It is thereby placed in such a way that, according to Afshar, Watkins and Yap's [1] variability data, each central contact has 100% probabilities to be located within the dentate nucleus.

Since acute stimulation produced a noticeable improvement, the electrode was externalized for a period of trial stimulation. After 10 weeks of percutaneous testing, during which different electrode combinations and parameters of stimulation were first clinically and then electrophysiologically evaluated, the system was permanently implanted. Under general anaesthesia, the percutaneous extension was removed, and the chronic electrode was connected to a receiver subcutaneously placed in the infraclavicular region, where it is transdermally activated by an inductively coupled radiofrequency transmitter.

Pre- and post-operative neurological, psychiatric, physiatric and speech assessments were independently made. Psychological testing was performed before and repeated serially after surgery, both with and without ongoing stimulation. Neurophysiological studies were sequentially performed (*cf.* 19, 20, 23). Although data germane to the selection of electrodes and parameters of stimulation are discussed, they will be fully reported elsewhere.

Results

Chronic stimulation of the dentate nucleus, typically with capacitatively coupled waves, 100 Hz, 0.25 milliseconds duration pulses, 2 V, produced first a marked improvement in speech quality and then, a significant relief of spasticity, allowing voluntary movements that were not performed before or without stimulation. At the

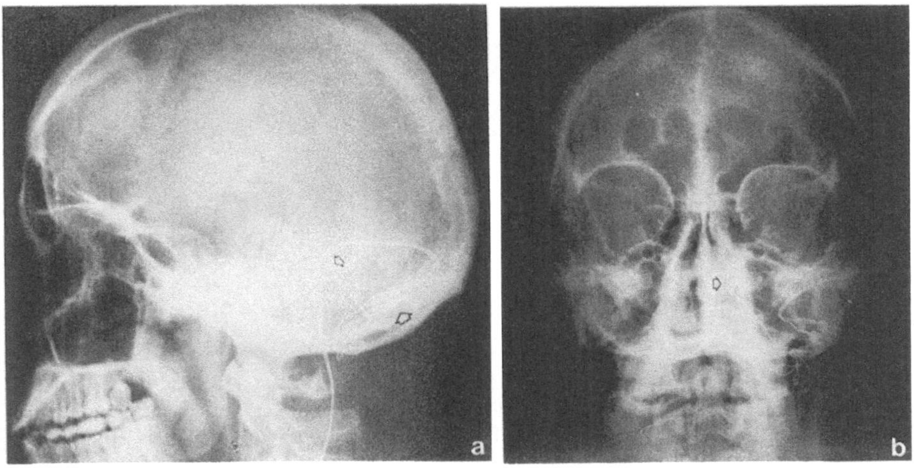

Figs. 1 a and b. Lateral and anteroposterior radiographs demonstrating the implanted system (small arrow: indwelling electrode; large arrow: extracranial connector)

same time, both he and his family reported a definite improvement in his contralateral hand, mainly as regards relaxation, which was difficult to evaluate.

There was, however, a clear cumulative result, with a progressively longer post-effect. The contralateral deviation of the head induced by right upper limb movement disappeared. A significant improvement in both posture and balance was produced, and ambulation became practically normal. His spasticity has diminished, and he can now perform complex voluntary movements, such as those associated with feeding and dressing, and more recently, with handwriting. His speech has also remarkably improved. There was no definite differential effect as regards upper or lower extremity with

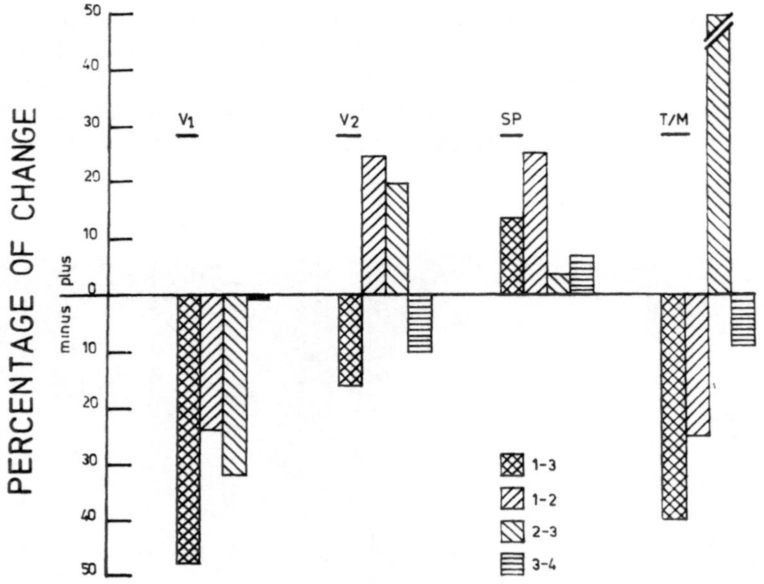

Fig. 2. Mean changes in the V_1 and V_2 responses, the silent period (*SP*) and the T/M ratio induced by stimulation of the dentate nucleus with different electrode couplings. Results are expressed as percentage of change of the prestimulation value/M ratio but for SP, which is expressed as percentage of its own previous value. Measurements are after 2 hours of stimulation. Each value is the average of 40 consecutive V_1 and V_2 waves and 20 consecutive SP and T/M readings, but each set of results represents the mean of two such experiments

different electrode combinations. Placebo sham stimulation consistently failed to induce clinical changes.

Clinical improvement was produced by coupling either electrodes 1–2, 2–3 or 1–3, but the latter seemed to be the best combination. They also produced the maximal reduction in the amplitude of the V_1 and V_2 responses and in the H/M and T/M ratios, and a submaximum increase in the electrically induced silent period (Fig. 2), as well as the most striking changes in the recovery curve of the H reflex conditioned by a preceding stimulus (Fig. 3). They were obtained after 2 hours of stimulation, when the patient's curve was within one standard deviation of the mean value of the control group.

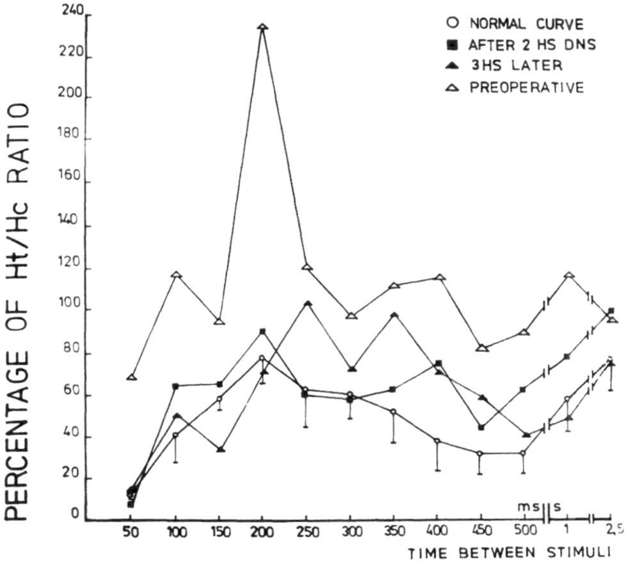

Fig. 3. Sequential changes in the H reflex recovery curve induced by stimulation of the dentate nucleus with electrodes 1–3. Results are expressed as percentage of the Hc/Ht ratio. Hc is the response elicited by the conditioning stimulus/M ratio and Ht is the response elicited by the test stimulus/M ratio. ○ Normal control-group curve. Standard deviation is indicated by vertical bars, though only towards one side; ■ immediately after 2 hours of stimulation; ▲ without further stimulation, 3 hours later. Recovery curves at 6, 12, 24, and 36 hours are ommited, but the latter closely resembled the □ pre-operative curve

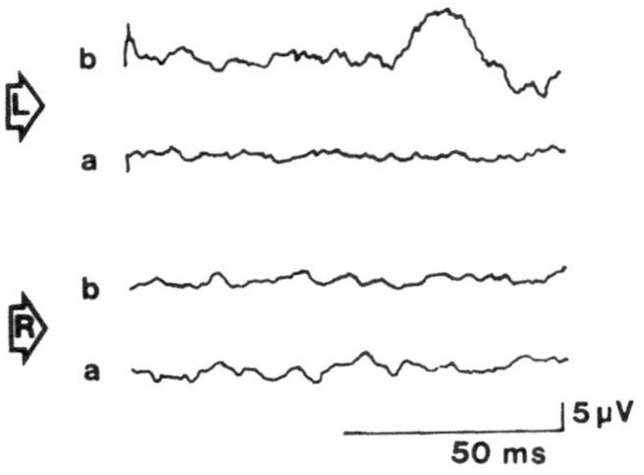

Fig. 4. Changes in cortical somato-sensory evoked potentials induced by stimulation of the dentate nucleus. Each trace represents 200 averaged potentials evoked by 2 Hz stimulation of the right median nerve and recorded from the C 2–C 3 positions of the International 10–20 system, with Fz reference. *b* Before; *a* after dentate nucleus stimulation

It then remained more or less unchanged beyond the actual stimulation, up to about 3 hours. Thereafter, the post-effect began to gradually fade off, until 36 hours later, the recovery curve was quite similar to the preoperative one. On this basis, the present regime of 2 hours on/3 hours off, was scheduled.

Also a lasting, significant depression in both the early and late components of the contralateral cortical somatosensory evoked potentials was induced by stimulation (Fig. 4).

Psychological testing after chronic stimulation showed an improved psychological status. Higher intellectual performances were improved. Alertness and concentration abilities were increased, and the verbal output was significantly enhanced. Also affective control became more adequate, and anxiety and tension were diminished.

Discussion

Cooper [8, 9] introduced chronic cerebellar cortical stimulation for the treatment of spasticity, via surface silicone-mesh electrode plates bearing 8 platinum-iridium contacts, each array having a 45 mm^2 stimulating surface [10]. Bilateral placement over the cortex of both the anterior and posterior cerebellum is currently considered the combination of choice, and passage of current across the superior and inferior cerebellar surface is recommended [10, 15, 18]. The rationale of the procedure is the activation of Purkinje cells, with subsequent inhibition of the deep cerebellar nuclei.

This has led to several investigations on the possibility of cortical damage induced by stimulation. Severe cerebellar lesions in monkeys have been reported [12, 21], but others doubted the suitability of the monkey for these experiments and concluded that lesions were more likely to be caused by mechanical injury than by the application of current [14]. Also pressure-related destruction subjacent to the electrodes has been reported in autopsy cases [24].

However, Ulrich, Watkins, Amin *et al.* [24] have demonstrated diffuse, widespread cerebellar lesions, in biopsy material obtained prior to electrode placement from 30 patients undergoing cerebellar implant, 18 of whom had motor disorders. A severe loss of Purkinje cells, ranging from 50 to 100%, was observed in 83.3% of the patients with motor disturbances (*i.e.*, between 50 and 75% in 53.3% and between 90 and 100% in 46.6% of the specimens). Similarly, 100% of the cases with epilepsy showed identical abnormalities. Although highly selected, this group is representative in every aspect of the patients undergoing cerebellar cortical stimulation. Hence, considering the already present significant cortical damage, further discussion re injuries induced by electrical stimulation seems to be rather irrelevant.

Nevertheless, the consistently demonstrated Purkinje cell devastation may preclude, or at least minimize, their prosthetically induced activation. Indeed, even in a normal cortex, the relatively crude, widespread excitation elicited by several multicontact surface electrode arrays may activate any number of neural elements of the cortical complex rather than only one specific cellular type. Other alternative mechanisms may therefore be considered.

Bantli, Bloedel and Tolbert [4] have demonstrated that cerebellar cortical stimulation can antidromically activate cerebellar afferent fibers, can synaptically activate neurons in the dentate nucleus, and can transsynaptically activate neurons in the reticular formation. The antidromic activation of cerebellar afferents was demonstrated by single cell recording at their site of origin, *i.e.*, at the inferior olivary nucleus for climbing fibers and at the medial reticular formation for mossy fibers [5, 11]. Since most of the cerebellar afferents give off collaterals to the cerebellar nuclei [5], their antidromic excitation by cortical stimulation resulted in synaptic activation of neurons in the dentate nucleus. The antidromic activation of cerebellar nucleocortical pathways activated neurons in the dentate nucleus too, but as they are often collaterals of efferent fibers, it can also excite dentatofugal pathways orthodromically. Neurons in the reticular formation were synaptically activated by collaterals of antidromically activated cerebellar afferent fibers [5], but also transsynaptically by projections from the dentate nucleus, probably mediated by the descending branch of the brachium conjuntivum [6, 17]. Caudally projecting reticulo-spinal pathways [3] as well as rostrally projecting reticulo-mesencephalo-thalamic fibres [4] were activated from the dentate nucleus. It also projects directly onto the intralaminar nuclei, centromedianum, parafascicularis, zona incerta and ventralis anterioris [6, 13], in addition to the classic, mainly facilitatory projection onto the ventralis lateralis [2, 16]. Many different complex though conceivably inter-related feedback circuits may then be simultaneously activated.

Chronic stimulation of the dentate nucleus with the electrodes located as to presumably produce the larger activation of dentatofugal fibres induced a significant improvement in motor function. An immediate but cumulative relief of spasticity was obtained, thereby enabling voluntary movements which were not performed prior to stimulation. They included certain complex skillful acts related to daily activities or, *e.g.*, handwriting. Posture, balance and gait were improved, and the quality of speech was markedly enhanced. Sequential studies consistently demonstrated a decrease in the amplitude of the V_1 and V_2 responses and in the H/M and T/M ratios, an increase in the electrically induced silent period, and significant changes in the H reflex recovery curve.

Although electrophysiological changes do not necessarily reflect the degree of clinical improvement, they provided objective evidence of stimuli-related modifications in the excitability of spinal motoneurons. Furthermore, they strongly suggest a change in supraspinal mechanisms acting upon spinal motoneurons whereby both a decreased facilitation and an enhanced inhibition are involved. Thus, the effects on V_1 and V_2 responses and on the H reflex recovery curve conceivably indicate a decreased descending facilitation, and the effect on the silent period an increased descending inhibition, both acting onto alpha-motoneurons, whereas the reduced T/M ratio conceivably indicates a diminished facilitation acting onto gamma-motoneurons.

So far, this case seems to suggest that the clinical effects of cerebellar cortical stimulation are not due to prosthetically induced inhibition of the dentate nuclei. Contrariwise, it further implies that, in selected cases, chronic self-stimulation of the dentate nucleus, an elegant and presumably a more direct and precise way of activating the neoçortical outflow pathways, may be a rational approach to relieve spasticity and to improve motor function, warranting therefore further exploration.

References

1. Afshar, F., Watkins, E. S., Yap, J. C., Stereotactic atlas of the human brainstem and cerebellar nuclei. A variability study. New York: Raven Press. 1978.
2. Angaut, P., Bases anatomo-fonctionnelles des interrelations cérébello-cérébrales. J. Physiol. *67* (1973), 53—116.
3. Bantli, H., Bloedel, J. R., Monosynaptic activation of a direct reticulo-spinal pathway by the dentate nucleus. Pfluegers Arch. *357* (1975), 237—242.
4. Bantli, H., Bloedel, J. R., Tolbert, D., Activation of neurons in the cerebellar nuclei and ascending reticular formation by stimulation of the cerebellar surface. J. Neurosurg. *45* (1976), 539—554.
5. Bloedel, J. R., Cerebellar afferent systems: a review. In: Progress in Neurobiology, Vol. II, pp. 3—68 (Kerkut, G., Phillis, J. W., eds.). Oxford: Pergamon Press. 1973.
6. Carrea, R., Mettler, F. A., The anatomy of the primate brachium conjuntivum and associated structures. J. Comp. Neurol. *101* (1954), 565—689.
7. Carrea, R., Reissig, M., Mettler, F. A., The climbing fibers of the simian and feline cerebellum. Experimental inquiry into their origin by lesions of the inferior olives and deep cerebellar nuclei. J. Comp. Neurol. *87* (1947), 321—365.
8. Cooper, I. S., Effect of chronic stimulation of the anterior cerebellum on neurological disease. Lancet *1* (1973), 206.
9. Cooper, I. S., Effect of chronic stimulation of the posterior cerebellum on neurological disease. Lancet *1* (1973), 1321.

10. Cooper, I. S., Some technical considerations of cerebellar stimulation. In: Cerebellar Stimulation in Man, pp. 13—18 (Cooper, I. S., ed.). New York: Raven Press. 1978.
11. Eccles, J. C., Ito, M., Szentágothai, J., The Cerebellum as a Neuronal Machine. Berlin-Heidelberg-New York: Springer. 1967.
12. Gilman, S., Dauth, G. W., Tennyson, V. M., Kremzner, L. T., Chronic cerebellar stimulation in the monkey. Arch. Neurol. *32* (1975), 474—477.
13. Hassler, R., Hexapartition of inputs as a primary role of the thalamus. In: Corticothalamic Projections and Sensorimotor Activities, pp. 551—579 (Frigiesi, T., Rinvik, F., Yahr, M. D., eds.). New York: Raven Press. 1972.
14. Larson, S. J., Sances, A., Cusick, J. F., Myklebust, J., Millar, E. A., Boehmer, R., Hemmy, D. C., Ackmann, J. J., Swiontek, T. L., Cerebellar implant studies. IEEE Trans. Biomed. Eng. *23* (1976), 319—328.
15. Larson, S. J., Sances, A., Hemmy, D. C., Millar, E. A., Physiological and histological effects of cerebellar stimulation. Neurosurg. *1* (1977), 212—213.
16. Massion, J., Intervention des voies cérébellocorticales et corticocérébelleuses dans l'organisation et la régulation du mouvement. J. Physiol. *67* (1973), 117—170.
17. Pompeiano, O., Reticular Formation. In: Handbook of Sensory Physiology, Vol. II, pp. 381—488 (Iggo, A., ed.). New York: Springer. 1973.
18. Sances, A., Larson, S. J., Myklebust, J., Swiontek, T., Millar, E. A., Cusik, J. F., Hemmy, D. C., Jodat, R., Ackmann, J. J., Studies of electrode configuration. Neurosurg. *1* (1977), 207—212.
19. Sica, R. E., McComas, A. J., Upton, A. R., Impaired potentiation of H reflexes in patients with upper motoneuron lesions. J. Neurol. Neurosurg. Psychiat. *34* (1971), 712—717.
20. Sica, R. E., Sanz, O. P., Some speculations on the normal silent period evoked in the small muscles of the hand. Medicina *35* (1975), 483—497.
21. Tennyson, V. M., Kremzner, L. T., Dauth, G. W., Gilman, S., Chronic cerebellar stimulation in the monkey. Neurology *25* (1975), 650—654.
22. Tolbert, D., Bantli, H., Bloedel, J. R., Anatomical and physiological evidence for a cerebellar-nucleo-cortical projection in the cat. Neuroscience *1* (1976), 205—217.
23. Upton, A. R., McComas, A. J., Sica, R. E., Potentiation of late responses evoked in muscles during effort. J. Neurol. Neurosurg. Psychiat. *34* (1971), 699—711.
24. Urich, H., Watkins, E. S., Amin, I., Cooper, I. S., Neuropathologic observations on cerebellar cortical lesions in patients with epilepsy and motor disorders. In: Cerebellar Stimulation in Man, pp. 145—159 (Cooper, I. S., ed.). New York: Raven Press. 1978.

Section IV

Advances and New Techniques

Acta Neurochirurgica, Suppl. 30, 363—366 (1980)

Experimental Percutaneous Approach to the Trigeminal Ganglion in Dogs with Histopathological Evaluation of Radiofrequency Lesions

Y. Kanpolat* and **B. Onol****

With 3 Figures

Summary

A percutaneous approach via the foramen ovale to the trigeminal ganglion of dog was developed and used to produce radiofrequency lesions analogous to those made for the treatment of trigeminal neuralgia. Histological studies over 14 post-lesion days indicated that neural destruction is more extensive than previously concluded.

Keywords: Trigeminal ganglion; percutaneous approach; radiofrequency lesion; histopathological evaluation.

Introduction

The percutaneous approach to the human trigeminal ganglion via the foramen orale was first described by Harris[2]. A modification of that procedure is in wide clinical use to treat trigeminal neuralgia by radiofrequency (RF) lesion of the trigeminal ganglion[4, 5]. In the present study we developed a simple, non-traumatic analogue in dog of the human method and examined the histopathological changes that occurred up to 14 days after RF lesion of the trigeminal ganglion.

Methods and Material

Experiments were performed in 20 adult mongrel dogs (two others were discarded because of accidental puncture of the internal carotid artery). Two needle electrode systems (Radionics Inc.) were tested: cordotomy electrodes with 5 mm active tips and temperature-monitoring (TM) electrodes. The approach was made by inserting the needle just medial to the mandible and 3-to-4 cm rostral to the

* Department of Neurosurgery, Faculty of Medicine, University of Ankara, Ankara, Turkey.

** Department of Pathology, Faculty of Medicine, University of Hacettepe, Ankara, Turkey.

0065-1419/80/Suppl. 30/0363/$ 01.00

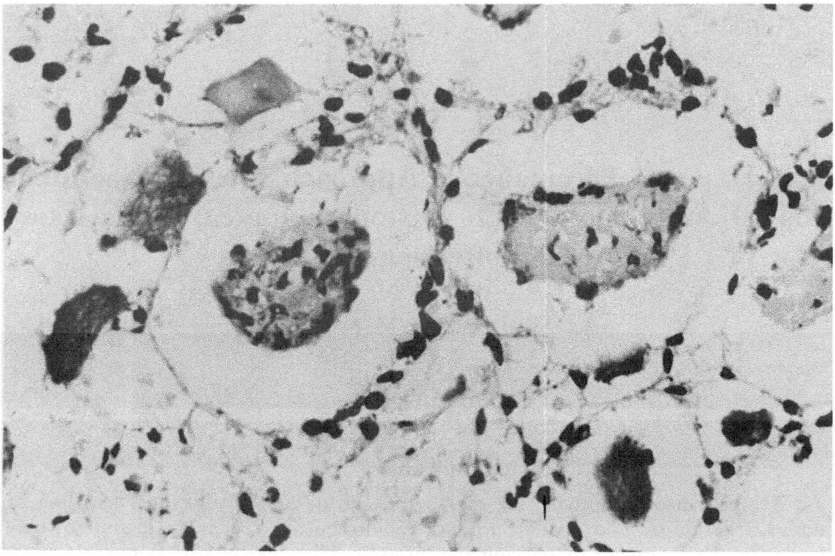

Fig. 1. 12 hours post-lesion: Mononuclear cells had infiltrated massively, including into ganglion-cell cytoplasm. ×480

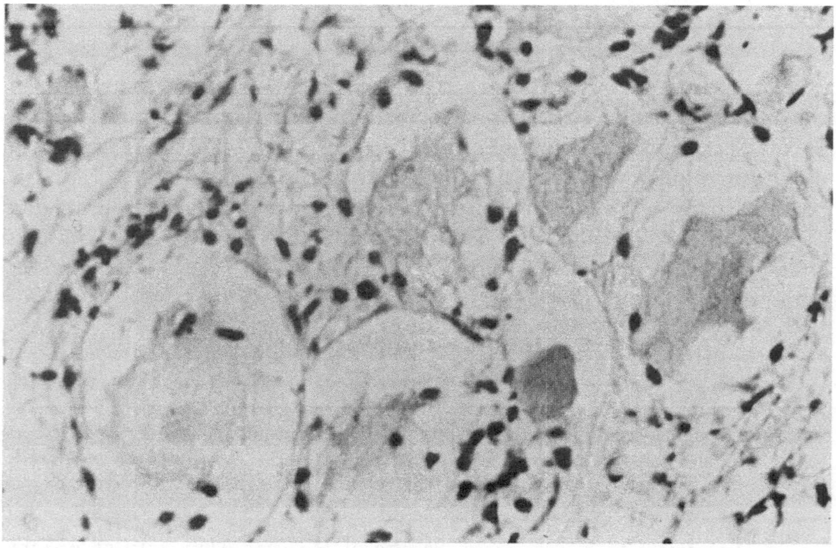

Fig. 2. 24 hours post-lesion: Mononuclear-cell infiltration continued, ganglion-cell necrosis (vacuolization, homogenization, nucleolysis) had appeared, and axons had swollen. ×480

angular process, guiding it to the pterygoid hamulus, and then inserting it into the nearby oval foramen and adjacent Trigeminal ganglion. Active electrodes for both needle systems were inserted 10 mm into the foramen; locations were confirmed with X-ray pictures and electrical stimulation. RF thermocoagulation lesion parameters were those in standard clinical use. A total of 28 lesions (8 bilateral, 12 unilateral) were made. The cordotomy system was used with the right

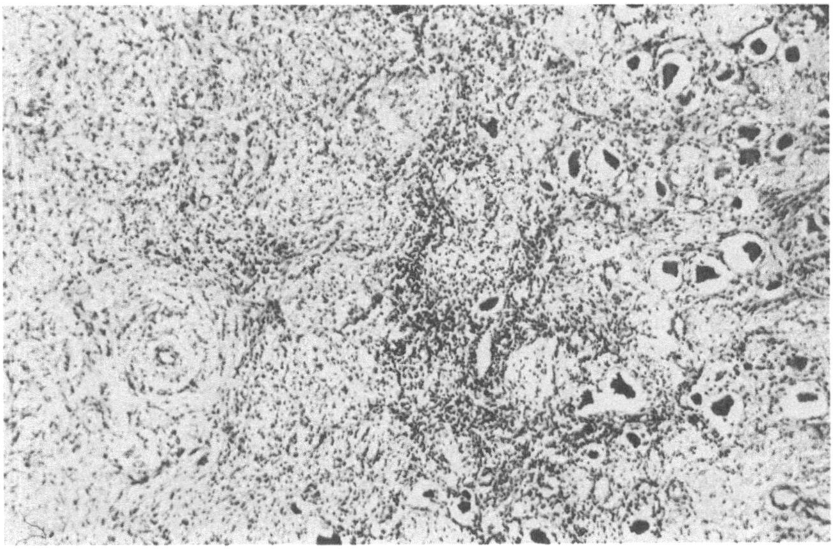

Fig. 3. 14 days post-lesion: At 3 and 5 days there were progressive necrosis, continued axon swelling, development of ghost cells devoid of Nissl substance, destruction of cell bodies, and increases in neutral fat particles. At 7 days there had been disappearance of ganglion cells, satellite-cell and smallvessel proliferation, increases of neutral fat particles, and continuation of other destructive processes. At 14 days (×80), granulation tissue had developed, other destructive processes continued, and large amounts of neutral fat particles (not shown) were present

trigeminal ganglion; the TM system was used with the left. Intact ganglia from dogs with unilateral lesions were used as control materal. Animals were sacrificed at 12 hours (2 dogs), 24 hours (2), 3 days (2), 5 days (2), 7 days (8), or 14 days (4). Trigeminal ganglion were removed with microtechniques and prepared with hematoxylin-eosin, Nissl, and fat stains.

Results

Significant pathological changes were aparent in lesioned areas throughout the post-lesion interval, as shown in Figs. 1–3 (all Nissl stains) and described in the accompanying legends. The two types of electrodes produced similar changes.

Discussion

The percutaneous approach to the trigeminal ganglion and the RF-lesion parameters used here in dogs duplicated the clinical procedure for treatment of trigeminal neuralgia. Earlier studies [1] suggested that damage following RF lesion of the TG is limited to A delta and C sensory fibres. By contrast, our histopathological examination over a two-week post-lesion period indicated that such lesions produce, in the lesioned area, massive necrosis in ganglion cells and subsequent granulation; the scar tissue invades the entire area of the lesion and is not limited to selected fibres. These results demand reassessment of the mechanisms by which RF lesions of the TG relieve trigeminal neuralgia. Further, the relatively simple, non-traumatic animal procedure developed for this study will permit important long-term studies of TG function and dysfunction.

Acknowledgements

We thank Ms. Patricia J. Salis for her creative editing and assistance in the preparation of our final manuscript.

References

1. Frigyesi, T. L., Siegfried, J., Broggi, G., The selective vulnerability of evoked potentials in the trigeminal sensory root to graded thermocoagulation. Exp. Neurol. *49* (1975), 11—21.
2. Harris, W., Alcohol injection of the Gasserian ganglion for trigeminal neuralgia. Lancet *1* (1912), 218—221.
3. Miller, M. E., Anatomy of the dog. Philadelphia: W. B. Saunders. 1964.
4. Siegfried, J., 500 percutaneous thermocoagulations of the Gasserian ganglion for trigeminal pain. Surg. Neurol. *8* (1977), 126—131.
5. Sweet, W. H., Wepsic, J. G., Controlled thermocoagulation of trigeminal ganglion and rootlets for differential destruction of pain fibers. Part 1: Trigeminal neuralgia. J. Neurosurg. *40* (1974), 143—156.

Acta Neurochirurgica, Suppl. 30, 367—370 (1980)

Stereotaxic Aspects of Percutaneous Trigeminal Gangliolysis

L. M. Modesti* and **T. Perl****

With 4 Figures

Summary

The authors describe the technique of fluoroscopically guided percutaneous trigeminal thermogangliolysis. In 20 consecutive cases this method has proved effective, safe and expeditious.

Keywords: Tic douloureux; trigeminal neuralgia; percutaneous trigeminal gangliolysis; radiofrequency coagulation.

Over a one-year-period, we have treated 20 cases of trigeminal neuralgia by a precisely placed radiofrequency lesion in the trigeminal root. We have adapted the radiographic guidance technique for alcohol injection developed by Ecker and Perl [1] to the thermocoagulative technique introduced by Sweet and Wepsic [5] and now widely used by others. The intimate anatomic relationship of the trigeminal root to the trigeminal notch of the petrous ridge and the mandibular nerve to the foramen ovale [4] allows us to determine the direction of the electrode insertion stereotactically. Hartel [2] has described the trigeminal axis as the line extending from the centre of the trigeminal notch through the centre of the foramen ovale to the entry point on the skin of the cheek. If the electrode is inserted in this axis it may be advanced safely to the correct depth in the trigeminal root.

Method

The patient is placed supine on the radiographic table with the body elevated on a mattress and the head extended and tilted toward the contralateral side

* Department of Neurosurgery, SUNY, Upstate Medical Center, Syracuse, NY 13210, U.S.A.

** Department of Radiology, Veterans Administration Medical Center, Syracuse, NY 13210, U.S.A.

0065-1419/80/Suppl. 30/0367/$ 01.00

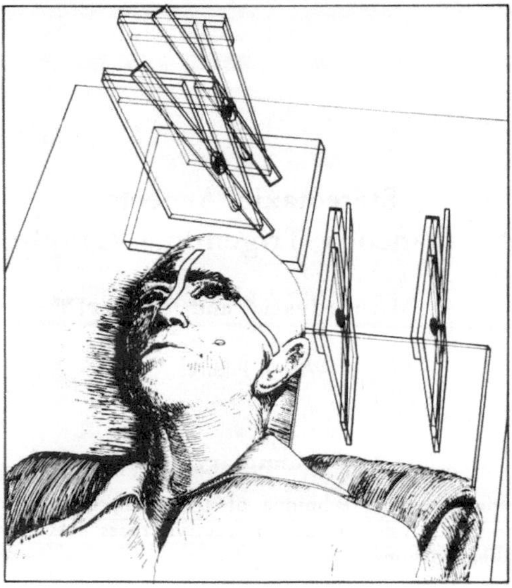

Fig. 1. Patient's head is extended and rotated controlateral to involved side. The foramen ovale and trigeminal notch are seen fluoroscopically through the cheek. The orbito-meatal and sagittal lines are marked for simultaneous observation through protractors

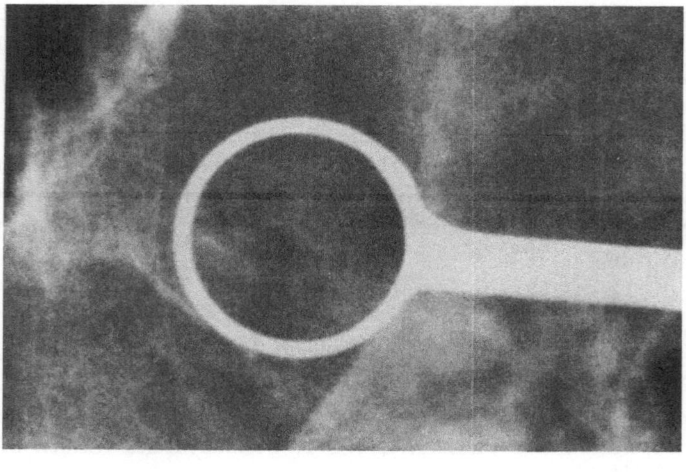

Fig. 2. A circular marker is placed over the fluoroscopically aligned foramen ovale and trigeminal notch to mark the entry point on the cheek

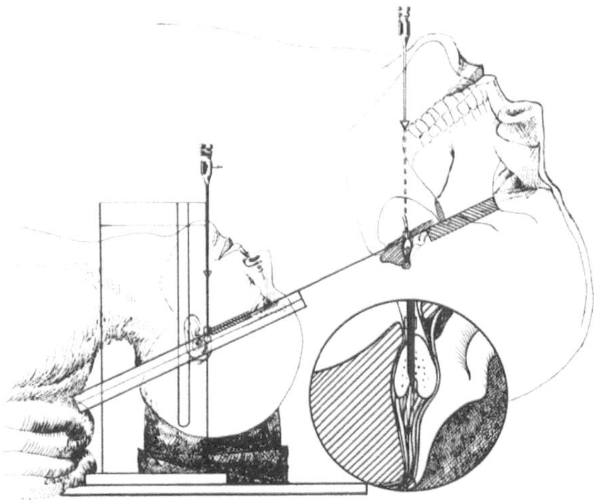

Fig. 3. Under biplane guidance through protractors the needle is inserted vertically into foramen ovale. View from side

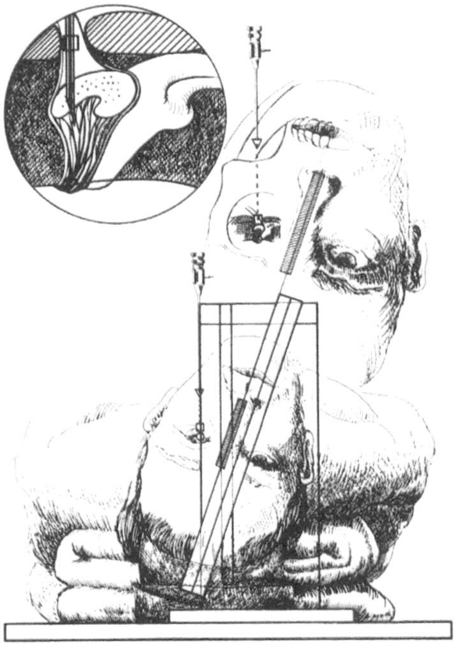

Fig. 4. Same, from head-end

(Fig. 1). The degree of extension is controlled by observation of the orbitomeatal line from the side through a transparent protractor; the degree of tilting is controlled by observation of the mid-sagittal line from the head-end of the table. The foramen ovale is observed fluoroscopically through the cheek and aligned to the trigeminal notch by adjusting the patient's head position. A circular marker is placed over the fluoroscopically aligned foramen ovale and trigeminal notch and the needle entry point is marked on the cheek at the centre of the ring (Fig. 2). The head is held in this position without fluoroscopy. Continuous visual guidance is maintained by means of the protractors as the electrode is inserted in the vertical trigeminal axis through the foramen ovale (Fig. 3–4).

Submento-vertical radiographs are utilized to determine precisely the depth of the tip in relationship to the posterior margin of the foramen ovale. Because of the variations of the intracranial length of the mandibular nerve and of the size of the ganglion, the target area varies [3]. Therapeutic radiofrequency lesions sufficient to produce localized profound analgesia and slight hypesthesia are made only after electrical stimulations confirm the correct placement of the electrode by inducing paraesthesiae in the painful trigeminal division.

Discussion

This technique is based upon the following principles: 1. Precise radiographic control of the trajectory and depth of the electrode. 2. Neurophysiological verification of the electrode position. 3. Controlled incremental thermocoagulative lesions. 4. Verification of effectiveness of the procedure by physiological testing.

This method has proved to be effective, safe, expeditions and well tolerated even by elderly and debilitated patients.

Reliance on precise radiological control avoids a "free-hand" approach and possible injuries to intracranial neural and vascular structures. In 20 consecutive cases, complete pain relief was achieved in all patients with no complications or undesirable side effects.

References

1. Ecker, A., Perl, T., Selective gasserian injection for tic douloureux. Technical advances and results. Acta Radiologica *9* (1969), 38—48.
2. Hartel, F. F., Röntgenologische Darstellung des Foramen ovale des Schädels und ihre Bedeutung für die Behandlung der Trigeminusneuralgie. Dtsch. Med. Wschr. *61* (1935), 1069.
3. Henderson, W. R., The anatomy of the gasserian ganglion and the distribution of pain in relation to injections and operations for trigeminal neuralgia. Ann. Roy. Coll. Surg. (Engl.) *37* (1965), 346—373.
4. Penman, J., A simple radiological aid to gasserian injection. Lancet *2* (1979), 268—274.
5. Sweet, W. H., Wepsic, J. G., Controlled thermocoagulation of trigeminal ganglion and rootlets for differential destruction of pain fibers. Part I. Trigeminal neuralgia. J. Neurosurg. *40* (1974), 143—156.

Acta Neurochirurgica, Suppl. 30, 371—376 (1980)

The Effectiveness of Trigeminal Thermocoagulation for Recurrent Paroxysmal Trigeminal Neuralgia After Previous Intra-Cranial Surgery

J. W. Turner*

With 2 Figures

Summary

Six patients are described in whom recurrent trigeminal neuralgia was treated by thermocoagulation. Their initial symptoms had been relieved by intra-cranial operation usually many years previously. In the majority, cerebro-spinal fluid was obtained and physiological corroboration of probe placement was satisfactory. Symptoms were relieved in all cases. Trigeminal thermocoagulation is safe and effective in relieving recurrent trigeminal neuralgia in patients who have had a previous intra-cranial operation for their symptoms.

Keywords: Trigeminal neuralgia; intra-cranial surgery; thermocoagulation.

Introduction

After intra-cranial operation for trigeminal neuralgia, pain recurs in 5 [1] to 40% [4] of patients. In many centres, trigeminal thermocoagulation is now the method of choice in the surgical treatment of paroxysmal trigeminal neuralgia. The paper describes its use and the results in patients with recurrent trigeminal neuralgia, all of whom had previously been treated by intra-cranial operation.

Patients and Methods

Six patients are described with recurrent trigeminal neuralgia following previous intra-cranial operation who have been treated by thermocoagulation since 1971 by me. Clinical data have been collected prospectively and the patients followed up at regular intervals for between five months and five years. The surgical method used was similar to that described by Sweet and Wepsic [3] (1976), and particular attention was paid to the threshold voltage [5].

---

* Institute of Neurological Sciences, Southern General Hospital, Glasgow G51 4TF, Scotland.

0065-1419/80/Suppl. 30/0371/$ 01.20

Results

Previous Surgery

As might be expected, most patients were female (Table 1) and right-sided pain predominated generally in the second and third divisions of the trigeminal distribution. The average age at the time of the first operation was forty nine years and the average duration of pain was eight and a half years. In four cases, decompressive or

Table 1. *Clinical Picture at Time of Previous Surgery*

Patient	Sex	Age at 1st operation	Site of pain	Duration of pain (years)	Type of operation	Sensory changes	Pain relief (years)
M. W.	f.	38	l. v. 2, v. 3	8	decompression	none	5
K. H.	f.	60	r. v. 3	½	decompression	none	15
A. McG.	m.	46	l. v. 2, 3	1½	decompression and heat	v. 3 analgesia	11
J. D.	f.	46	r. v. 2	20	v. 2 section	v. 2 anaesthesia	18
L. C.	f.	52	r. v. 3, 2	6	v. 2, 3 section	anaesthesia 1, 2, 3	4
			r. v. 1	5	total section	anaesthesia 1, 2, 3	several
A. M.	m.	50	r. v. 2	10	decompression and trauma to v. 2	v. 2 hypalgesia	10

compressive surgery [2] was undertaken, and in two cases the root was partially sectioned. In one case (L. C.) total section was performed, six years after previous partial section. Following decompressive surgery, sensation was normal in two patients (M. W., K. H.) but there was hypalgesia or analgesia in another two patients (A. G., A. M.) in whom heat or mild trauma had been applied during the operation. More profound deficits were noted in patients in whom the root had been sectioned. With time, the deficits tended to fade and when the pain recurred the trigger spots tended to be located at patchy areas of returning sensation.

Thermocoagulation

The interval between intra-cranial surgery and trigeminal thermocoagulation ranged from 8 to 19 years with an average of 15 years (Table 2). Pain generally recurred at the original site. It is noteworthy that cerebro-spinal fluid was obtained easily in the majority of procedures in spite of the previous intra-cranial surgery, repeated in one case. It is also noteworthy that physiological corroboration by electrical stimulation at the probe tip during the procedure was satisfactory. The threshold for evoking tingling sensation in the pain or trigger area ranged from 40 to 280 mV. In those patients who showed a patchy return of sensation, electrical stimulation evoked a tingling sensation at these points which were then rendered analgesic by thermocoagulation. Sensory changes following coagulation covered the pain area and trigger spots in all patients. In all patients,

Table 2. *Trigeminal Thermocoagulation*

Patient	Site of pain	Duration (years)	C.S.F. obtained	Minimum threshold mV	Sensory change	Pain relief (years)
M. W.	l. v. 2	3	n.r.	200	analgesia v. 1, v. 2	3 +
	l. v. 2/v. 3	1/6	yes	70	analgesia v. 2, v. 3	1½
K. H.	r. v. 3	½	yes	190	analgesia v. 3	3 +
A. McG.	l. v. 2/v. 3	4	no	250	analgesia v. 2, v. 3	2 +
J. D.	r. v. 2 (1)	1	yes	100	analgesia v. 2	¾ +
L. C.	r. v. 2/v. 3 lips	several	yes	280	analgesia v. 2, v. 3	2/3 +
A. M.	r. v. 2	5	yes	40	analgesia v. 2	½ +

+ Pain relief continues to present time.
(1) Left sided trigeminal neuralgia relieved by thermocoagulation in 1977.
n.r. Not recorded.

pain was abolished. In one case (M. W.) unwanted sensory depression occurred in the ophthalmic division as well as in the pain area of the maxillary division. Pain relief was then maintained for three years but pain recurred in the second division and developed in the third division. Further thermocoagulation has relieved the pain up to the present time. In another case (J. D.) neuralgia developed in the second and third divisions on the opposite side of the face, and again this was successfully relieved by thermocoagulation.

The following are two typical cases:

Case 1—(K. H.)

In 1960, this sixty years old lady developed paroxysmal trigeminal neuralgia in the right mandibular region with an associated trigger area. In November 1960 via an extra-dural approach the dura was incised over the ganglion and radially along the second and third divisions. Postoperatively there was no sensory deficit and the patient remained pain free for fifteen years. In 1975, the pain recurred and was not relieved by large doses of Carbamazepine which in addition produced side effects. In June 1976, trigeminal thermocoagulation was performed and clear, colourless cerebro-spinal fluid was obtained. The minimum threshold voltage for stimulation was 190 mV. Post operatively there was analgesia over the mandibular region and no trigger spot. The lady remains pain free up to the present time, more than three years post operatively.

Case 2—(L. C.)

In 1953, this lady presented with trigeminal neuralgia affecting the lower jaw, cheek and tongue with some pain radiating towards the eye. At operation through a temporal extra-dural approach, it was noted that the rootlets were very adherent and tougher than usual. The fibres of the third division and some of the second division were partially divided. Post operatively the patient was pain free but subsequently developed further pain in the forehead and nose. In 1959, prior to further surgery, analgesia was noted over the second and third divisions with preservation of some sensation in the ophthalmic area. At re-operation, all sensory fibres were divided with relief of most of her pain. In 1978, she presented again with a patchy area of sensation particularly medially over the lower and upper lips, where trigger spots were situated. At trigeminal thermocoagulation clear cerebrospinal fluid was obtained. The threshold voltage, 280 mV, at which electrical stimulation produced tingling in the trigger areas, was rather high. Thermocoagulation abolished the trigger area and the pain.

Two patients not tabulated above developed anaesthesia or analgesia dolorosa in addition to recurrent trigeminal neuralgia after previous intra-cranial surgery for trigeminal neuralgia. One patient (E. D.) who had a complete section at the original operation in 1966, developed anaesthesia dolorosa, a facial palsy and keratitis. The trigeminal neuralgia eventually returned. Thermocoagulation appeared to relieve the neuralgic pain and had no effect on the anaesthesia dolorosa. In another patient (S. D.) analgesia dolorosa developed after a selective section. Five years later, thermocoagulation was performed for recurrent neuralgia with some success and without exacerbating the analgesia dolorosa. The analgesia dolorosa has subsequently shown improvement with other treatments.

Discussion

It would be expected that intra-cranial surgery directly on the ganglion and retro-gasserian rootlets would disturb and distort the anatomy in that region with consequent difficulty at attempted thermocoagulation. However, the finding that it was possible in the majority of cases to obtain cerebro-spinal fluid during subsequent thermocoagulation clearly demonstrated that adhesions were not so severe as to obliterate the sub-arachnoid space. That the anatomy was not disturbed in a major way, was demonstrated by the ability to obtain good physiological corroboration of the tip of the electrode. In addition, the production of analgesia and hypalgesia by thermocoagulation showed that the lesion was created in the appropriate

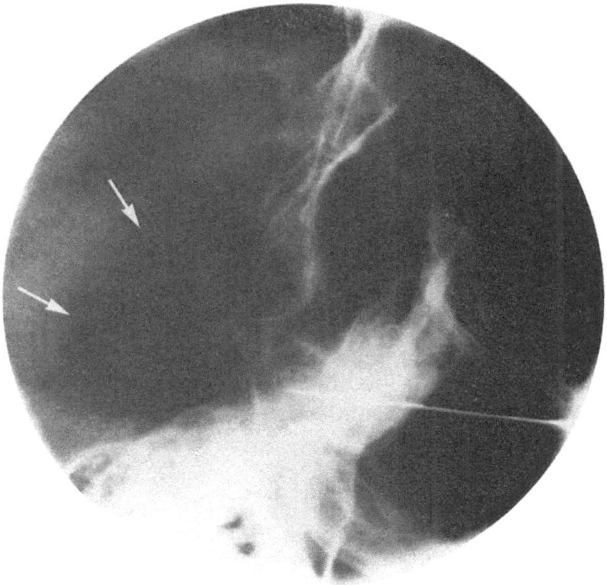

Fig. 1. Radiograph showing craniectomy of previous decompression. Thermocoagulation probe in position (1976)

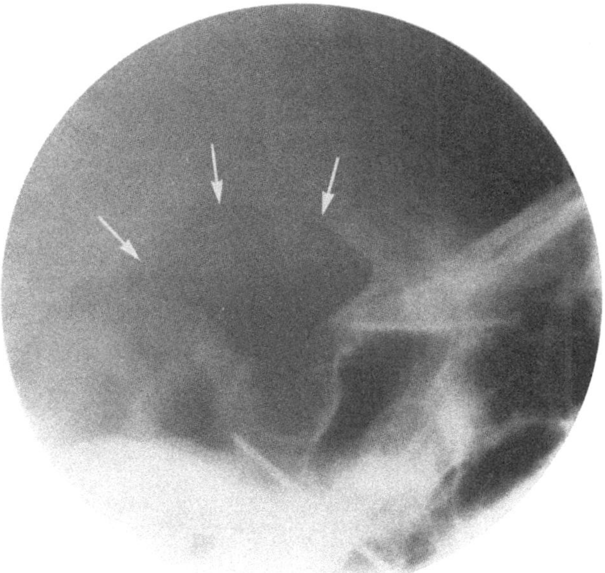

Fig. 2. Radiograph showing craniectomy defect from previous intra-cranial surgery. Thermocoagulation probe in position (1978)

anatomical site. While the follow-up period is fairly short in some of the cases, it is likely from prediction studies that the long-term results will be good, especially in those patients where there was a low threshold voltage, a good flow of cerebro-spinal fluid and analgesia covered the trigger zone [5]. Thermocoagulation would be undertaken in patients with dolorosa symptoms only when there is very clear cut evidence of neuralgic pain with identifiable trigger spots. The risk of exacerbating the dolorosa symptoms particularly in the ophthalmic area is high.

Conclusion

Thermocoagulation is technically satisfactory and gives good results in recurrent paroxysmal trigeminal neuralgia after previous intra-cranial operation.

References

1. Peet, M. M., Schneider, R. C., Trigeminal neuralgia. A review of six hundred and eighty nine cases with a follow-up study on sixty five per cent of the group. J. Neurosurg. *9* (1952), 367—377.
2. Shelden, C. H., Pudenz, R. H., Freshwater, D. B., Crue, B. J., Compression rather than decompression for trigeminal neuralgia. J. Neurosurg. *12* (1955), 123—126.
3. Sweet, H., Wepsic, J. G., Controlled thermocoagulation of trigeminal ganglion and rootlets for differential destruction of pain fibres. J. Neurosurg. *40* (1974), 143—156.
4. Taarnhøj, P., The place of decompression of the posterior root in the treatment of trigeminal neuralgia. J. Neurol. Neurosurg. Psychiat. *24* (1961), 294—296.
5. Turner, J., The results of trigeminal thermocoagulation in the treatment of trigeminal neuralgia. J. Neurol. Neurosurg. Psychiat. *41* (1978), 187—188.

Acta Neurochirurgica, Suppl. 30, 377—381 (1980)

First Results with Extralemniscal Myelotomy

J. Eiras*, J. Garcia, J. Gomez, L. I. Carcavilla, and **S. Ucar**

With 4 Figures

In the past thalamic lesions have been practised in our clinic to treat deep medial pain in cancer patients in the advances stages. Such lesions centred on the CM-Pf complex resulted in considerable pain relief without any objective sensory loss. However the frequent recurrence of pain and the accompanying psychic disturbances called for a critical analysis of their indications [2].

Since 1970, Hitchcock has carried out centromedullary stereotactic lesions on the spinomedullary junction obtaining bilateral analgesia without encroachment of the respiratory pathways [1]. Schvarcz [3] performed a similar lesion at the base of the dorsal funiculi obtaining good results in dealing with deep pain and hyperpathy common in cancer patients. This lesion termed "extralemniscal myelotomy" (EM) only produces subjective analgesia as it seems to interrupt the paleospinothalamic tracts. A percutaneous technique to perform EM is reported and compared with results obtained after stereotactic lesions in the postero-medial thalamus.

Clinical Material and Method

Since 1977, 12 patients all complaining of medial or bilateral pain due to malignancy in advanced stages have been submitted to E. M. Treatment with opiates had previously been started in 8 cases.

The first two patients were operated on using the Riechert-Mundinger frame and following Hitchcock's technique. The long duration of the stereotactic procedure and the difficulty encountered in controlling the electrode in the A-P projection prompted the search for a technique to overcome these problems.

A percutaneous technique using the Rossomoff Kit for lateral cordotomy was carried out on the other ten patients. Under local anaesthesia a cisternography

* Department of Neurosurgery of the Social Security, Zaragoza, Spain.

0065-1419/80/Suppl. 30/0377/$ 01.00

with emulsified Pantopaque was performed with the patient lying prone. The radiologic equipment allowed us to obtain simple X-rays in the A-P and lateral projections plus fluoroscopy in the lateral (Fig. 1). The target point was placed on the mediosagital plane referred to the dens and 5 mm under the dorsal border of spinal cord (Figs. 2 and 3). The Rossomoff needle-holder was attached to a rigid support on the operating table over the patient's neck. Electrodes with a 2 mm bare tip were used for stimulation and lesion. The patients complained of

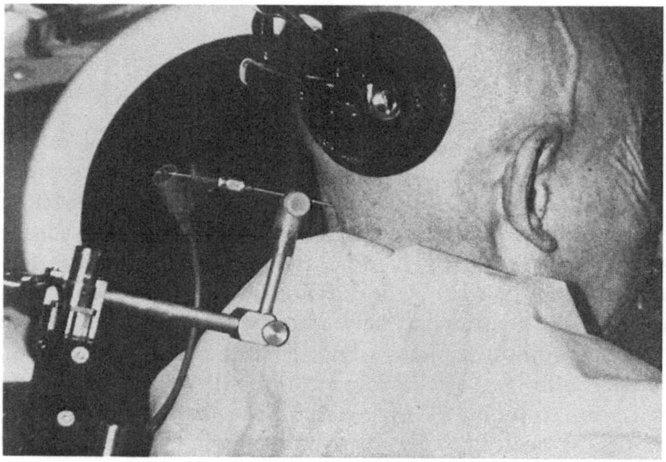

Fig. 1. Percutaneous E.M. is being performed. General view

a brief shock-like sensation as the electrode pierced the cord. Electrical stimulation and clinical testing were carried out until the target point was reached with parameters of 0.2–1 Volt and 50–75 Hz and ms. Sensations of pinpricks and burning and/or throbbing feelings in the lower limbs were the most commonly elicited responses. Occasionally burning sensations in the thoracic or abdominal areas and other trigeminal responses were noted. These responses did not differ in any way from those described by Hitchcock and Schvarcz: in our patients however stimulation over 1 volt was always followed by nausea.

A radio-frequency lesion of 50 mA and of 60 seconds was made in front of the point where the most distal responses in the lower limbs were obtained. Further lesions were performed on 4 patients in the same position at 75 and 100 mA until they felt considerable relief from pain. Persistent unilateral responses were obtained in some cases in spite of a correct radiological position; but the tract of the electrode however could-be modified very easily with our procedure.

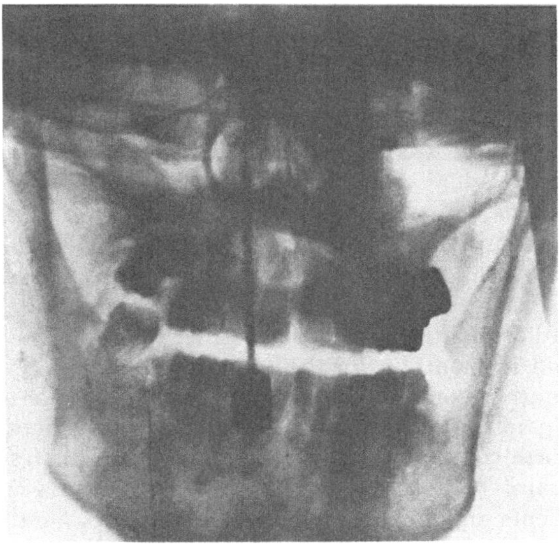

Fig. 2. Spinal needle is directed towards the dens

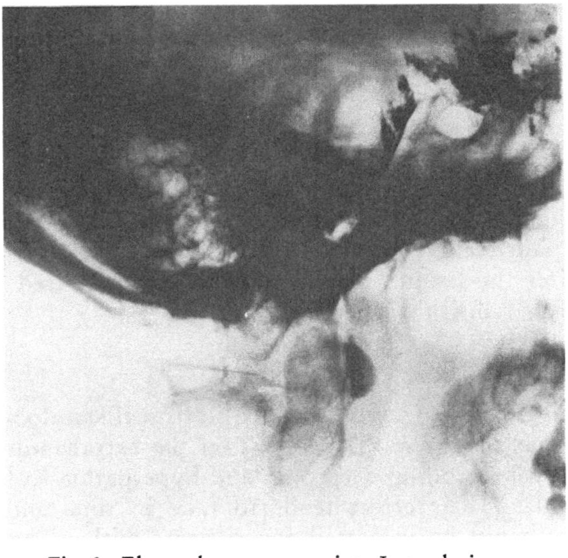

Fig. 3. Electrode at target point. Lateral view

Results

The post-operative follow-up ranged from 2 to 22 months (Fig. 4). Eight patients are now dead, 3 lost from follow up and only 1 patient remained alive at the last follow up 14 months after the operation. All the patients obtained good pain-relief. Total alleviation of pain was achieved in 7 for periods of from 3 to 14 months. Residual pain needing non-narcotic erase analgesics persisted in 5 cases. A progressive recurrence of pain was observed in 5 patients but this only reached the pre-operative level in 3 cases: 8, 9 and 20 months after the operation. Only three patients did not need to take analgesics in the post-operative follow-up, in one case until his death 7 months later and the other two until we lost control of them 6 and 13 months after the operation.

Post-operative complications common to all patients were dysmetria and gait disturbances that in no case lasted more than two weeks but these complaints caused the patients no distress because of relief from pain. Non-dermatomal areas of hypoalgesia were detected in three patients and four others complained of paraesthesias in the soles for periods of 2 to 8 days. Neither sphinter nor motor weakness appeared.

Results After Thalamotomy

In the past cryogenic lesions centred on the CM-Pf complex were carried out by the authors on 11 similar cases of malignant pain due to malignancy and the results have been reviewed in order to compare both techniques.

One patient died two days after the operation because of ventricular haemorrhage. The remaining patients obtained immediate pain relief. Three patients did not require analgesics for a period of from 3 to 8 months. Six others needed non-narcotic analgesics. In 5 cases the pain recurred reaching its pre-operative level from 3 to 9 months after the lesion. Mental disturbances appeared in 7 cases, which in 2 lasted until their death.

Conclusions

While this is a small series from the statistical standpoint, certain conclusions can be drawn. The lesions on the extralemniscal system are effective in controlling deep pain and hyperpathia so frequent in cancer patients. Their effect tends to fade in time and therefore these lesions should be indicated for patients with a short life expectancy. The interruption of this pathway in the spinomedullary junction by means of stereotactical procedures obtain satisfactory results without the side effects caused by thalamic lesions. In spite of radiological accuracy the results of stimulations are of paramount importance for target identification. The percutaneous technique described by the authors cuts down the operating time considerably an important factor to be taken into account when dealing with patients in bad general conditions.

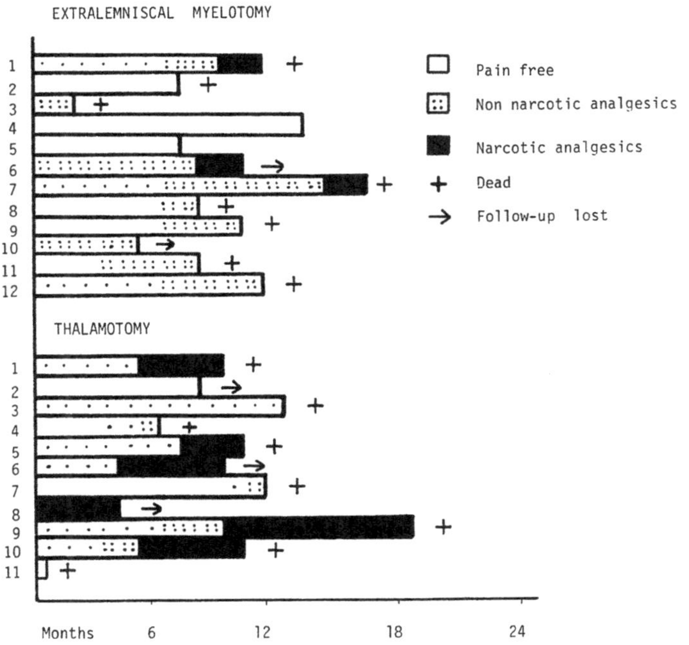

Fig. 4. Graph showing evolution after E.M. in 12 patients and comparative results with thalamotomy

References

1. Hitchcock, E. R., Stereotactic cervical mielotomy. J. Neurol. Neurosurg. Psychiat. *33* (1970), 224—230.
2. Pagni, C. A., Place of stereotactic technique in surgery for pain. Advances in Neurology, Vol. 4, pp. 699—706. New York: Raven Press. 1974.
3. Schvarcz, J. R., Functional exploration of the spinomedullary junction. Advances in Stereotactic and Functional Neurosurgery, pp. 179—185 (Gillingham, F. J., Hitchcock, E. R., eds.). Acta Neurochir. Suppl. 24. Wien-New York: Springer. 1977.

Acta Neurochirurgica, Suppl. 30, 383—389 (1980)

Pain Relief After Dorsal Root Entry Zone Lesions

B. S. Nashold Jr.* and **R. H. Ostdahl**

With 1 Figure

Pain is an early symptom following avulsion of the brachial plexus in 70% of patients, but only 20% develop intractable disabling pain requiring surgical intervention. In the past neurosurgical treatment has consisted of rhizotomy, cordotomy, dorsal column stimulation and stereotactic mesencephalotomy all of which have been largely unsuccessful [1, 2]. Recently 18 patients with intractable pain from brachial plexus avulsion lesions were treated with a new surgical technique using radiofrequency coagulation of the dorsal root entry zone (DREZ) of the cervical cord in the region of the avulsed nerve root. Since the initial clinical results in the brachial plexus avulsion patients were encouraging, we have applied the treatment to three additional patients with intractable pain from other causes. These include one man with a gunshot injury to the brachial plexus, a woman suffering from a gunshot wound to the spine with involvement of the spinal word and a third man with intractable chronic pain due to a pelvic tumour.

Of the 18 patients in this series with partial or complete avulsion of the brachial plexus, 8 have been injured in motorcycle accidents, 5 have been involved in automobile accidents and 3 have sustained industrial crush avulsion injuries. One was involved in a bicycle mishap and another was the victim of a speedboat accident. The onset of the pain usually appears between 10 to 20 days after the avulsion injury. The pain involves the dermal distribution related to those roots demonstrated to be avulsed at the time of the subsequent surgery. The patients described the pain in various ways such as "severe", "sharp", "burning", "throbbing", "aching" or "pulling". Several patients experienced phantom sensation in the

* Duke Hospital, Durham, North Carolina, U.S.A.

0065-1419/80/Suppl. 30/0383/$ 01.40

denervated limb. The phantoms described were reminiscent of those associated with limb amputation due to other forms of trauma. The pain could be either constant or intermittent and various external stimuli would intensify the pain. Some patients noted the pain intensified after physical exhaustion, anxiety, changes in temperature, especially cold weather, and excessive exercise. The diagnosis and evaluation of brachial plexus avulsion injuries is not difficult. Depending on the extent of the injury, varying degrees of motor paralysis may be encountered, such as a flail and paralyzed extremity, which is the most common finding in our series. The sensory loss often involves the entire limb up to the shoulder girdle. At times the motor or sensory deficits at the time of injury extend beyond the distribution of the avulsed nerve, suggesting additional infraganglial damage to the plexus and/or injury to the spinal cord. The physical forces producing the avulsion are complex and every one of our 18 patients was found to have an abnormal appearing spinal cord at surgery. An ipsilateral Horner's syndrome was noted in 12 patients. Prior to the treatment using the dorsal root entry zone coagulation, patients had undergone surgical procedures including rhizotomy, dorsal column stimulation, cingulotomy, stereotactic mesencephalotomy, stellate block and sympathectomy. None of these treatment methods had relieved the patient's pain.

The myelographic signs following avulsion of the brachial plexus have been well described in the literature. It is important to recognize that the abnormal myelographic appearance does not necessarily indicate the extent of the injury, a finding pointed out by other observers in the past. However, it is important that all patients, prior to any decision for surgical treatment, have a complete cervical myelogram.

Surgical Technique of DREZ Coagulation

The patient is placed in the sitting position for the operation and central venous pressure is monitored using doppler techniques. Laminectomy is carried out over the cervical spine usually from C 5 through T 1, and the dura is exposed. On several occasions, posterior meningoceles were noted when the dura was exposed which were not seen on the preoperative myelogram. If large meningoceles are encountered, they are dissected free and the dural defects are closed. Magnification is essential when examining the cord prior to the production of the lesion. The arachnoid is often thickened with numerous arachnoidal bands crossing the subarachnoid space to the spine and these require careful dissection.

The cervical spinal cord in the region of the avulsion injury appeared abnormal in all patients. The cord was shrunken on the side of the injury with thickening of the pia arachnoid. The cervical roots were absent and in some cases both dorsal and ventral roots were missing. In several patients small radicular blood vessels remained intact even though the dorsal root was absent, and it appeared to us that the dorsal surface of the spinal cord may have been hypervascularized. Careful palpation of the cord revealed small cystic areas often associated with softening and yellowish discoloration. The area of the DREZ is inspected under magnification to verify the external landmark on the cord. The most important landmark for the production of the lesion is the intermediolateral sulcus on the side of the avulsion. It courses along the dorsal surface of the cord at the lateral edge of the dorsal column and on the normal side of the cord the dorsal roots can be seen originating from the sulcus as they pass out to the foramen. An insulated

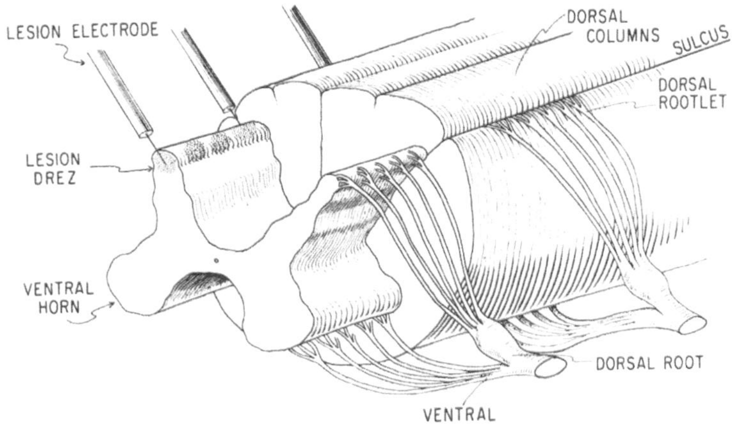

Fig. 1

stainless steel electrode (0.018 inches) with a tapered uninsulated 2 mm tip is used for the coagulation. It is introduced at a 25° angle into the lateral medial direction through the intermediolateral sulcus, and it penetrates the cord for approximately 2 mm (Fig. 1). A Radionics radiofrequency coagulator is used at 70 ma for 15 seconds. Spacing of the radiofrequency lesions is approximately 2–3 mm along the longitudinal extent of the sulcus and the number of lesions are determined by the number of roots that are avulsed. Coagulations may vary between 10 to 20, depending on the extent of the nerve root avulsion. As the coagulation is formed, one notes a circular whitening of the coagulated area around the tip of the electrode which usually extends 1 to 2 mm and we believe that the final lesion consists of an elongated strip of coagulation extending throughout the area of the avulsion. The upper lesion is made just below the attacked rootlet on the avulsed side and the lowest lesion is made just above the lowest intact rootlet on the avulsed side. At the time that the lesions are being produced, intravenous steroids are given and are continued for several days postoperatively. The cord does not appear grossly abnormal following this procedure nor is there any evidence of significant swelling. It is usually possible to identify the lesions clearly. The dura and the remainder of the wound are then closed.

Results

The 18 patients with the DREZ coagulations were all male. Postoperative pain relief was defined as a good result signifying 75% or greater relief of pain, a fair result was equivalent to pain relief of 25 to 75%, a poor result meant relief of less than 25%. By these criteria, 10 of the 18 patients with avulsion injuries and the patient with the upper extremity gunshot wound experienced not only good but lasting pain relief. In most of these patients the pain relief has been greater than 90%. Two patients with lower extremity pain also continue to be pain-free. Thus, a total of 13 of 21 patients (67%) continue to experience relief of pain of at least 75%. Postoperative morbidity is noted to be mild or moderate consisting of weakness in the ipsilateral extremity plus certain postoperative changes. At the most recent follow-up examination, 11 of the 21 patients continue to experience some degree of residual weakness barely detectable but not resulting in any functional change in gait. Equally important are the postoperative sensory changes. Six of the 21 patients had no new postoperative sensory findings, however, 15 patients experienced sensory abnormalities attributable to the surgical procedure. These included a variety of intriguing sensory symptoms and signs. The most severe and consistent change noted had been a proprioceptive deficit of the ipsilateral lower extremities in which position sense was affected but not vibration sense. Some patients experienced an alteration of pain and temperature for three dermatomal segments below the level of the last lesion—in other words, in areas in which the nerve roots are perfectly intact. This usually disappears within a matter of weeks. There has been no evidence of postoperative dysaesthesia as a result of the lesions up to this time with the longest follow-up four years.

Discussion

We believe that the pain of brachial plexus avulsion is central in nature related to pathophysiologic changes occurring in the DREZ as a result of traumatic afferent disconnection of the cervical dorsal roots. In the medical literature we found only one report on a post mortem examination of a patient with a brachial plexus avulsion injury occurring 52 years before [3]. At the time of examination of the spinal cord there was evidence of gray matter destruction and pseudocyst formation associated with a traumatic meningocele. There have been no post mortem examinations in our patients.

We believe that there are three possible neurophysiological mechanisms responsible for the development of central pain in this group of patients. 1. Hypersensitive neuronal pools of the injured DREZ due to deafferentation, 2. injury to the spinothalamic and spinoreticular pathways, and 3. local dysfunction of the neuronal pools of the dorsal root entry zone due to facilitory or inhibitory influences on the tract of Lissauer.

Denervation hypersensitivity is a well known neurophysiological phenomenon described both in experimental animals and humans. The deafferented neuron becomes hyperactive and discharges paroxysmally, possibly resulting in painful dysaesthesia [4, 5]. It is now well recognized that the networks of cell masses of the dorsal root entry zone form an exceedingly complex neuronal conglomerate in a synaptic environment modulated by peripheral afferent input and regional influences from surrounding spinal cord activity [6]. Thermal coagulation of the DREZ in our patients will destroy areas with hyperactive neurons and, thereby, abolish pain analogous to the resection of an epileptic cortical tissue to abolish seizure activity. Some workers conclude that the phenomenon of central pain is due primarily to the pathophysiologic changes along the afferent sensory pathways irrespective of whether the cells or the fibers are destroyed [7]. Two important afferent pathways that could be involved in cervical avulsion injuries are the spinothalamic and spinoreticular tracts whose cells of origin to some extent are in the dorsal root entry zone. Support for this idea lies in the fact that intractable pain of avulsion injury has been relieved by high cervical cordotomy, mesencephalic tractotomy, and, now, localized coagulation of the DREZ. Pain relief after DREZ coagulation simply may be due to destruction of the cells of origin in these two important pathways. Detailed postmortem and histopathologic studies of the spinal cords of patients with avulsion injuries treated in this fashion will be required to settle this question. The tract of Lissauer has gained importance in regard to its possible role in central dysaesthesia [10]. Ranson suggested in 1913 that the tract was responsible for the transmission of pain and temperature and later, Hyndman carried out differential section of the tract of Lissauer in patients with a variety of painful conditions and was able to show that pain and temperature were abolished over an area of several dermatomes adjacent to the level of the Lissauer tract section in the human spinal cord [6, 8]. These alterations in pain and temperature are similar to those noted in our patients which extend below the level of the coagulations. The tract of Lissauer extends throughout the length of the spinal cord with 25% consisting of afferent fibers of central origin and the remaining 75% of fibers arising from neurons located in the substantia gelatinosa. Lissauer's tract lies in the dorsal portion of the dorsal root entry zone with its fibers bifurcating and running up and down the cord for several segments, making rich connections with cells throughout the DREZ. The influence of this structure on cutaneous dermatomes was illustrated by observations of the monkey by Denny-Brown which are differential Lissauer tract sections [5]. Denny-Brown noted that selected section of the medial division of the tract of Lissauer tended to abolish the debilitating effect of the neighboring roots on the dermatomal representation of the test root while section of the lateral division interferred with a strong inhibitory influence on the test root. The pain relief experienced in our patients could be related to a modification of the influences of Lissauer's tract on the spinal segment adjacent to the injury level.

At present one can only speculate regarding the possible neurophysiological mechanisms responsible for intractable central pain in certain patients with brachial plexus avulsion injury. It is becoming more evident from neurophysiological and clinical observations in humans and animals, however, that afferent input to dorsal roots exerts a potent influence on segmental spinal cord activity. Deafferentation in some fashion modulates the message conveyed centrally such as is consciously experienced as pain. In 1966 Kerr [11] demonstrated the experimental feasibility of destruction of the trigeminal spinal nucleus caudalis and theorized on the possible treatment of intractable craniofacial pain. It is particularly intruiguing to us that patients with chronic pain from other causes other than root avulsion have obtained significant benefit from DREZ destruction. We believe that future neurosurgical operations can be designed with smaller and more precise lesions localized to various structures of the human spinal cord for the relief of a variety of symptoms.

References

1. Falconer, M. A., Surgical treatment of intractable phantom limb pain. Brit. Med. J. *1* (1953), 299—304.
2. Zorub, D. S., Nashold, B. S., Jr., Cook, W. A., Jr., Avulsion of the brachial plexus. I. A review with implications on the therapy of intractable pain. Surg. Neurol. *2* (1974), 347—353.
3. Tillman, B., Engel, H., Clinical and late pathoanatomical findings after brachial plexus avulsion. Fortschr. Neurol. Psychiatr. *42* (1974), 28—37 (Ger).
4. Loeser, J. D., Ward A. A., Jr., Some effects of deafferentation on neurons of the cat spinal cord. Arch. Neurol. *17* (1967), 629—636.
5. Loeser, J. D., Ward, A. A., Jr., White, L. E., Jr., Chronic deafferentation of human spinal cord neurons. J. Neurosurg. *29* (1968), 48—50.
6. Denny-Brown, D., The importance of steady-state equilibria in small-celled reticular systems. In: The Neurosciences. Paths of Discovery, pp. 295—308 (Warden, F. G., Swagery, J. P., Adelman, G., eds.). Cambridge, Mass./London: MIT Press. 1975.

7. Pagni, C. A., Central pain and painful anesthesia: Pathophysiology and treatment of sensory deprivation syndromes due to central and peripheral nervous system lesions. In: Progress in Neurological Surgery, Vol. 8, pp. 132—257 (Krayenbühl, H., Maspes, P. E., Sweet, W. H., eds.). Basel: S. Karger. 1976.
8. Ranson, S. W., The course within the spinal cord of the non-medullated fibers of the dorsal roots: A study of Lissauer's tract in the cat. J. Comp. Neurol. *23* (1913), 259—281.
9. Hyndman, O. R., Lissauer's tract section. A contribution to chordotomy for the relief of pain (preliminary report). J. Int. Coll. Surg. *5* (1942), 394—400.
10. Denny-Brown, D., Kirk, E. J., Yanagisawa, N., The tract of Lissauer in relation to sensory transmission in the dorsal horn of spinal cord in the macaque monkey. J. Comp. Neurol. *151* (1973), 175—199.
11. Kerr, F. W. L., Spinal V nucleolysis: intractable craniofacial pain. Surg. Forum *17* (1966), 419—421.

Acta Neurochirurgica, Suppl. 30, 391—393 (1980)

Rostral Mesencephalic Reticulotomy for Pain Relief

Report of 15 Cases

K. Amano*, H. Iseki, M. Notani, H. Kawabatake, T. Tanikawa, H. Kawamura, and **K. Kitamura**

Summary

Rostral mesencephalic reticulotomy was performed for relief of intractable pain in 15 patients. The target was 14 mm posterior to the midpoint of the AC-PC line, 5 mm below the AC-PC line and 5 mm lateral from the centre of the aqueduct. The rationale and clinical results of this procedure are discussed briefly.

Keywords: Endorphin; pain relief; midbrain reticular formation; central gray matter.

Introduction

Since 1974 the authors [1] have performed rostral mesencephalic reticulotomy (RMR) for relief of intractable pain based on the fact that the medial mesencephalic reticular formation (paleospinothalamic projection) bordering the periaqueductal gray matter is more significant than the lateral spinothalamic tract at the midbrain level (neospinothalamic projection) in the central conduction of nociceptive impulse in man. The present report is concerned with the clinical results of this procedure for pain relief.

Material and Methods

Fifteen patients (12 males and 3 females) with intractable pain had stereotactic rostral mesencephalic reticulotomy using a Todd-Wells stereotactic frame under local anesthesia with additional intravenous administration of Diazepam and Pentazocin. The target of RMR was 14 mm posterior to the midpoint of the AC-PC line, 5 mm below the AC-PC line and 5 mm lateral from the centre of the aqueduct. The target was located at the border between the periaqueductal gray matter and the medial end of the mesencephalic reticular formation at the level between the superior colliculus and the posterior commissure. In order to avoid postoperative Parinaud's syndrome, the burr hole for electrode insertion was made more frontally than the usual burr hole position for stereotactic operations

* Department of Neurosurgery, Neurological Institute, Tokyo Women's Medical College, 10 Kawada-cho, Shinjuku-ku, Tokyo, Japan.

0065-1419/80/Suppl. 30/0391/$ 01.00

such as those for involuntary movement. The burr hole was made at 30% frontal point of glabella—inion distance, thus the trajectory to the midbrain never penetrated the pretectal area or the superior colliculus. Intraoperative single neuron recording of the target zone was made with tungsten microelectrode. Homovanillic acid and endorphin were measured in the third ventricular cerebrospinal fluid before and after the electrical stimulation of the target zone.

Results

Out of 15 patients, 11 patients had good results of pain relief. The follow-up period for pain relief was 3 months to 5 years (Table 1). All of these 15 patients had unilateral operations contralateral to the side of pain. Bilateral operation was not performed in order to avoid excessive surgical intervention to the rostral mesencephalon and because the result of the unilateral operation was enough to produce satisfactory pain relief in many of these patients. Postoperative Parinaud's syndrome was avoided because of the new target and trajectory to the midbrain. Intraoperative single neuron recording with tungsten microelectrode showed the presence of many nociceptive neurons in the target zone of RMR. These nociceptive neurons were characterized by large receptive fields and delayed firing in response to peripheral pin-prick stimulation. High frequency electrical stimulation of the medial mesencephalic reticular formation produced severe pain mostly contralateral to the side of stimulation. High frequency electrical stimulation of the periaqueductal gray matter produced evidence of neither pain relief nor pain reproduction but produced autonomic response characterized by pupillary dilatation, tachycardia, flushing of the face and fear sensation. Marked increase in endorphin as well as homovanillic acid [3] in the third ventricular cerebrospinal fluid was observed after high frequency electrical stimulation of the periaqueductal gray matter.

Discussion

First of all, rostral mesencephalic reticulotomy is essentially different from classical mesencephalic tractotomy by Walker [7] or Spiegel and Wycis [6] in which the lateral spinothalamic tract was considered to be the principal pathway conducting pain sensation in the midbrain level. The target of RMR is much more medial than the classical tractotomy [1]. The medial mesencephalic reticular formation bordering the periaqueductal gray matter was chosen for stereotactic target for pain relief [2]. Postoperative Parinaud's syndrome [4, 5] was avoided in cases of RMR using the new trajectory and target. Although the significance of an increase in homovanillic acid [3] and in endorphin in the third ventricular cerebrospinal fluid after the periaqueductal stimulation is still to be further investigated, these neurochemical alterations in the cerebrospinal fluid may be relevant to the mechanism of pain perception.

Table 1. *Rostral Mesencephalic Reticulotomy (RMR) for Pain Relief. Etiology of Pain and Results of the Procedure in 15 Patients*

Cases	Age	Sex	Site of pain	Type of pain	Cause of pain	Results
1. O. Y.	62	m	l. face and arm	thalamic syndrome	CVD	relief
2. W. Y.	47	m	l. leg	thalamic syndrome	CVD	relief
3. O. K.	48	m	l. face and neck	cancer pain	carcinoma	relief
4. H. J.	65	m	l. face	cancer pain	carcinoma	relief
5. M. K.	50	f	r. face	thalamic syndrome	CVD	partial relief
6. K. S.	59	m	l. face and arm	thalamic syndrome	CVD	relief
7. A. K.	60	f	l. face and arm	thalamic syndrome	CVD	relief
8. T. Y.	63	m	r. face and arm	thalamic syndrome	CVD	partial relief
9. K. M.	64	m	r. face and arm	thalamic syndrome	CVD	relief
10. O. T.	47	m	l. face and arm	thalamic syndrome	CVD	partial relief
11. E. K.	50	m	r. arm and leg	thalamic syndrome	CVD	relief
12. K. K.	62	f	r. arm and leg	thalamic syndrome	CVD	relief
13. W. I.	51	m	l. arm and leg	thalamic syndrome	CVD	relief
14. K. S.	49	m	l. arm and face	cancer pain	carcinoma	relief
15. S. T.	64	m	l. trunk and leg	tabes dorsalis	syphilis	partial relief

References

1. Amano, K., Kitamura, K., Sano, K., Sekino, H., Relief of intractable pain from neurosurgical point of view with reference to present limits and clinical indications. A review of 100 consecutive cases. Neurol. Medico-chirur. *16* (1976), 141—153.
2. Amano, K., Tanikawa, T., Iseki, H., Kawabatake, H., Notani, M., Kawamura, H., Kitamura, K., Single neuron analysis of the human midbrain tegmentum. Rostral mesencephalic reticulotomy for pain relief. Appl. Neurophysiol. *41* (1978), 66—78.
3. Amano, K., Notani, M., Iseki, H., Kawabatake, H., Tanikawa, T., Kawamura, H., Kitamura, K., Homovanillic acid concentration of the third ventricular CSF before and after electrical stimulation of the midbrain central gray and the periventricular gray in human. In: Modern concepts in psychiatric surgery, pp. 65—76 (Hitchcock, E. R., *et al.*, eds.). Amsterdam: Elsevier. 1979.
4. Nashold, B. S., Jr., Wilson, W. P., Slaughter, D. G., Sensation evoked by stimulation in the midbrain of man. J. Neurosurg. *30* (1969), 14—24.
5. Nashold, B. S., Jr., Wilson, W. P., Slaughter, D. G., Stereotaxic midbrain lesions for central dysesthesia and phantom pain. J. Neurosurg. *30* (1969), 116—126.
6. Spiegel, E. A., Wycis, H. T., Mesencephalotomy in treatment of intractable facial pain. Amer. Med. Ass. Arch. Neurol. Psychiat. *69* (1953), 1—13.
7. Walker, A. E., Relief of pain by mesencephalic tractotomy. Arch. Neurol. Psychiat. *48* (1942), 865—883.

Acta Neurochirurgica, Suppl. 30, 395—400 (1980)

Stereotactic Lesions Studied by Computer Tomography

G. Kullberg*, **S. Cronqvist**, and **J. Brismar**

With 9 Figures

Repeated CT examinations were performed following stereotactic placement of radiofrequency lesions in 25 patients in order to study the appearance of the lesions.

Methods

10 patients had bipolar coagulation performed in the amygdala, anterior internal capsule or cingulate white matter (Leksell coagulator; paired electrodes 6 mm apart, tip length 6 mm; 65° for 40 seconds). 15 patients had monopolar coagulation in the ventrolateral thalamus (Wyss coagulator; electrode tip 2 × 4 mm; 120–150 mA for 40 seconds). 8 of these patients received peroperative steroid treatment. Electrode position was checked by X-ray. A total of 60 CT examinations were performed at varying time intervals after the operation.

Results

CT changes following amygdalotomy, capsulotomy or cingulotomy were often difficult to define, due to interference from neighbouring anatomical structures. Only 4 out of 9 amygdalotomies were detectable, one is shown in Fig. 1. Following some of the white matter coagulations unexpectedly large areas of decreased attenuation were seen, as exemplified in Fig. 2.

CT changes following thalamotomy were more consistent and the study was therefore focused on this group. The typical thalamic lesion appeared as a rounded area of decreased attenuation with a more or less marked central core of higher density (Fig. 3).

The low density area tended to increase during the first postoperative week, then diminished in size. The central core gradually resolved (Figs. 4 and 5).

---

* Departments of Neurosurgery and Neuroradiology, University Hospital, S-221 85 Lund, Sweden.

0065-1419/80/Suppl. 30/0395/$ 01.20

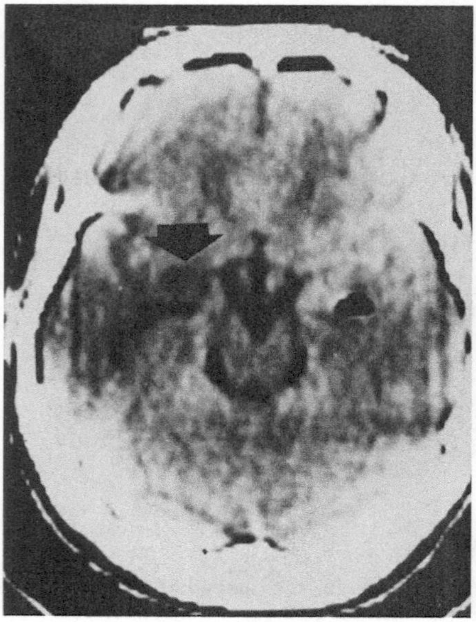

Fig. 1. Amygdalotomy

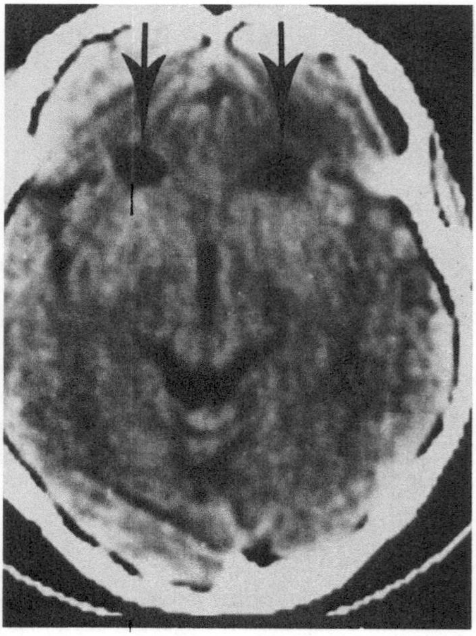

Fig. 2. Capsulotomy

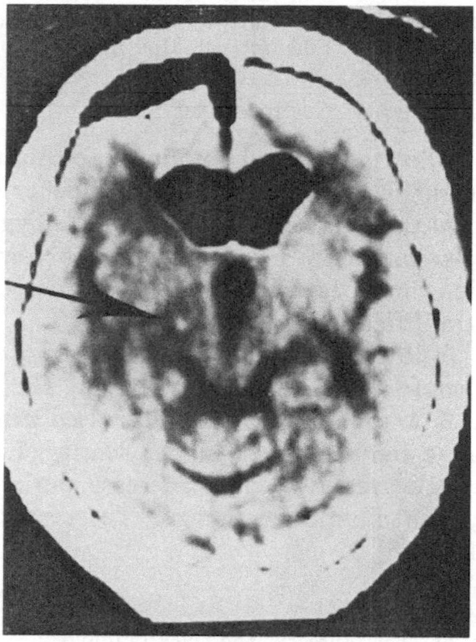

Fig. 3. Thalamotomy

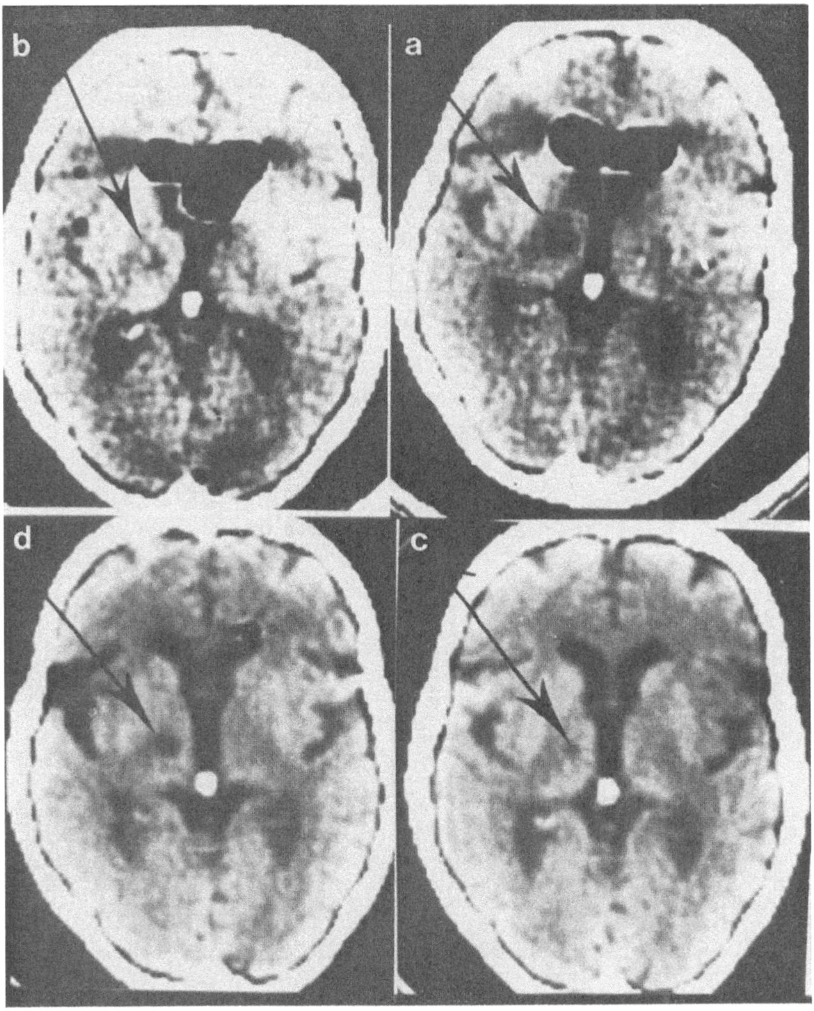

Fig. 4. Serial CT scans days 1 (b), 3 (a), 15 (d), and 50 (c) illustrating the typical temporal course of a thalamic lesion

The relation between the coagulation variable and the size of the lesion, as appearing in CT one week after the operation, is shown in Fig. 6. As expected, lesion size rose with increasing current intensity.

The correspondence between actual and intended localization of the lesions was examined by plotting distance from the midline to

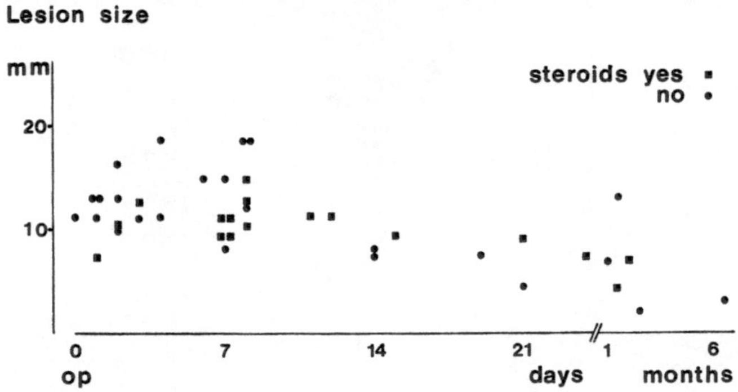

Fig. 5. Size of the talamic lesions as appearing in repeated CT scans in 15 patients

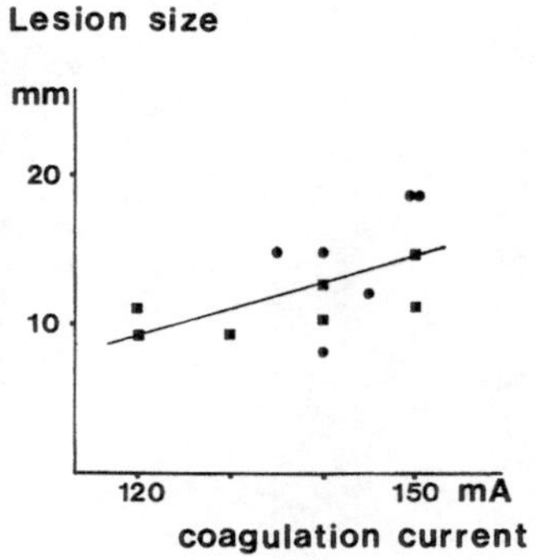

Fig. 6

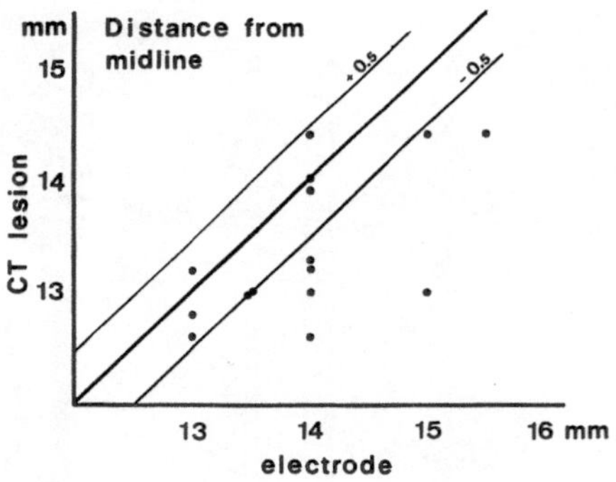

Fig. 7

Fig. 6. Lesion size in CT one week postop in relation to the coagulation variable

Fig. 7. Relation between actual and intended localization of the thalamic lesions

the centre of the CT lesions against electrode position (Fig. 7). There was a fairly good agreement in most cases. Deviations from planned position tended to be in the medial direction.

Damage to the brain along electrode tracks was disclosed by the CT scans in 2 patients. Fig. 8 shows a small haemorrhage above the thalamic target area. Fig. 9 shows rather extensive changes after the introduction of four electrodes on each side towards the amygdala region.

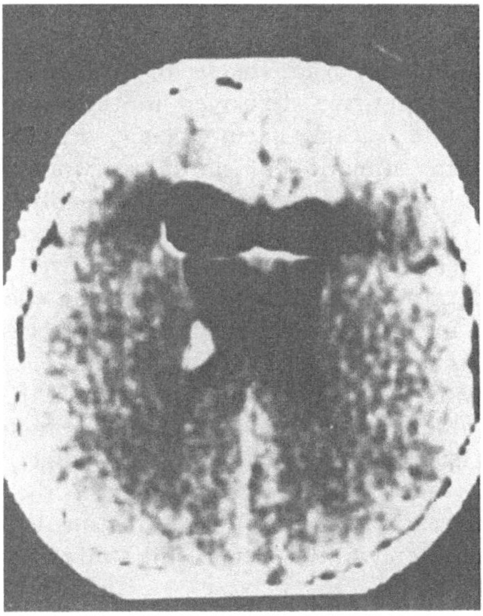

Fig. 8. Haemorrhage above the thalamic target area

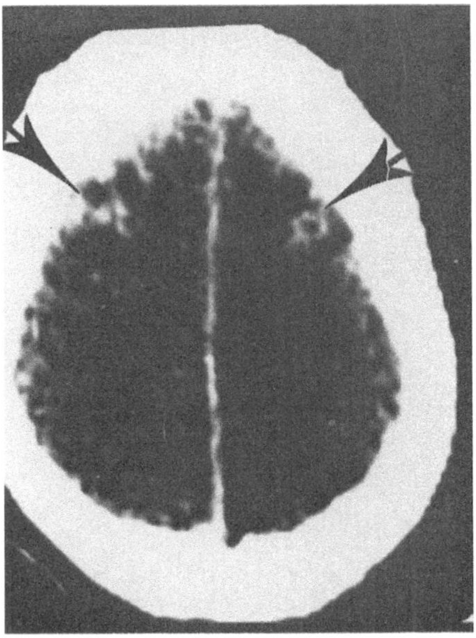

Fig. 9. Extensive changes around electrode tracks

Comments

CT does not provide an exact answer to the question: How large is the portion of brain tissue destroyed in these procedures? The central dense area, often clearly haemorrhagic, may be considered to represent a minimum estimation of the destruction. The maximum size of the surrounding low density area is probably an overestimation of the lesion. Its change in size over time suggests development and regression of oedema—which would also fit well with the common occurrence of transient neurological deficit in the postoperative period. At what time the CT picture accurately reflects the size of the destroyed area cannot be stated. However, CT can be used for relative measurements, for example in comparing different coagulation procedures, if due attention is paid to the time factor.

In the present study the size of the CT changes, including the presumed oedema, tended to be somewhat lower in the steroid treated group but the difference from no steroid treatment was not significant. It is planned to extend this part of the study further.

Acta Neurochirurgica, Suppl. 30, 401—403 (1980)

Long Term Effects of Stereotaxic Thalamotomy on Parameters of Cognitive Functioning

L. M. Modesti* and **A. E. Blumetti****

Summary

Extensive pre- and post-operative neuropsychological evaluation, performed on ten dyskinesic patients undergoing single radiofrequency ventrolateral thalamotomy showed no residual long term loss in cases of familial tremor. All other cases showed minimal to moderate loss of neurobehavioral cognitive abilities.

Keywords: Dyskinesia; cognitive functions; thalamus; stereotaxic thalamotomy.

Introduction

Past research has consistently shown that there are indeed effects of surgically placed thalamic lesions on cognitive functions as measured by psychological tests [2, 3]. The strongest relationship found to date has been between the alteration of language function and left hemisphere thalamotomy [5]. It is also apparent that the measured loss is dependent on the nature of the task and the lesion site. Very little emphasis however, has been placed on the contribution of the medical condition necessitating surgery and the differential post-operative cognitive losses resulting. Previous investigations deal mostly with patient groups suffering from Parkinson's disease, seizure disorders or pain from advanced cancer. In addition, the psychological tests employed are usually standard test of intellectual, personality and motor functioning and not suitable primarily to measure adaptive cognitive abilities dependent on organic brain function. The present research is an initial study attempting to differentiate the long-term effects on neurobehavioural adaptive functions of thalamic lesion in patients with dyskinesiae of differing etiologies.

---

* Department of Neurosurgery, SUNY Upstate Medical Center, and Veterans Administration Medical Center, Syracuse, NY 13210, U.S.A.

** Department of Psychiatry (Psychology), SONY Upstate Medical Center, Syracuse, NY 13210, U.S.A.

0065-1419/80/Suppl. 30/0401/$ 01.00

Method

Ten patients, ranging in age from 31 to 65 years underwent unilateral stereotaxic thalamotomy with a single radiofrequency lesion placed in the ventro-lateral (VL) nucleus of the thalamus for relief of dyskinesia. Three patients were diagnosed as having heredofamilial tremor while the other patients had a diagnosis of Parkinsonism, and multiple sclerosis. Stereotaxic surgery was carried out in two stages as described by Andrew *et al.* [1]. After preliminary single unit microelectrode recording or monopolar stimulation, or both under local anaesthesia, radiofrequency lesion is made with an electrode tip of 5 mm and with a current up to 65–70 °C for 150 seconds. The average size of our lesion is 6–7 mm in length and 3–4 mm in diameter.

A single left VL nucleus lesion was made in 3 patients, while the remaining 7 patients had right VL lesions.

All patients underwent extensive neuropsychological testing at least one week prior to surgical intervention, within 3–4 weeks post-operatively and again 12 to 24 months after surgery. In addition to a Mental Status Examination, the Wechsler Adult Intelligence Scale, the Wechsler Memory Scale and the Halstead-Reitan Neuropsychological Test Battery [4] were administered.

Results

Test data indicate deterioration of both receptive and expressive verbal performances and attention immediately after surgery in all cases, with more loss noted after left VL lesions and with significant improvement over time. Non-verbal memory impairment in terms of both recollection and recall was noted more after (R) VL lesions with improvement over time. Classifying adaptive cognitive ability as measured by the various tests into the four categories of processing, memory, attention and emotion [6], it was found that only in the three cases of familial tremor (two right and one left) was there no residual loss on long-term evaluation in any of the functions with consistent improvement post-operatively. In all other cases, minimal to moderate impairment was found in at least two categories in this classification. Most severe impairment was found in cases of Parkinsonism while minimal residuals were found in patients with disseminated sclerosis.

Discussion

It is clear that extremely sophisticated measures of cognitive functioning indicate involvement of the VL nuclei of the thalamus in higher level adaptive abilities. Although the number of cases in this initial study is small, the interaction effect of disease entity and perhaps premorbid level of cerebral integrity play an important role in long-term effect in cognitive skills when surgery is performed to relieve a primary motor disturbance.

References

1. Andrew, J., Rice Edwards, J. M., de M. Rudolf, N., The placement of stereotaxic lesions for involuntary movements other than in Parkinson's disease. Acta Neurochir. (Wien) Suppl. *21* (1974), 39—47.
2. Andy, O. J., Jurko, M. F., Giurintano, L. P., Behavioral changes correlated with thalamotomy site. Confin. Neurol. *36* (1974), 106—112.
3. Jurko, M. F., Andy, O. J., Psychological changes correlated with thalamotomy site. J. Neurol. Neurosurg. Psychiat. *36* (1973), 846—852.
4. Reitan, R. M., Davidson, L. A., Clinical neuropsychology, current status and application. Washington, D.C.: V. H. Winston. 1974.
5. Riklan, M., Cooper, I. S., Psychometric studies of verbal functions following thalamic lesions in humans. Brain and Language *2* (1975), 45—64.
6. Watson, R. T., Heilman, K. M., The differential diagnosis of dementia. Geriatrics *29* (1974), 145.

Acta Neurochirurgica, Suppl. 30, 405—412 (1980)

Stereotaxic Clipping of Arterial and Arteriovenous Aneurysms of the Brain

E. I. Kandel* and **V. V. Peresedov***

With 5 Figures

Summary

A new method of stereotaxic clipping of arterial and AV aneurysms has been developed. The surgical technique and the special clipping device are briefly described. Successful results have been obtained in 30 clipping operations performed on 27 patients with arterial or AV aneurysms at different locations with follow-up ranging from 6 months to 6 years. There was one fatal outcome not directly related to the clipping operation.

Keywords: Arterial aneurysms; arteriovenous aneurysms; stereotaxic surgery; stereotaxic clipping.

Introduction

In spite of remarkable improvement in the results of direct attack on arterial and arterio-venous (AV) aneurysms the technical difficulties and rate of complications remain unsolved problems. An intensive search for new surgical treatment of the aneurysms is continuing in an effort to reduce the rate of serious complications and mortality. With this aim several years ago we developed a new technique of stereotaxic clipping of cerebral aneurysms through a burr hole [4, 5].

Method and Material

After a 3 or 4 vessel angiographic study and exact diagnosis of arterial or AV aneurysms the preoperative calculations on angiograms were made. The aim of the calculations was the choosing of the point of clipping of the feeding vessel or the aneurysmal neck, the location of burrhole and the plane of clip opening. The geometrical methods used permitted us to find the interrelations between the axis of the artery or the neck, the plane of clip opening and the axis of the device for stereotaxic clipping. The preoperative calculations were also used to perform clipping on a special model of the brain arteries.

---

* Neurosurgical Clinic, Institute of Neurology, Moscow D-367, USSR.

0065-1419/80/Suppl. 30/0405/$ 01.60

Our special device for stereotaxic clipping (Fig. 1) was constructed for use with our stereotaxic apparatus previously described [3]. The device is a stainless steel tube 17 cm long and 3.2 mm in outer diameter. At the outer end of the device is a special structure for controlling clip movements and disconnecting the clip from the device. The special removable stainless steel clips of different size permit the clipping of vessels from 1 to 7 mm in diameter.

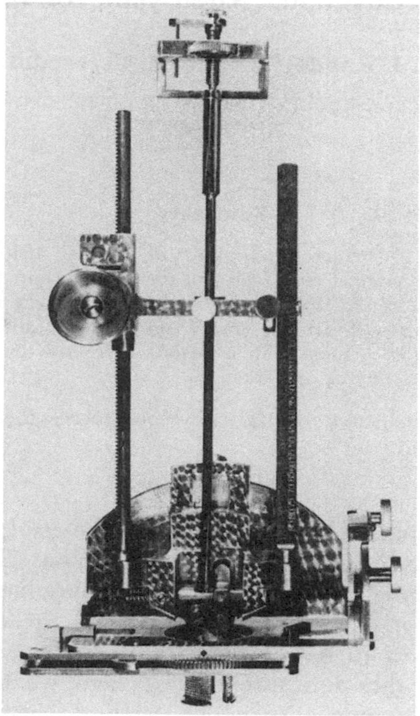

Fig. 1. Device for stereotaxic clipping combined with stereotaxic apparatus

All operations were carried out under general anaesthesia or neuroleptoanalgesia. A plastic catheter was inserted percutaneously into the carotid artery for repeated intraoperative angiography. The patient's head was placed supine in a headholder. The clipping device was attached to the stereotaxic apparatus fixed in a burrhole at the previously choosen point (more often near the coronal suture).

The target point was transferred from the angiograms to the plain films taken on the operating table. Stereotaxic calculation was made for the correct orientation of the clipping device. All operations were made under the control of a image amplifier with TV monitoring.

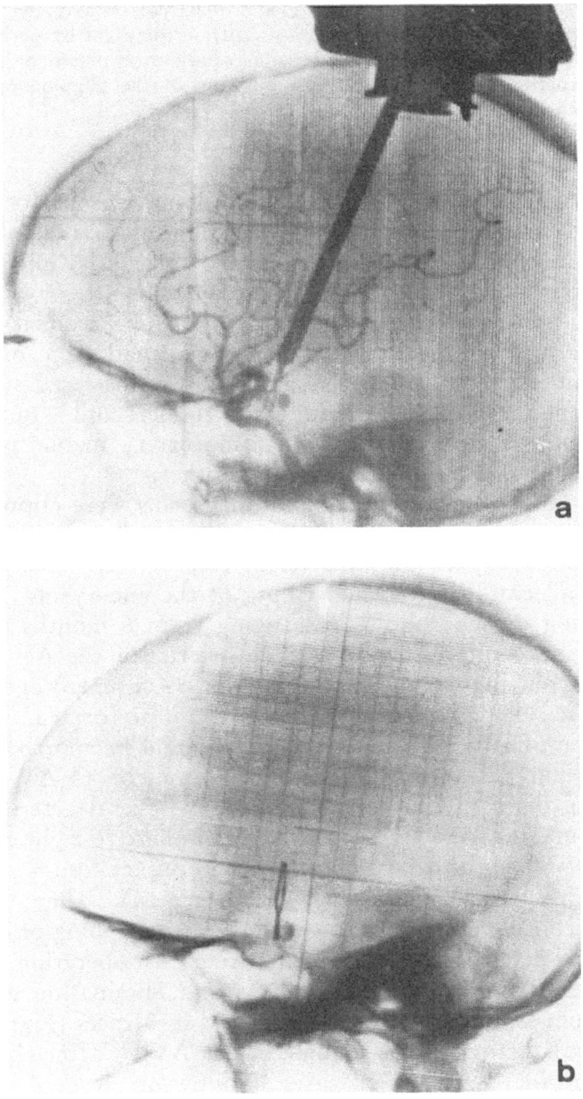

Fig. 2. Supraclinoid internal carotid aneurysm during the operation. a) angiogram before clipping through burrhole; b) plain film shortly after operation. Note the remains of contrast medium in the sac after clipping of the neck of the aneurysm

After the tip of the pivot touched the target point the clip was opened, put on the vessel or aneurysmal neck and closed. The correct clipping was checked by control angiography. The clip was released from the pivot by pushing a button on the outer part of the device. If it is necessary to clip two or more vessels, the entire procedure was repeated. The duration of the clipping operation was between 1.5 and 2 hours.

Results

The first operation of stereotaxic clipping was performed by us in 1973. To date we have done 30 operations on 27 carefully selected patients—14 operations on 13 patients with arterial aneurysms and 16 operations on 14 patients with AV aneurysms.

Patients with arterial aneurysms (5 men and 8 women) were aged between 22 and 53 years. All patients have had from one to three subarachnoid haemorrhages. The angiography disclosed supraclinoid aneurysms of the ICA in 11 cases (7 on the left and 4 on the right), aneurysm of the anterior communicating artery in one patient and aneurysm of the frontopolar artery in another.

The necks of the 11 supraclinoid aneurysms were clipped (Figs. 2 and 3); in two other cases the clips were put on the dominant anterior cerebral and the pericallosal arteries respectively. Control angiography in all cases showed non-filling of the aneurysms. There was no rebleeding during follow-up, ranging from 6 months to 6 years.

Stereotaxic clipping of the feeding arteries of the AV aneurysms was carried out in 14 patients (10 men and 4 women) aged from 13 to 45 years. 16 clipping operations were performed. The main clinical symptoms in all cases were intracranial haemorrhages and/or epileptic seizures, severe headache, etc. 12 out of 14 AV aneurysms were of big or giant size and were fed by several arterial systems. 11 AV aneurysms were located in the hemisphere (6 right and 5 left), 2 in the region of third ventricle and corpus callosum and one in the interhemispheric fissure (frontobasal region). They were deep-seated and considered as radically inoperable. Clipping of one or two main feeding arteries was performed during each operation.

Control angiography showed that total elimination of AV aneurysms from the circulation was achieved in 3 cases (Figs. 4 and 5). Significant reduction of the volume of the AVA's after clipping was disclosed in the majority of cases. Follow-up from 4 months to 6 years has shown substantial clinical improvement in 13 out of the 14 patients (cessation of the intracranial haemorrhages, disappearance of epileptic fits, headache, etc.).

There were 3 complications after 30 operations: in one case there was moderate hemiparesis lasting several days and after two operations the clips slipped. In both cases a second successful clipping

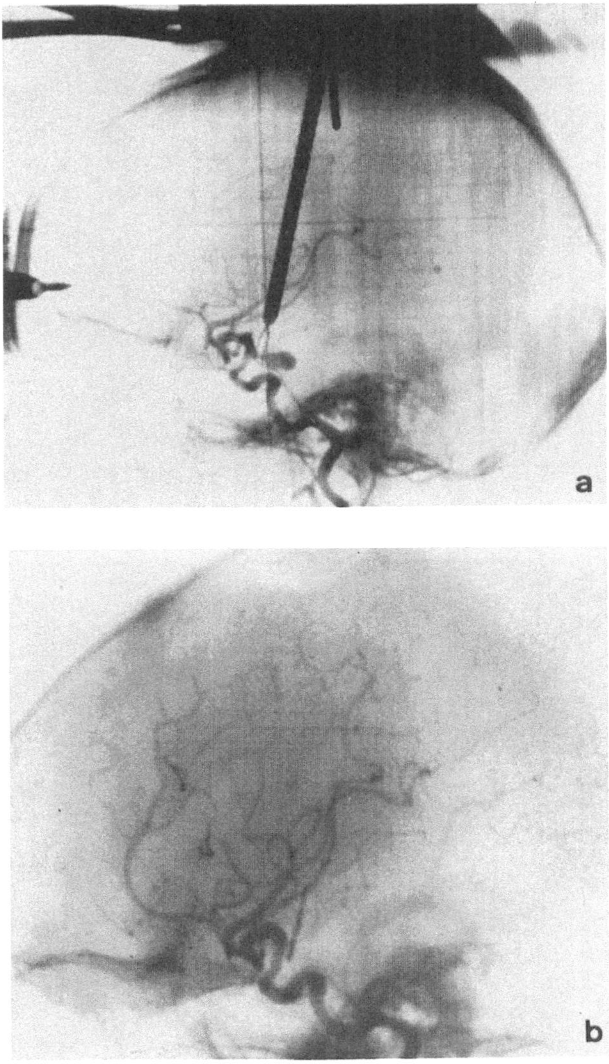

Fig. 3. Supraclinoid internal carotid aneurysm. a) Just before stereotaxic clipping during the operation; b) 2 weeks after operation

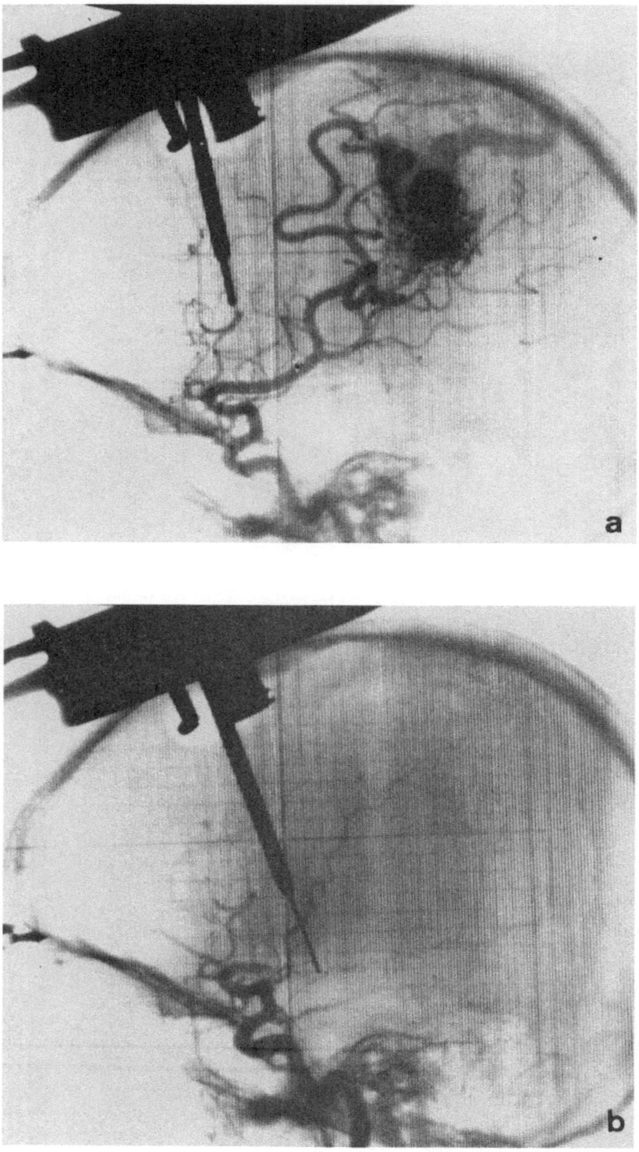

Fig. 4. Angiograms showing a big AVA, supplied by hypertrophic branch of the middle cerebral artery during the operation. a) The stereotaxic direction of the clipping device to the choosen target point on the artery. b) After clipping the aneurysm did not fill

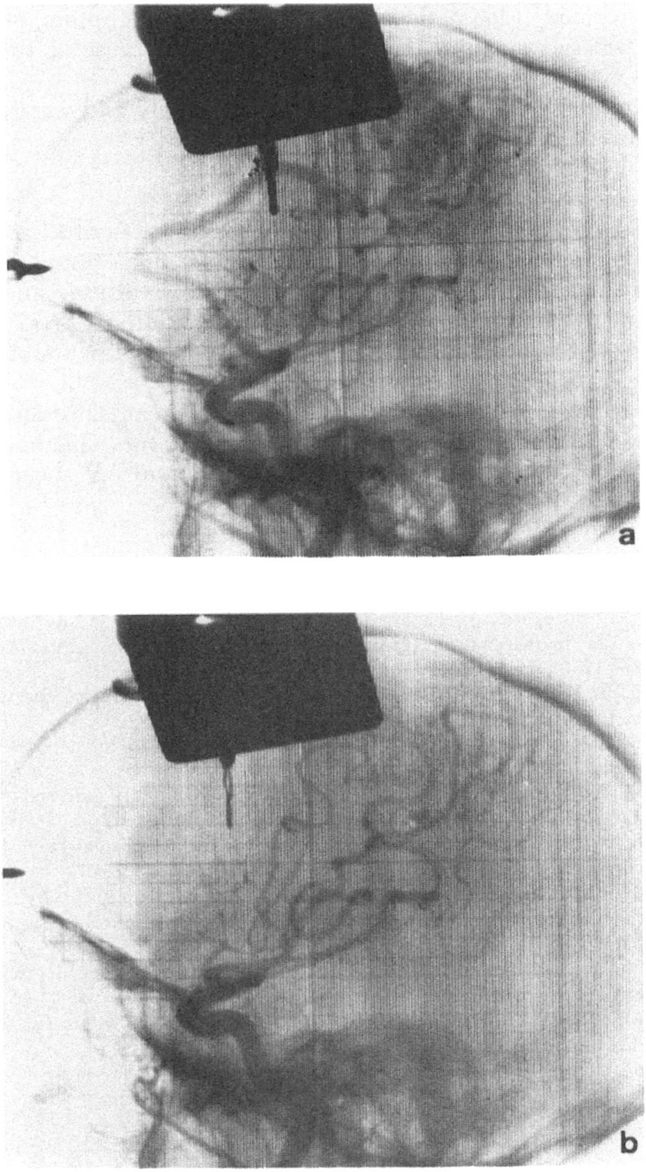

Fig. 5. Angiograms of the big AVA, supplied by an enlarged pericallosal artery. a) During the operation before clipping of the artery. b) Nonfilling of the aneurysm after clipping

was performed. One patient died after successful clipping of a supraclinoid arterial aneurysm from haemorrhage because of the rupture of an AV aneurysm in the same hemisphere.

All patients endured the operation very easily and were ambulant 2 to 4 days after surgery.

Discussion

Guiot *et al.* [2] and Riechert and Mundinger [8] described a combination of stereotaxic technique and the classic open craniotomy used in several cases of arterial and AV aneurysms. Alksne and Rand [1], Rand and Mosso [7], Mullan [6], Samotokin and Hilko [9] used the technique of stereotaxic puncture of the arterial aneurysms for thrombosis by using a suspension of iron or electric current.

We believe that stereotaxic clipping has some substantional advantages. It is reasonable to suppose that the new method will be rational and useful in selected cases of arterial and AV aneurysms.

References

1. Alksne, J. F., Progress on the magnetically controlled stereotactic thrombosis of intracranial aneurysms. Confin. Neurol. *34* (1972), 368—373.
2. Guiot, G., Rougerie, J., Sachs, M., Hertzog, E., Molina, P., Repérage stéréotaxique de malformations vasculaires profondes intracérébrales. Sem. Hôp. Paris *36* (1960), 1134—1143.
3. Kandel, E. I., New stereotactic apparatus and cryogenic device for stereotactic surgery. Confin. Neurol. *37* (1975), 128—132.
4. Kandel, E. I., Peresedov, V. V., Stereotactic clipping of an arterial aneurysm of the brain. Vopr. Neirokhir. *39* (1975), 13—15 (Rus.).
5. Kandel, E. I., Peresedov, V. V., Stereotaxic clipping of arterial aneurysms and arteriovenous malformations. J. Neurosurg. *46* (1977), 12—23.
6. Mullan, S., Experiences with surgical thrombosis of intracranial berry aneurysms and carotid cavernous fistulas. J. Neurosurg. *41* (1974), 657—671.
7. Rand, R. W., Mosso, J. A., Treatment of cerebral aneurysms by stereotaxic ferromagnetic silicone thrombosis. Bull. Los Angeles Neurol. Soc. *38* (1972), 21—23.
8. Riechert, T., Mundinger, F., Combined stereotaxic operation for treatment of deep-seated angiomas and aneurysms. J. Neurosurg. *21* (1964), 358—363.
9. Samotokin B. A., Hilko, V. A., Aneurysms and arteriovenous fistulas of the brain. Leningrad: Meditsina. 1973 (Russ.).

Acta Neurochirurgica, Suppl. 30, 413—416 (1980)

Combined Approach (Stereotactic-Microsurgical) to a Paraventricular Arteriovenous Malformation

Case Report

R. Garcia de Sola*, J. Cabezudo, E. Areitio, and **G. Bravo**

With 3 Figures

Summary

The authors present one case of a 42 years old male patient who had a small right paraventricular arteriovenous malformation. At operation the patient was placed in the Talairach's stereotactic frame and, after performing a right carotid angiogram to locate the lesion exactly, a flexible cannula was inserted stereotactically, through a previous trephine hole, until the tip reached the AVM. Using a microsurgical technique and through a 1–2 cm corticotomy the cannula pathway was followed easily reaching the AVM. Total removal of the AVM was confirmed by a carotid angiogram, the patient was discharged without symptoms 7 days later.

The authors propose that due to the special design of the Talairach's stereotactic frame, its application as a locating system for small and deep AVM's would greatly facilitate their removal using microsurgical techniques.

Keywords: Paraventricular arteriovenous malformation.

Introduction

Complete surgical removal without producing deficits is the ideal treatment of intracranial arteriovenous malformation (AVM). Some present formidable technical difficulties. Small paraventricular AVM's are included in this group and are usually regarded as inoperable [6] or likely to lead to considerable morbidity and mortality after attempts at surgical excision [3], which are frequently incomplete.

Considering the special design of the Talairach's stereotactic frame, we suggest its application as a localizing procedure for small

---

* Service of Neurosurgery, Clinica Puerta de Hierro, Universidad Autonoma de Madrid, Spain.

0065-1419/80/Suppl. 30/0413/$ 01.00

and deep AVM's which facilitates the removal of these AVM's using microsurgical techniques.

Case Report

Our presentation concerns a 42-year-old man who developed an acute clinical syndrome of headaches, vomits, left hemiparesis and progressive coma. A CT scan showed a massive intraventricular haemorrhage but the patient recovered from

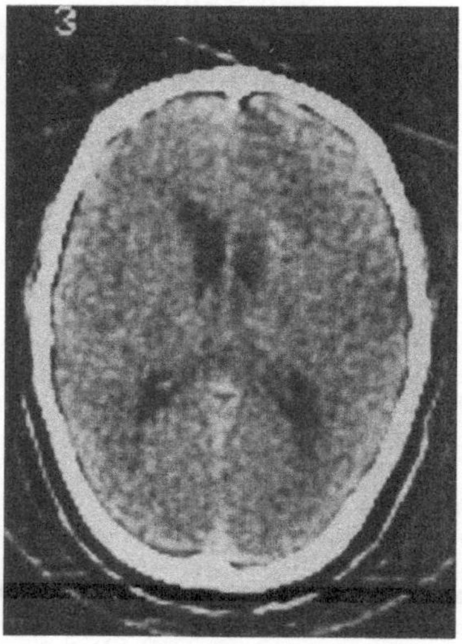

Fig. 1. CT scan showing the right paraventricular AVM as a nodular impression with positive enhancement in the outer wall of the frontal horn

coma and hemiparesis with conservative measures. A new CT scan showed a small nodular impression with positive enhancement in the outer wall of the frontal horn of the right ventricle (Fig. 1). A right carotid angiogram revealed a small AVM with its feeder vessels coming from a branch of the anterior cerebral artery and draining to the internal cerebral vein.

The patient was placed in the Talairach's stereotactic frame and a carotid angiogram was performed by direct carotid puncture, using a G-18 Abocath catheter which was left in place (Fig. 2), the AVM was stereotactically localized. After performing a paramedial trephine hole in front of the coronal suture, a flexible cannula was inserted through the oblique grid, until the tip was placed at the target point of the AP and lateral grids, which corresponded to the location of the AVM. Using microsurgical techniques, and through a 1–2 cm cortical excision, the course of the cannula was followed. It was not difficult to reach the AVM and totally remove it, a control angiograms showed the total excision of the AVM (Fig. 3). The patient was discharged from hospital seven days later without any neurologic sequelae.

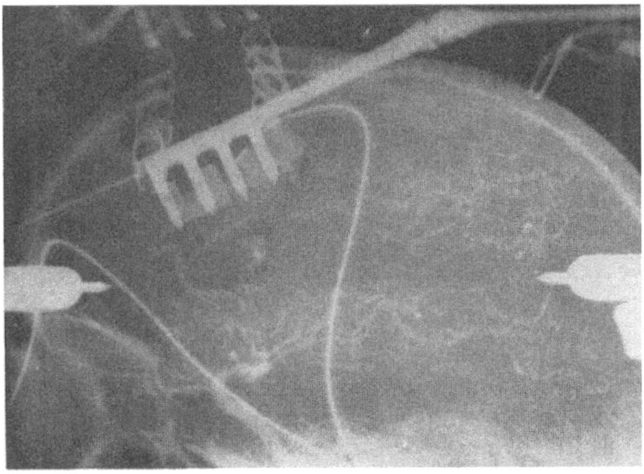

Fig. 2. Stereotactic carotid angiogram. The small paraventricular (frontal horn) AVM

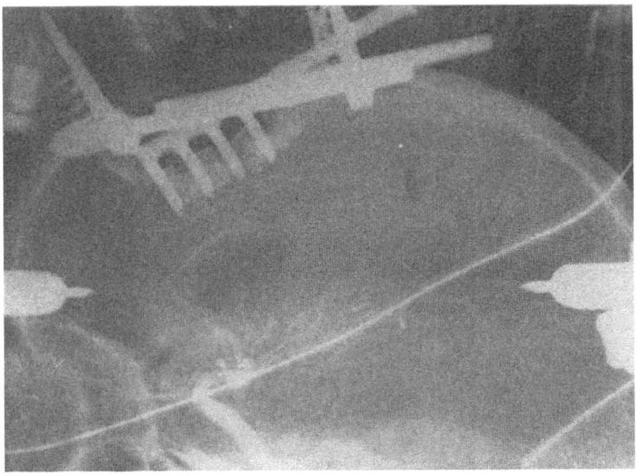

Fig. 3. Control angiogram shows the total removal of the AVM and an air-level in the frontal horn which was opened at the moment of the excision of the AVM

Discussion

Different stereotactic approaches have been used (radiosurgery [9], coagulation [2] and clipping of feeders [5] to overcome some of the difficulties in the surgical treatment of small paraventricular AVM's.

We think that the approach used in our case (described originally by Guiot *et al.* (1960) and later used by other authors [1, 7, 8] guarantees the total removal of the small and deep AVM's with the minimum of complications, combining the exact localization of the AVM with the stereotactic system and the accuracy of the microsurgical technique.

References

1. Bushe, K. A., Bockhorn, J., Schäfer, E. R., Macro- and Microsurgery of Central Angiomas. In: Cerebral Angiomas. Advances in Diagnosis and Therapy, pp. 123—128 (Pia, H. W., *et al.*, eds.). Berlin-Heidelberg-New York: Springer. 1975.
2. Cahan, L. D., Rand, R. W., Stereotactic coagulation of a Paraventricular Arteriovenous Malformation. Case Report. J. Neurosurg. *39* (1973), 770—774.
3. Discussion in Chapter V. In: Cerebral Angiomas. Advances in Diagnosis and Therapy, pp. 178—182 (Pia, H. W., *et al.*, eds.). Berlin-Heidelberg-New York: Springer. 1975.
4. Guiot, G., Rougerie, J., Sachs, M., Herzog, E., Molina, P., Repérage stéréotaxique de malformations vasculaires profondes intracérébrales. Sem. Hôp. Paris *36* (1960), 1134—1143.
5. Kandel, E. J., Peresedov, V. V., Stereotaxic Clipping of Arterial Aneurysms and Arteriovenous Malformations. J. Neurosurg. *46* (1977), 12—23.
6. Perret, G., The Epidemiology and Clinical Course of Arteriovenous Malformations. In: Cerebral Angiomas. Advances in Diagnosis and Therapy, pp. 21—26 (Pia, H. W., *et al.*, eds.). Berlin-Heidelberg-New York: Springer. 1975.
7. Riecher, T., Mundinger, F., Combined stereotaxic operation for treatment of deep-seated angiomas and aneurysms. J. Neurosurg. *21* (1964), 358—363.
8. Riechert, T., Stereotactic Treatment of Central Angiomas. In: Cerebral Angiomas. Advances in Diagnosis and Therapy, pp. 129—135 (Pia, H. W., *et al.*, eds.). Berlin-Heidelberg-New York: Springer. 1975.
9. Steiner, L., Leksell, L., Forster, D. M. C., Greitz, T., Backlund, E. D., Stereotactic Radiosurgery in Intracranial Arteriovenous Malformations. Acta Neurochir. (Wien) Suppl. *21* (1974), 195—209.

Acta Neurochirurgica, Suppl. 30, 417—421 (1980)

Investigations Concerning Motor Control in Patients Suffering from Various Lesions of Sensory-Motor Systems*

A. Struppler, F. Erbel, C. H. Lücking,** and **F. Velho**

With 7 Figures

Summary

Motor control in patients following thalamotomy and subthalamotomy as well as in patients with ataxia due to dorsal column lesion or spino-cerebellar degeneration was compared with the results in normal subjects. Responses to external forces applied to the elbow joint and their compensation were analysed. The results give evidence for loss of adaptive functions to compensate for external disturbances in patients with hypotonia.

Stereotaxic interventions give the opportunity to investigate motor control in alert human subjects following well defined subcortical lesions. Our interest in the control mechanisms of different kinds of motor performances, encouraged investigation of the muscles of the arm which are important for both supporting reactions (posture) and goal directed movements.

Keywords: Thalamotomy; subthalamotomy; hypotonia; functional stretch reflexes.

Methods

The investigations were done simultaneously on the normal and the affected side to compare motor performance on an identical background of alertness. The effect of concentrating on the performance of one arm could be studied.

The external forces were applied to the elbow joints by two identical torque machines electrically coupled in series. The points could be either extended or flexed. The patients were asked to innervate the flexors isometrically against an initial torque and were instructed to resist any additional externally applied torque and to compensate for the displacement. The EMG of the brachialis and triceps muscles as well as the angular displacements were recorded on both sides (Struppler *et al.* 1978 a and 1978 b).

---

* Supported by: Deutsche Forschungsgemeinschaft (SFB 50 Kybernetik).

** Neurologische Klinik der Technischen Universität, Möhlstrasse 28, D-8000 München 80, Federal Republic of Germany.

0065-1419/80/Suppl. 30/0417/$ 01.00

Results

When the isometrically innervated muscle of a normal subject is suddenly stretched, the EMG shows 3 distinct synchronized peaks of activity with characteristic latencies (Hammond 1956).

The first peak has the latency of the proprioceptive reflex (20–25 milliseconds) on a segmental level. The second peak has a latency of about 60 milliseconds. This is shorter than the shortest

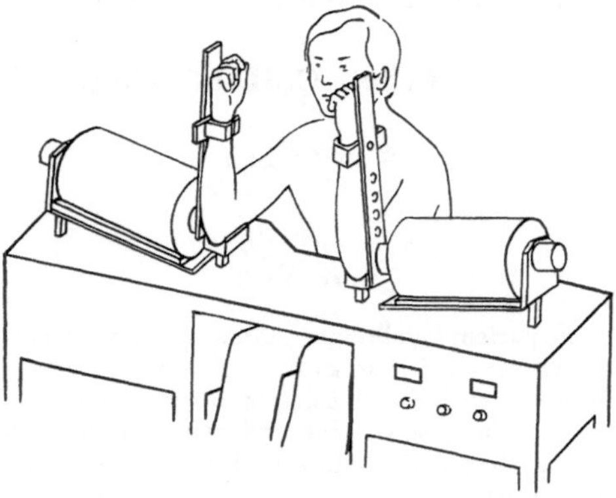

Fig. 1. Initial torque: 2–6 Nm. Disturbance torque: 4–14 Nm. EMG: brachial m. + triceps m. Muscle spindle afferents recording in musculocutaneous nerve mechanogram of the elbow joint

reaction time to kinaesthetic stimuli. This response is probably mediated by supraspinal systems. The third peak appears after 90 milliseconds. It seems obvious that it is transmitted via the cerebral cortex (long-loop reflex).

In patients following thalamotomy and subthalamotomy these 3 short latency components showed a deficiency.

The compensation of the external disturbance was mainly achieved by voluntary activity which by itself led to an overshooting movement.

Following active unloading the arm of the operated side swang back farther.

The EMG showed two phenomena: there was no stretch reflex in the antagonist and the activity in the agonist following the silent period was decreased.

A different type of hypotonia could be studied in a patient with spino-cerebellar degeneration combined with areflexia. When the patient was asked to compensate for an externally applied stretch to the muscle, he showed none of the 2 short latency components (Fig. 5).

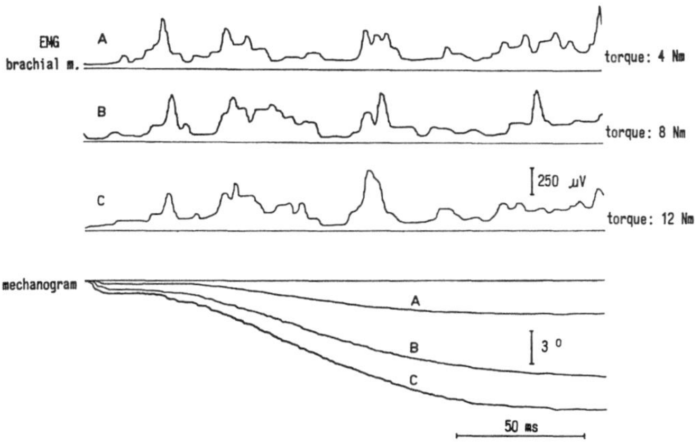

Fig. 2. Load compensation of a torque induced disturbance of an isometrically contracted muscle

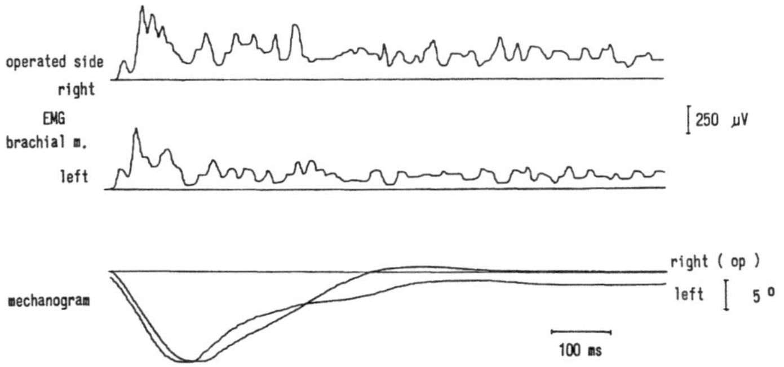

Fig. 3. Load compensation of a torque induced disturbance of isometrically contracted muscles. Hemiparkinsonism, following stereoencephalotomy. Simultaneously bilaterally applied disturbance

The compensation was achieved only by voluntary activity. Following unloading there were two phenomena (Fig. 6):

As in patients with stereotaxic lesions, there was no stretch reflex in the antagonist, unlike patients with stereotaxic lesions, however, there was no silent period (unloading reflex) in the agonist. In a patient with an unilateral lesion of the dorsal column the displacement of the arm by the external force was always larger on the affected side. Following stretching of the muscle, the EMG showed a relatively unaffected first component whereas the second and third components were distinctly decreased (Fig. 7).

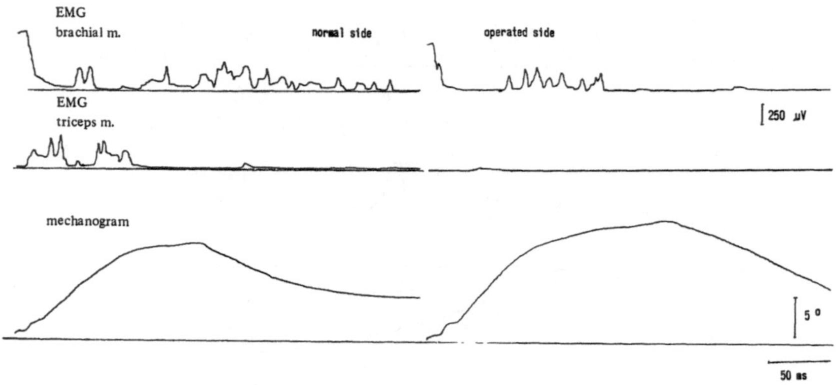

Fig. 4. Effect of active unloading on isometrically contracted muscles. Hemi-parkinsonism, following stereoencephalotomy

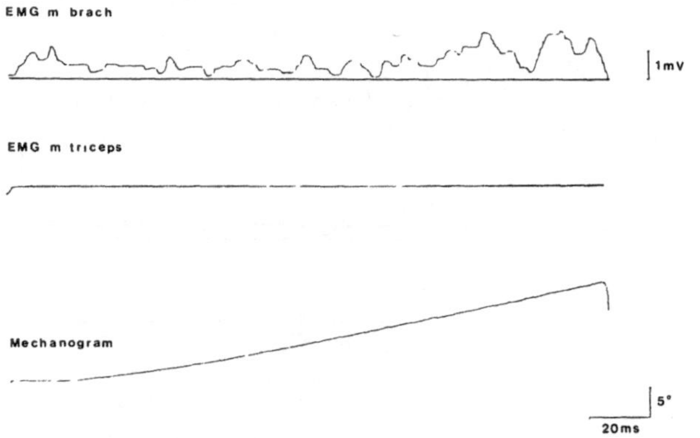

Fig. 5. Hypotonia-areflexia (M. W. ♂). Compensation from disturbance load (unloading)

Discussion

The decrease of the tonic component of motor control is clinically known as hypotonia. It can be found in the following conditions. 1. Spinal deafferentation (tabes dorsalis): the spindle drive is diminished; 2. cerebellar lesions: this type of hypotonia is possibly caused by a deficit of gamma drive; 3. selective blockade of gamma fibres in the peripheral nerve (differential block) which decreases the sensitivity of the spindle receptors; 4. thalamotomy and subthalamotomy for which, there is only indirect evidence on the role of the gamma loop in this type of hypotonia.

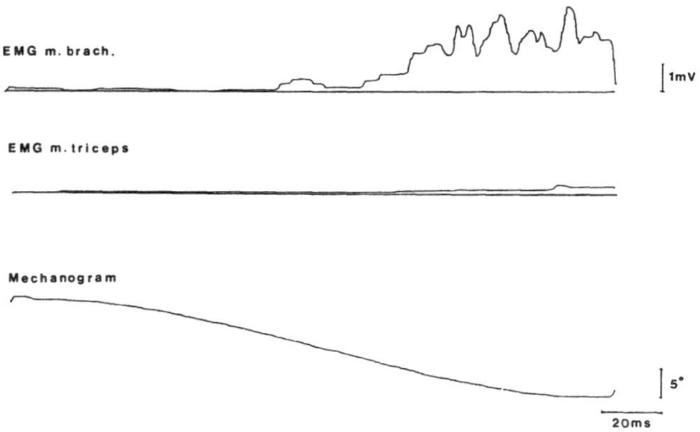

Fig. 6. Hypotonia-areflexia (M. W. ♂). Compensation from disturbance load (stretch)

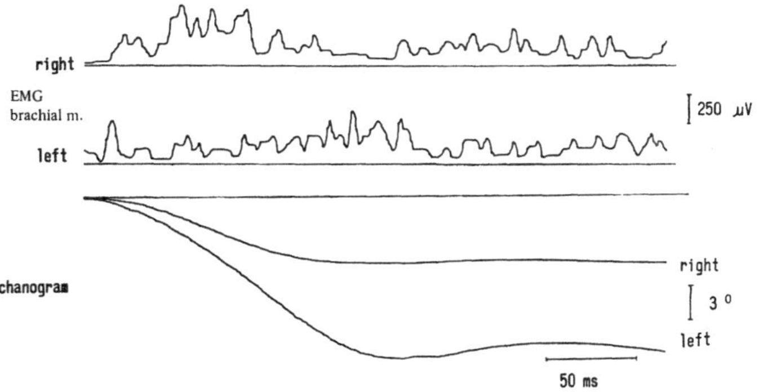

Fig. 7. Load compensation of a torque induced disturbance of isometrically contracted muscles. Left dorsal column lesion

Acknowledgement

The torque machine was constructed in cooperation with Prof. Dr. Lorenzen, Technische Universität München.

References

Hammond, P. H., The influence of prior instruction to the subject on an apparently involuntary neuromuscular response. J. Physiol. (London) *132* (1956), 17.

Struppler, A., *et al.*, Mode of innervation following stereoencephalotomy. Contemp. Clin. Neurophysiol. (EEG Suppl. No. 34), pp. 494—500. Amsterdam: Elsevier.

— Motor control analysis during stereoencephalotomy. Advances in Neurosurgery (in press). Berlin-Heidelberg-New York: Springer.

Acknowledgement

References

Acta Neurochirurgica, Suppl. 30, 423—428 (1980)

Evoked Responses by Physiological Sensory Inputs in Human Central Motor Structures

J. Vajda*, Sz. Tóth, and A. Sólyom

With 5 Figures

Summary

In human with chronic implanted electrodes physiological evoked responses could be detected from those structures they were thought to be parts mainly of central motor system. Investigating the functional changes of evoked responses to motor states and attention the results have suggested the responses do not sign the centres to treat as directly the sensory inputs *i.e.* auditory, visual, somatosensory stimuli as motor stimuli.

Keywords: Central motor system; implanted electrodes; sensory evoked responses; functional dependency.

The nature, localization, functional changes of scalp auditory (AER), visual (VER) and somatosensory (SSER) evoked responses are commonly investigated and could be considered as a well known problem. Though stereotactic implantation of chronic electrodes in different diseases is relatively common, the question of these physiological evoked responses from different structures is rarely put forward in the literature. Haider *et al.*[3], Wilson and Nashold[6], Fukushima *et al.*[2], Ervin and Mark[1] have written about AER, VER and SSER from thalamic, middle temporal and midbrain areas that were thought to be specific responses of registered structures, and the result of these investigations has become emphasized as necessary for determination of proper position of implanted electrodes. In our material these evoked responses, occurred so widely in the central motor system that we believe they may not necessarily be a function of the registered structure alone.

We considered three mechanisms which could be involved in development of these responses: 1. registered region takes part in

* National Institute of Neurosurgery, Budapest, Hungary.

0065-1419/80/Suppl. 30/0423/$ 01.20

the treatment directly of these stimuli but was not obvious before. 2. Registered area does not treat the stimuli, the evoked potentials pass through only, "passive behaviour". 3. There is a centre near to the observed structure that is a part of the system specific to the very input.

Table 1. *Latencies in Milliseconds*

AER

Component of responses	Motor cortex	VL	AD-VPL	Pall.	Dent.	Cerebel. cortex
Early		30	60	40 50	60	40
Middle	100 180	95	110 160	100 150	100	90
Late	250	300		280 360		240

VER

Component of responses	Motor cortex	VL	AD-VPL	Pall.	Dent.	Cerebel. cortex
Early	80	90	80 100		80	60
Middle	120	150	125 180	150	130 160	150
Late	220			220 300	400	260

SSER

Component of responses	Motor cortex	VL	AD-VPL	Pall.	Dent.	Cerebel. cortex
Early	40	35	25	30	40	
Middle	80 130	100	60 120	70 160	70 150	
Late		220	220			

Previously investigating the motor system we observed a marked functional dependence of evoked responses stimulating within the motor system [4]. In the active areas the evoked answers particularly their reflex correlated potential-parts (between 30 and 80 milliseconds latency) show remarkable increase during voluntary contraction and decrease elsewhere [5].

Material and Methods

Chronic electrodes were implanted in the motor cortex, pallidum, ventrolateral thalamic nucleus, anterior dorsal-ventrolateral posterior nucleus-complex of thalamus, and in other sided cerebellar cortex as well as brachium conjunctivum—dentate nucleus complex in 53 patients with various disorders (motor disturbances, pain syndrome, epilepsy). A tone pip (60 dB and 90 dB, 1,000 Hz, 20 ms) was applied to patients through loudspeaker at a distance of 20 cm. Two ranges of flash-light (20 ms) was applied to the patients with closed eyes. The appropriate sided hallux was stimulated as a somatosensory stimulus with square-wave impulses (200 V, 0.3 ms). 40 or 100 evoked responses were averaged. These procedures were repeated during different functional states as voluntary contraction, reading, counting, or applying touch on both legs.

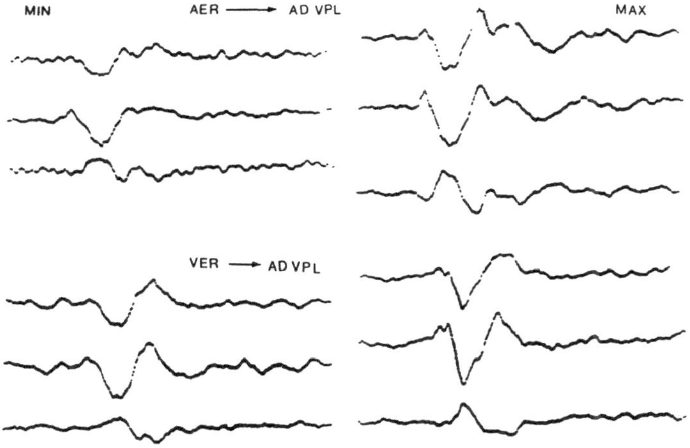

Fig. 1. 40 averaged auditory and visual responses from left thalamus (dwell time: 600 ms). Upper two traces are from *VPL*, lower trace from *AD*. Each evoked responsepart is uniformly dependent to stimulation-level

Results

In the vast majority of our cases AER, VER, SSER with various amplitudes and latencies could be observed. They were usually the early, middle and late component about 30–80, 100–180 and 220–360 milliseconds respectively. The shortest latencies are shown in the cases of somatosensory stimulation, being just the half of visual responses (Table 1).

Amplitudes increased passively or were unchanged on higher level of stimulation (Fig. 1). Few differences appeared between auditory and visual responses in the same registered structure. Comparing the sensory evoked responses from motor cortex and from dentate nucleus obtained in rest with those obtained during voluntary contraction marked reduction of all parts of evoked responses could be detected (Fig. 2), while evoked responses from ventrolateral thalamus and pallidum did not show functional changes (Fig. 3). Marked decrease occurred, however, when the patient was asked to read (Fig. 4), as well as to count or to attend to examination of graphaesthesia on legs (Fig. 5).

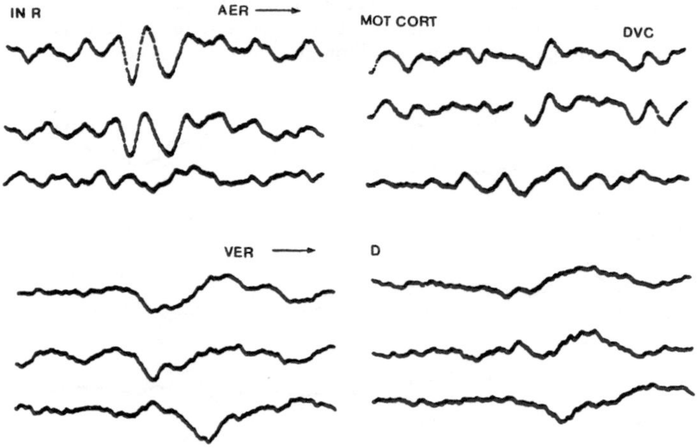

Fig. 2. Upper part shows 100 averaged auditory evoked responses from right motor cortex in rest (*INR*) and during voluntary contraction (*DVC*) of left biceps muscle. Below visual evoked responses are demonstrated from left brachium conjunctivum (upper trace) and dentate nucleus (lower traces). Dwell time: 600 ms. The evoked responses show marked decrease in the new functional state

Discussion

Our previous finding that voluntary contraction enhances evoked responses within central motor system particularly their reflex-correlated middle part [5] was not observable at all in cases of sensory input stimulation.

The functional feature of these responses was characterized by decrease, which could be thought to be one sign of desynchronization; even reading which requires real concentration was able to minimize the evoked responses. In addition the decrease as a functional change is usual in those centres where desynchronization to other stimulus would develop such as in the motor cortex. Another question arises from the fact, that the same decrease occurs in the cerebellum where many types of activation cause synchronization, so the functional

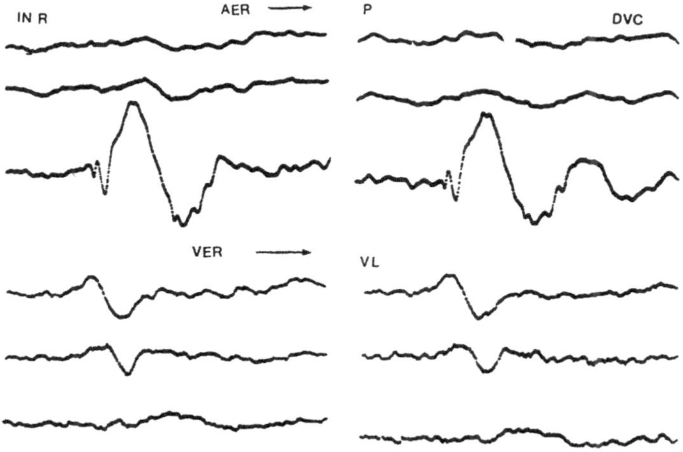

Fig. 3. 40 averaged auditory evoked responses (above) and visual responses (below) from three points of right pallidum (above) and right ventrolateral nucleus (below). Dwell time: 600 ms. Comparing responses under voluntary innervation (*DVC*) of left biceps muscle with resting state (*INR*) no significant functional change can bee seen

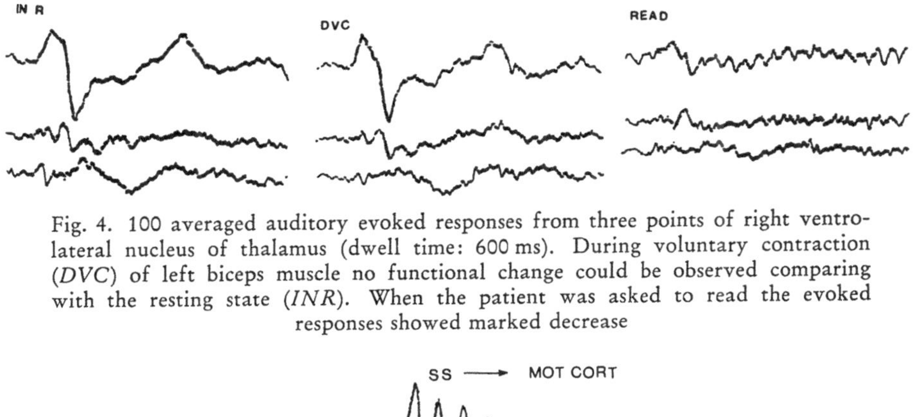

Fig. 4. 100 averaged auditory evoked responses from three points of right ventrolateral nucleus of thalamus (dwell time: 600 ms). During voluntary contraction (*DVC*) of left biceps muscle no functional change could be observed comparing with the resting state (*INR*). When the patient was asked to read the evoked responses showed marked decrease

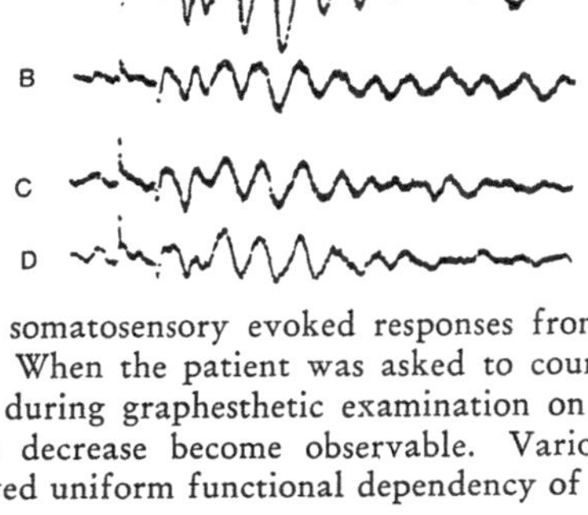

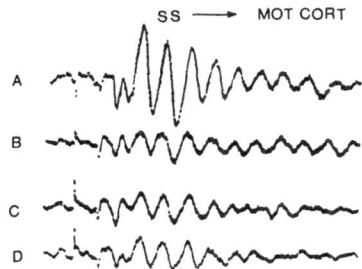

Fig. 5. 100 averaged somatosensory evoked responses from the left motor cortex (dwell time: 600 ms). When the patient was asked to count the responses showed marked decrease (*B*), during graphesthetic examination on left (*C*), later on right (*D*) leg the previous decrease become observable. Various types of functional states showed uniform functional dependency of the responses

behaviour of responses as well as of electrical activity could be different.

Though evoked responses are relative to function our investigations of the expressed physiological sensory evoked responses from different points of central motor system—are not in close correlation with the function of registered centres. This opinion is based on the passive—one way—behaviour of sensory evoked responses under different circumstances. This result could be, however, the consequence of the experimental approach used.

References

1. Ervin, F., Mark, V. H., Stereotactic thalamotomy in the human II. Physiologic observations on the human thalamus. Arc. Neurol. *3* (1960), 368—380.
2. Fukushima, T., Mayanagi, Y., Bouchard, G., Thalamic evoked potentials to somatosensory stimulation in man. Electroenceph. clin. Neurophys. *40* (1976), 481—490.
3. Haider, M., Ganglberger, J. A., Groll-Knapp, E., Computer analysis of slow potential phenomena in humans. Confin. Neurol. *34* (1972), 224—229.
4. Tóth, Sz., Vajda, J., Zaránd, P., The study of recovery and modification of the evoked potentials and motor answers of the motor system. Acta Neurochir. (Wien) Suppl. *24* (1977), 151—157.
5. Tóth, Sz., Vajda, J., Zaránd, P., Sólyom, A., Motor regulation in patients with chronic deep electrodes. In: Recent Developments of Neurobiology in Hungary, Vol. 8, pp. 73—91 (Lissák, K., ed.). Budapest: Akademia. 1979.
6. Wilson, W. P., Nashold, B. S., Evoked photic responses from the human thalamus and midbrain. Confin. Neurol. *35* (1973), 338—345.

Acta Neurochirurgica, Suppl. 30, 429—433 (1980)

Pisces Stimulation for Motor Neurone Disease

R. Plotkin*

Summary

Electrical stimulation of the spinal cord using the Pisces system (Medtronic Inc.) has been used for treating five patients with motor neurone disease. A short clinical description is given of each case, together with results of stimulation. In all five patients improvement was dramatic, but in two of them the progress of the disease was not halted. One, with advanced bulbar symptoms and signs, died two months after the implantation of the stimulating electrodes, although there had been initial improvement in her condition. One patient was lost to follow up. The period of stimulation in the remaining four patients ranged from eleven to six months. No medication was given other than antibiotics during the initial test phase, and all patients had physiotherapy. The results in these patients warrants continuation of this form of treatment in suitably selected patients.

Keywords: Motor neurone disease; electrical stimulation; spinal cord; neuro-augmentative surgery.

Introduction

Electrical stimulation of the spinal cord to improve function in multiple sclerosis has been well documented by Cook [1, 2, 4], and these results have been confirmed in the author's own series of twenty cases. As reduction of spasticity in this disease seems to be the most marked effect of stimulation, it was thought that this might be equally well applied in patients with spasticity resulting from lateral sclerosis or motor neurone disease. A perusal of the literature revealed only one reference, from the same worker, Cook [3], in which he reports on spinal cord stimulation in three cases of motor neurone disease. The author therefore felt justified in proceeding with the introduction of a Pisces system into a woman with moderately advanced motor

* Senior Consultant Neurosurgeon, Johannesburg Group of Teaching Hospitals and The University of the Witwatersrand, 3 Wycombe Medical Mews, 25 Bruce Street, Hillbrow, Johannesburg, 2001, South Africa.

0065-1419/80/Suppl. 30/0429/$ 01.00

neurone disease following a strong request from her that something be done to help her deteriorating condition.

Methods and Material

The results of this first case were so encouraging that a further four patients presenting over the ensuing six months were also treated with electrical stimulation. All five patients had been previously diagnosed as suffering from motor neurone disease by reputable neurologists. All of these patients had seen at least two, and sometimes more, neurologists on different occasions, and all had been fully investigated along the way. The diagnosis in each case was confirmed by clinical examination, but patients were not subjected to any further special investigations. In all the cases the diagnosis was quite clearcut, and there was no dissenting opinion from any of the neurologists who had seen these patients previously. Four of the patients could be described as being moderately advanced in the course of their disease, and two of them were confined to wheel chairs. The fifth patient was markedly advanced and clearly had a short prognosis. It was agreed to treat her for two reasons: firstly because the patient and her family were insistent that anything be done to help, and secondly because it would be useful to determine if electrical stimulation in any way halted or slowed the progression of the disease.

Electrodes were of the Medtronic Sigma type introduced into the epidural space via Tuey needles under radiographic control. Patients were placed in either the left lateral position or supine with two pillows under the chest on a screening table with image intensifier. Lignocaine 2% was infiltrated into the skin and subcutaneous tissues overlying the spines of D 5, D 6, and D 7, and between the spinous processes of these vertebrae. A longitudinal skin incision was made as far as deep fascia, as it is necessary to have sufficient tissue for burying the electrodes and their anchoring clips. The first Tuey needle was introduced between the spines of D 5 and 6 until the epidural space was encountered, confirmed by the vacuum saline drop test. The second needle was introduced between the spines of D 6 and D 7 to the same space. The electrodes were then passed through the needles and as far as they would travel freely. Their position was confirmed with X-ray control, the upper electrode lying at the level of C 3, and the lower at C 5. They came to lie most often in the mid-position posteriorly, but it was not considered important if they did not lie in the mid-line plane. The electrodes were then connected to a pulse generator, and the patient asked to report on any sensation, its nature and its situation. Invariably paraesthesiae are produced in one or other arm or shoulder, and this was considered a satisfactory position providing no pain was experienced. Pain on stimulation indicates that one of the electrodes approximates one of the nerve roots, and requires adjustment of position. Once satisfied that the electrodes were in correct position, they were anchored with the plastic clips supplied, and the leads were then passed subcutaneously with a tunneling instrument out of the right flank. The incision over the dorsal spines was then closed with a subcutaneous and skin suture. The patient was then submitted to a one week test period to determine effectiveness of the stimulation. As there was improvement in all five patients, chronic implantation was then undertaken in each case. Under general anaesthetic in the operating theatre, the Pisces radio receiver was implanted over the lower rib cage on the right anterior chest wall, the new leads connected to the electrodes, and the old leads discarded. Correct polarity of the electrodes was determined during the test period, and was selected on the basis of the most efficient stimulation with the least side effects. During this period all the patients underwent physiotherapy. Apart from the exhibition of antibiotics during the test period during which leads issued from the skin, no other medication was employed.

Results

The first patient had all four limbs affected, was confined to a wheel chair, and had some difficulty with swallowing. Her right hand in particular was severely wasted and completely paralyzed. Almost immediately after commencing stimulation on the X-ray table the patient announced that she was able to move her right thumb, which she had not been able to do for several months. By the next day all of her motor function had improved, and before the chronic implant she was able to walk unaided. Function in the right hand improved sufficiently for supportive movements and gripping small objects, and she was beginning to isolate movements in the fingers. Swallowing also improved. However, four months later she had fallen back somewhat in that her walking had again deteriorated although she still did not need a wheel chair. Her right hand had again become helpless and function of the left hand was not as good as previously. Swallowing was again becoming difficult.

The second patient was a middle aged man with mainly shoulder girdle involvement and difficulty in swallowing. He also improved significantly during the test period, and found that he was able to lift his arms to comb his hair, and that he no longer had to move his head from side to side while holding a tooth brush fixed in the one hand, but could now actively brush his teeth in a more normal manner. He was able to hold his head erect on his shoulders which he was quite unable to do previously, and swallowing improved. He has continued his improvement to date.

The third patient was the very advanced case with mainly bulbar symptoms and signs. She was no longer able to speak, could not move the tongue, and was reduced to eating mushy foods in that she could not cope with solids or swallow liquids. She was totally aphonic. After several days of stimulation she was again moving her tongue and could protrude it as far as the lips. She was again able to vocalize, although speech was difficult to understand. She could now cope with somewhat more solid food than previously. This patient maintained her improvement for one month, but then she suddenly deteriorated in a very short space of time. Her tongue again became paralysed, she was unable to talk, and swallowing deteriorated. She died within a period of several days after her sudden deterioration.

The fourth patient was a middle aged woman in whom all four limbs were affected, as well as speech and swallowing. All of her motor function improved, that is gait, hand movements, speech, and swallowing. She has maintained this improvement and has not yet fallen back.

The last patient was confined to a wheel chair and both hands were very weak. Spasticity was immediately relieved, and arm movements were much improved. However, she was not able to leave her wheel chair. Shortly after the chronic implant she returned to Europe where she is resident, and despite having been requested to keep us informed of her progress, she has not done so and is therefore lost to follow up.

The longest period of stimulation in this group of patients is eleven months, the shortest period six months apart from the patient who demised two months after the introduction of the stimulator. It is clear from these five patients that there is an immediate and dramatic improvement in function of all affected modalities. However, it is clear from two of the patients in this small series that progression of the disease is not halted, and is apparently not slowed to any appreciable degree. Apart from the patient who has died and the other that has been lost to follow up, the remaining three all feel that this form of treatment has been worthwhile, even though they understand that it is neither curative nor unlikely to increase their life span.

In this series there has been one complication and that in the patient with the shoulder girdle paralysis. The paravertebral and interscapular muscles are so wasted in this man that there has been difficulty in keeping the electrodes buried, and he has had a revision of the chronic implant without interfering with the electrodes. Since then he has had no problems.

Discussion

In Cook's series of three patients with "verified motor neurone disease", he claims: "Stimulation of the spinal cord has produced significant improvement in voluntary motor performance. This is not limited to isolated muscles but encompasses total synergistic activity. Speech, upper and lower limbs, and trunk all participate in the improved motor function." All five of our patients confirm these remarks and his findings. If Cook had any failed cases, he does not mention them. It would therefore seem that all three of his patients, and all five of ours have responded dramatically to this form of treatment.

The mechanism of improvement of function in motor neurone disease with this form of treatment is not clear, and would probably be difficult to determine with any degree of accuracy. It is obvious that not all motor units are non-functioning and that electrical stimulation presumably improves function by means of spatial summation and recruitment.

It might be argued, as it has been with the treatment of multiple sclerosis by this means, that the clinical improvement is due to the intensive physiotherapy that the patient is subjected to while in hospital. Certainly nearly all of the patients with multiple sclerosis, and none of this series of cases had been having physiotherapy of any consequence prior to the implantation of electrodes. But in these cases of motor neurone disease, there is no doubt whatever that the physiotherapy only plays a subsidiary and minor part. Improvement in at least one case was almost immediate on commencing stimulation, and in all the others the improvement was too rapid for the physiotherapy to have played any part. However, in the one case of bulbar motor neurone disease that was totally aphonic, physiotherapy, which included ice applications to the tongue and palate, may well have played a more important role.

Although electrical stimulation cannot be offered as anything more than palliative in the treatment of motor neurone disease, it is so far the only method of treatment that has been of any use whatever in this inexorably advancing dreadsome disease. It appears not to halt the progress, but does at least give significant improvement in function for a space of time. It is intended to continue with this method of treatment in suitably selected patients.

References

1. Cook, A. W., Weinstein, S. P., Chronic dorsal column stimulation in multiple sclerosis. N.Y. State J. Med. *73* (1973), 2868—2872.
2. Cook, A. W., Electrical stimulation of the spinal cord (letter to the editor). Lancet *I* (1974), 869—870.
3. Cook, A. W., Stimulation of the spinal cord in motor neurone disease (letter to the editor). Lancet *II* (1974), 230—231.
4. Cook, A. W., Electrical stimulation in multiple sclerosis. Hosp. Pract. *XI* (1976), 51—58.

be difficult to determine with any degree of accuracy. It is, however, likely that, if motor units are non-functioning and thus electrical stimulation presumably improves them by a process of sprout formation and reinnervation.

Though it is recognised [illegible] with the advent of multiple electrodes for this method, that the clinical improvement [illegible] intensive physiotherapy that the patient is subjected to while in hospital. Certainly nearly all of the patients with multiple electrodes [illegible]

[illegible]

References

1. [illegible]

2. [illegible]

3. [illegible]

4. [illegible]

Acta Neurochirurgica, Suppl. 30, 435—439 (1980)

Long-Term Results of Posterior Functional Rhizotomy

V. A. Fasano*, G. Broggi, S. Zeme, G. Lo Russo, and **A. Sguazzi**

With 1 Figure

Summary

The long-term results (2–7 years) of posterior functional rhizotomy (personal technique) in 80 cases of spastic cerebral palsy are presented. The lack of recurrencies, the minimal side effects, the effective improvement of spasticity in all cases, the actual suprasegmental improvement suggest posterior functional rhizotomy for the treatment of spastic cerebral palsy, associated with a physiotherapeutic rehabilitative treatment and orthopedic corrective treatment.

The long-term results of functional posterior rhizotomy, its side effects, recurrencies, segmentary and suprasengmentary effects and the functional results have been checked from the clinical point of view. Functional posterior rhizotomy is a personal modification of Foerster's rhizotomy [1, 4, 5]. The fundamental characteristics of this procedure is the selection of the fibres to be cut by intraoperative electrical stimulation of each root and rootlet from D 12 to S 1 bilaterally. The use of magnification and a complete, strict and careful examination of each root and rootlets is compulsory for this procedure. The different results from the Foerster's original operation is clearly demonstrated in a patient in whom a partial rhizotomy was first undertaken according to Foerster technique; two years later the hypertonia recurred most marked on the left leg. A functional posterior rhizotomy was then performed on the left side, with a noticeable and permanent reduction of spasticity lasting five years on the corresponding side.

Method

This procedure has been performed in 80 cases of cerebral palsy in which spasticity is the main symptom often associated with other symptoms namely motor deficit, dystonia (postural or motion) and bone or muscular alteration associated or subsequent to the primary disease [3].

* Istituto di Neurochirurgia, Universitá di Torino, Via Cherasco 15, I-10126 Torino, Italy.

0065-1419/80/Suppl. 30/0435/$ 01.00

Intraoperative electrical stimulation of posterior root or even rootlets in cases of cerebral palsy provokes abnormal responses grossly superimposable, characterized by a lack of the normal inhibition and a diffusion of the stimulus (Fig. 1). A section strictly restricted to these roots or even rootlets is capable of producing diffuse results beyond correspondent radicular areas. The effects are either segmentary (that is reduction of muscular hypertonia not only in the restricted territory related to the sectioned roots, but also in extensive spinal regional territories) and diffuse suprasegmentary effects (that is an overall improvement of

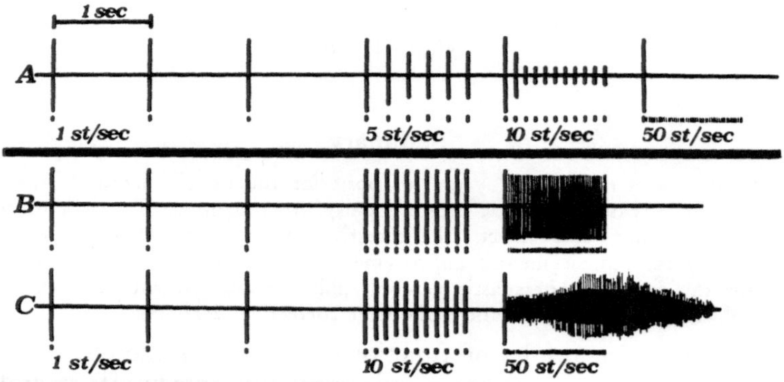

Fig. 1. Dorsal root stimulation and R.M.G. recordings: A) Normal inhibition: when the rate of stimulation is increased, the muscle contraction decreased: when 30 to 50 stimuli per second are applied, the muscle responds only to the first stimulus. B) Lack of inhibition: one potential appears after each stimulus at all rates of stimulation. C) Lack of inhibition: interferential recording with an afterdischarge at 50 stimuli per second. *St.sec* = stimuli (pulses) per second

hyertonia and motor performances up to a restoration of valid functional activity).

Clinical evaluation of our results is based upon the quantification of the spasticity obtained by clinical examination of muscular tone which includes: I. the study of the resting position, II. the study of passive mobilization of the limb and of the trunk with evaluation of the stretch reflexes, III. the study of the osteo-tendineus reflexes, the evaluation of clonic characteristics and pathological reflexes, IV. the study of active movement with evaluation of the amplitude of the movement, the muscular force and the motor coordination. In the content of this study we paid particular attention to the functional consequences: A) the standing reaction, B) the straightening reaction, C) the state of equilibrium in the sitting position, in the standing position and while walking. The various forms of dystonia and the influence of bone and tendineus alterations have been also checked. The follow-up is from two to seven years.

We consider as *poor* results the cases with improvement of pathologic characteristics between 10 and 30%; as *good* results the cases with an improvement between 30 and 70%; as *complete* results the cases with an improvement between 70 and 100%.

Table 1. *Side Effects*

	Permanent	Transitory
Sensory disorders (restricted area of a little hypoaesthesia in one leg)	2 (2.5%)	2 (2.5%)
Disorders of sphinteric control		1 (1.25%)
Marked and diffuse hypotonia		4 (5%)

Table 2

Segmentary results		No. case	Complete	Good	Moderate	Poor
Hypertonia		4	4 (100%)			
Hypertonia associated with orthopedic lesions	— no orthoped. treatment	57	5 (8.77%)	47 (82.45%)	5 (8.77%)	
	— orthoped. treatment	19	2 (10.52%)	7 (36.84%)	9 (47.36%)	1 (5.26%)
Dystonia		13		1 (7.69%)	5 (38.46%)	7 (53.85%)
Supra-segmentary effects		65	7 (10.76%)	18 (27.69%)	12 (18.46%)	28 (47.07%)

Table 3

Functional results	Poor	Moderate	Good	Complete
Sitting position	1 (1.53%)	25 (38.46%)	31 (47.69%)	8 (12.3%)
Standing position	4 (6.15%)	22 (33.84%)	32 (49.23%)	7 (10.76%)
Walking	24 (36.92%)	19 (29.23%)	15 (23.07%)	7 (10.76%)

Results

The surgical procedure has no mortality. The *side effects* (Table 1) are limited in some cases (2.5%) to a restricted area of sensory disturbances in one leg. We never registered a transient or permanent disturbance of motor function. Sphincter troubles and hypotonia are only transient. In the 5% of cases we observed a diffuse and marked hypotonia lasting from 2 to 6 months, which was followed in all cases by a complete recovery of muscular tone.

Preoperative hypertonia never recurred. The permanent diffuse hypotonia often produced by the Foerster operation was not seen. In Table 2 are presented the long-term results (2–7 years) in relation to the segmentary and suprasegmentary effects. A complete recovery has been obtained in all cases in which hypertonia was the only symptom. These cases therefore represent an elective indication for the procedure. In cases of hypertonia associated with tendineus retractions and articular lesions requiring orthopaedic treatment (the large majority of our cases) we observed: in 91% of the cases a good or complete resolution of tone not only on the restricted territories relating to the cut root and rootlets, but also to an extended spinal plurisegmental territory (*segmentary effect*) in 53% of the cases a remarkable improvement of trunk stability, a better use of the movement of the hand, a possibility of assuming a normal neck position, speech improvement, and a remarkable improvement in behaviour (*suprasegmentary effects*). In 39% of the cases the postural dystonia was also slightly influenced markedly in 8% of the cases. In 45% of cases the behaviour was also markedly improved. Table 3 shows the long-term results on postural and voluntary motor performances. We registered: for the sitting position: poor results (2% of cases) moderate results (38% of cases), good results (48% of cases), complete results (12% of cases); for the standing position: poor results (6%), moderate results (34%), good results (49%), complete results (11%); for walking: poor results (37%), moderate results (29%), good results (23%), complete results (11%). It must be pointed out that in the large majority of cases physiotherapeutic treatment was lacking or inadequate. Only one third of the cases had an orthopaedic treatment and it was seldom effective.

Discussion

In cases of spastic cerebral palsy, section from D 12 to S 1 bilaterally, limited to root and rootlets showing an anomalous response to electrical stimulation, has produced a permanent reduction of hypertonia not only in the territories related to the cut roots, but also in additional positive effects at segmentary and suprasegmentary levels.

We never saw permanent and diffuse sensory disorders nor any recurrence of the spasticity. These observations indicate that the procedure is not merely a "deafferentation", such as the Foerster operation, but rather a selective interruption of pathological spinal circuits [2]. Apart from the spasticity causing adaptative reactions, these also extend the inhibition of the local increase of muscle tone to the suprasegmentary level and also to the more integrated functions. In cases in which the spasticity is an isolated symptom, the result is complete; in the other cases the result is partial and conditioned, obviously, by the degree of preoperative motor involvement and by rehabilitation, whose goal should be the recovery from the selective "deafferentation" produced by the operation. Treatment of bone and articular alterations (associated or consequent to the spasticity) by orthopaedic procedures is also important.

In conclusion, the minimal side effects, the lack of recurrence and the real improvement of spasticity and of some suprasegmental motor and behavioural performances suggest that posterior functional rhizotomy is good treatment for hypertonic forms of cerebral palsy. An association with adequate physiotherapy and sometimes corrective orthopaedical treatment is mandatory.

References

1. Fasano, V. A., Barolat-Romana, G., Ivaldi, A., Sguazzi, A., La radicotomie postérieure fonctionnelle dans le traitement de la spasticité cérébrale. Neurochirurgie *22* (1976), 23—34.
2. Fasano, V. A., Barolat-Romana, G., Zeme, S., Sguazzi, A., Electrophysiological assessment of spinal circuits in spasticity by direct dorsal root stimulation. Neurosurgery *4* (1979), 146—151.
3. Fasano, V. A., Broggi, G., Barolat-Romana, G., Sguazzi, A., Surgical treatment of spasticity in cerebral palsy. Child's Brain, Vol. 4 (1978), 289—305.
4. Fasano, V. A., Urciuoli, R., Broggi, G., Barolat-Romana, G., Ivaldi, A., Benech, F., Sguazzi, A., New aspects of the surgical treatment of cerebral palsy. Acta Neurochir. Suppl. *24* (1977), 53—57.
5. Foerster, O., Über eine neue operative Methode der Behandlung spastischer Lähmungen mittels Resektion hinterer Rückenmarkswurzeln. Z. Orthop. Chir. *22* (1908), 202—223.

Acta Neurochirurgica, Suppl. 30, 441—444 (1980)

Intraneoplastic Administration of Bleomycin in Intracerebral Gliomas: A Pilot Study

D. A. Bosch*, Th. Hindmarsch, St. Larsson****, and **E.-O. Backlund****

With 1 Figure

Introduction

As human malignant gliomas of the brain cannot be treated successfully by conventional means, *i.e.*, bulk resection + radiotherapy, eventually combined with the systemic administration of cytostatic agents, we decided to start a trial consisting of stereotactic biopsy of the tumour and placement of a small catheter in the center of the tumour to administer chemotherapeutic agents. In contrast with those agents used in systemic administration that should be of small molecular size and lipid soluble to penetrate the CNS, for intraneoplastic drug delivery drugs could be used that do not pass the blood brain barrier. It seemed reasonable to chose a drug that will neither pass this barrier nor the brain-blood barrier. Besides that the drug should be a non-cell cycle specific drug as gliomas have a very low growth fraction [5] and should have shown at least some effectivity against glioma cells both in vivo and in vitro [7—9]. Bleomycin fulfilled all these criteria [2, 6] and has been taken as the first agent to test in this way.

Methods and Material

Bleomycin, a mixture of chemical similar glycopeptide antibiotics, has a molecular weight of about 1,400, is water soluble and does not penetrate the healthy blood-brain barrier. It has been proven to be a potent cytostatic agent in squamous cell carcinomas.

---

* Department of Neurosurgery, University Hospital, Groningen, The Netherlands.
** Department of Neurosurgery, Karolinska Sjukhus, Stockholm, Sweden.

0065-1419/80/Suppl. 30/0441/$ 01.00

Prior to the stereotactic intervention a CT-scan was performed for good localization of the process and served as a standard-picture for follow-up screening. Stereotactic biopsy with Leksell's technique was done under protection of Dexamethasone and a small catheter was placed at the target by the same route and fixed to the skin with a suture. When the pathologists confirmed the diagnosis and described the glioma as a malignant one (grade III-IV according to Kernohan) a start was made with the introduction of Bleomycin. Five mg was dissolved in 5 ml of NaCl (0.9%) and injected by way of a syringe-pump with a speed of 1 ml/hour. The same procedure was repeated two times with two days delay between the three administrations.

Results

The group consisted of three patients. In these cases an assessment of the possible distribution of Bleomycin was made by intraneoplastic injecting of only 400 μg of Bleomycin labelled with ^{111}Indium (500 μCi). Thereafter these three patients got 3 × 5 mg of Bleomycin by intraneoplastic route. One of them suffered of a sudden raise in ICP and was operated upon as an emergency. He thereafter did well for five months and died by a recurrence. The second patient died after three months due to tumour regrowth. The third patient, a man aged 60, who had suffered from a glioma grade II five years earlier and was then conventionally irradiated with 5,000 rad tumour dose had now a recurrent tumour in the left parietal region that proved to be a glioblastoma on stereotactic biopsy. He was treated with intraneoplastic Bleomycin (3 × 5 mg). He did very well and did not develop high pressure symptoms at all. Although his hemiplegia worsened and he became wheel-chair bound, follow-up CT-scan showed regression (Fig. 1). After one year he got the same treatment again (6 × 5 mg Bleomycin) and accepted it without complications. After two years his condition is now satisfactory and he has no complaints except for the hemiplegia and some difficulties in speaking.

Discussion

In malignant gliomas of the brain Bleomycin exchange between blood and tumour has been shown by various authors when the drug has been given the intravenous route. As inside the tumour there is an increased capillary permeability by opening of tight junctions in the endothelial wall [1, 5] Bleomycin enters the extracellular space (ECS) and moves by diffusion into the surrounding tumour tissues. In intraneoplastic administration of Bleomycin a significantly higher concentration of Bleomycin may be obtained in the ECS than after systemic or intrathecal administration. As movement of Bleomycin is dependent on concentration in the ECS it is affected by possible

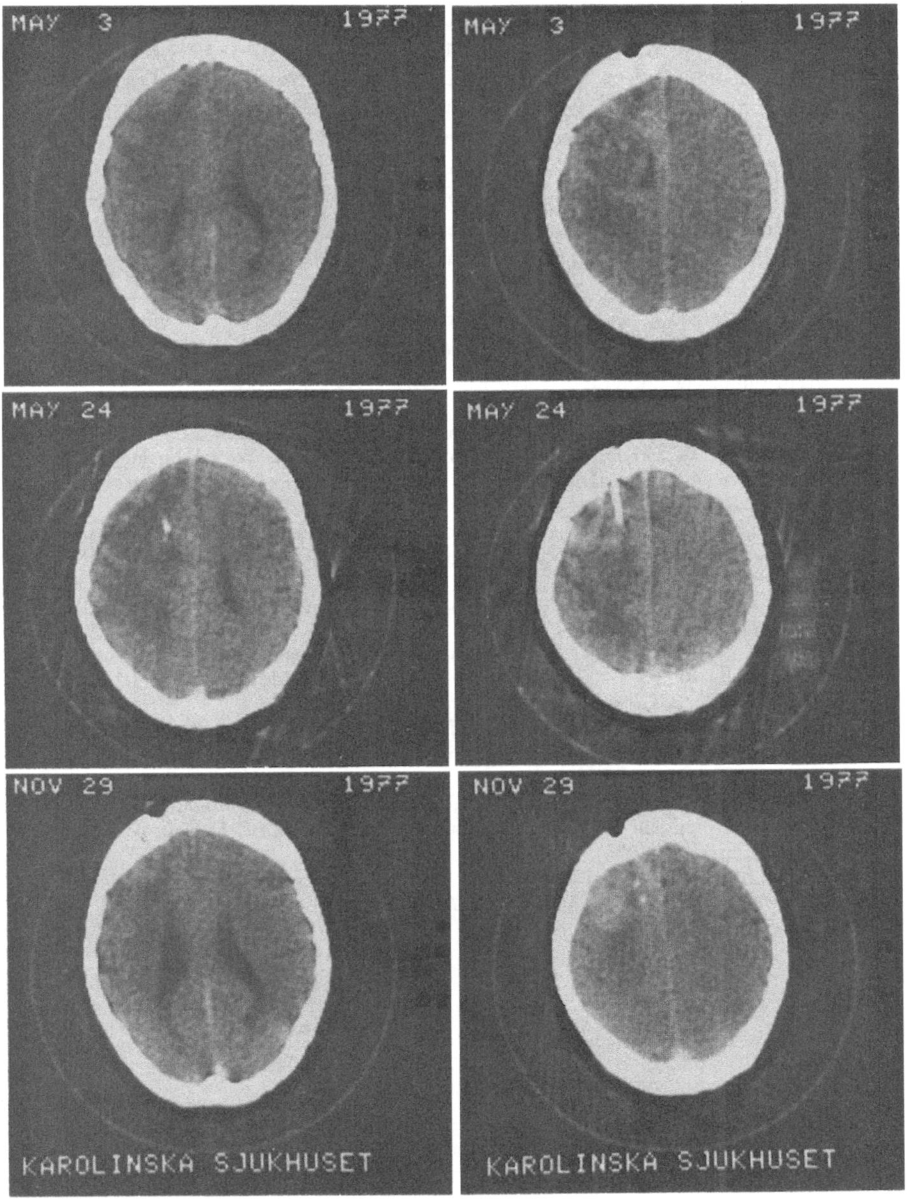

Fig. 1. Malignant glioma in the left parietal region: prior to biopsy, after stereotactic biopsy and placement of catheter inside the tumour, and half a year after intraneoplastic administration of 3 × 5 mg Bleomycin

transcapillary exchange and metabolism of the drug. Transcapillary loss of drug is higher with drugs that are more lipid soluble [3, 4] and will therefore be less than for BCNU or Methotrexate. Until now no data are available on these concentration limiting processes and therefore exact information on tumour/brain-tissue profiles of Bleomycin cannot be given. As transcapillary loss of Bleomycin should be much less than with the lipid soluble agents [1] the change in concentration with time is assumed to be due to the continuous diffusion through the ECS down the concentration gradient.

References

1. Ausman, J. I., Levin, V. A., Brown, W. E., Rall, D. P., Fenstermacher, J. D., Brain-tumor chemotherapy. J. Neurosurg. *46* (1977), 155—164.
2. Barranco, S. C., Bolton, W. E., Cell cycle phase recovery from Bleomycin-induced potentially lethal damage. Cancer Res. *37* (1977), 2589—2591.
3. Blasberg, R. G., Patlak, C., Fenstermacher, J. D., Intrathecal chemotherapy: brain tissue profiles after ventriculocisternal perfusion. J. Pharmacol. Exp. Ther. *195* (1975), 73.
4. Blasberg, R. G., Methotrexate, cytosine arabinoside, and BCNU concentration in brain after ventriculocisternal perfusion. Cancer Treat. Rep. *61* (1977), 625—631.
5. Fewer, D., Wilson, Ch. B., Levin, V. A., Brain tumor chemotherapy. Springfield, Ill.: Ch. C Thomas. 1976.
6. Hahn, G. M., Gordon, L. F., Kurkjian, S. D., Responses of cycling and non-cycling cells to 1.3-Bis(2-chloroethyl)-1-nitrosourea and to Bleomycin. Cancer Res. *34* (1974), 2373—2377.
7. Hayakawa, T., Ushio, Y., Mogami, H., Horibata, K., The uptake, distribution and anti-tumor activity of Bleomycin in gliomas in the mouse. Europ. J. Cancer *10* (1974), 137—142.
8. Hayakawa, T., Ushio, Y., Morimoto, K., Hasegawa, H., Mogami, H., Horibata, K., Uptake of Bleomycin by human brain tumours. J. Neurol., Neurosurg. Psychiat. *39* (1976), 341—349.
9. Takeuchi, K., A clinical trial of intravenous Bleomycin in the treatment of brain tumors. Int. J. Clin. Pharmacol. *12* (1975), 419—426.